Management of Pituitary Tumors
Second Edition

MANAGEMENT OF PITUITARY TUMORS

THE CLINICIAN'S PRACTICAL GUIDE

SECOND EDITION

Edited by

MICHAEL P. POWELL, MB, BS, FRCS
National Hospital for Neurology and Neurosurgery
London, UK

STAFFORD L. LIGHTMAN, MB, BChir, PhD, FRCP, FMedSci
University Research Centre for Neuroendocrinology
Bristol Royal Infirmary
Bristol, UK

EDWARD R. LAWS, JR., MD, FACS
Department of Neurosurgery
University of Virginia Health System
Charlottesville, VA

SPRINGER SCIENCE+BUSINESS MEDIA, LLC

Originally published by Humana Press Inc. in 2003
Softcover reprint of the hardcover 1st edition 2003

This publication is printed on acid-free paper. ∞
ANSI Z39.48-1984 (American National Standards Institute) Permanence of Paper for Printed Library Materials.

Cover design by Patricia F. Cleary.

Cover illustrations: Right: Dopamine agonist treatment of macroprolactinoma, an illustrative patient (*see* Fig. 2, p. 35, and discussion on pp. 33–35). Left: Stereotactic conformal radiotherapy of a small pituitary adenoma (*see* Fig. 2, p. 211, and discussion on pp. 208–210). Background: Dark-field photomicrograph of tissue fragments of a somatotroph adenoma (*see* Fig. 3 and discussion on p. 5).

10 9 8 7 6 5 4 3 2 1

Library of Congress Cataloging-in-Publication Data

Management of pituitary tumors : the clinican's practical guide / edited by Michael P. Powell, Stafford L. Lightman, Edward R. Laws Jr.--2nd ed.
p. ; cm.
Includes bibliographical references and index.
ISBN 978-1-61737-327-5 ISBN 978-1-59259-390-3 (eBook)
DOI 10.1007/978-1-59259-390-3
1. Pituitary gland--Tumors. I. Powell, Michael, MA. II. Lightman, Stafford L. III. Laws, Edward R.
[DNLM: 1. Pituitary Neoplasms--therapy. WK 585 M2664 2003]
RC280.P5 M36 2003
616.99'247--dc21

2002038810

Preface

Six years after the first edition, the target readership for *Management of Pituitary Tumors: A Clinician's Practical Guide, Second Edition* remains the trainee in the specialties that treat pituitary disorders. That trainee, possibly more than before, still needs a "user-friendly" guide to the many aspects of these complex conditions, and such a guide must be up to the minute in this rapidly changing field. We hope too that the specialist already treating one aspect of pituitary disease will find the book a helpful guide to keep abreast of advances in the associated specialties.

The book remains the combined view of a group of specialists in pituitary disease. Rather than the predominantly European views provided in the first edition, we have now taken a trans-Atlantic view and included the most up-to-date North American and European approaches to pituitary adenomas.

We still believe that centralized treatment improves the quality of care. In the UK and the US pituitary clinics/groups now regularly work together. It still holds true that this sort of interaction should hasten accurate diagnosis of such diseases as pituitary Cushing's and ensure the most appropriate treatment with the minimum of morbidity and delay.

Cost implications are of importance. Specialist groups may have greater "short-term" patient costs, but overall should be cheaper, with more appropriate investigational protocols and shorter stay, fewer complications, and better cure rate. Since fewer patients will require long-term replacement hormones, the overall cost is almost certainly lower. In the UK, it now seems easier to cross-refer patients out of health regions than it was five years ago, when the political quirks of the so-called "competitive market" were at their worst. In the US, however, managed health care systems often make this form of transfer to specialist groups outside their system financially unacceptable.

Endocrine management has undergone considerable change in the last decade. It would be almost unthinkable now to suggest surgery as primary treatment for prolactinomas, the argument for dopamine agonists having been won on grounds of both their effectiveness and their lack of side effects. The new territory for debate is the medical management of acromegaly. Nowadays some endocrinologists would favor the long-acting somatostatin analogs as first-line treatment. In the summer of 2000 at the European Workshop in Pituitary Adenomas, the debate on treatment was won by surgery, but only on a 70/30% vote. Interestingly, the same debate a few months later by the British Endocrine

Society was comfortably won by surgery—but will we be so comfortable in another six years? Similarly, the diagnosis and definition of cure in pituitary Cushing's disease continues to attract vigorous debate.

Pituitary surgery is still a highly specialized art. Ciric's audit from 1997 showed what can go wrong, even for those who consider themselves experienced, with between 200 and 500 cases *(1)*. Even these surgeons have a higher complication rate than those with 500 or more. It would theoretically be preferable if microadenoma surgery were carried out in centers that perform a minimum of 50 cases per year, but in practice very few units annually carry out even 50 transsphenoidal cases overall. With the incidence of endocrine-active tumors, this would mean that in the UK only six units would need to be considered as "endocrine pituitary surgery specialists." Yet there are still units with tiny experience declaring an interest. One UK neurosurgeon declares a special interest in pituitary surgery on eight operative procedures per year! Similar situations exist in the US, where some neurosurgery units with limited experience readily accept patients for transsphenoidal surgery.

Medical politics and patient groups will probably play an important part in the foreseeable future. Shalet *(2)* reported the experience in Manchester, UK, over a defined period when no single surgeon specialized in pituitary surgery; an average of eight cases were operated on per surgeon in the ten-year study period yielding a 17% cure rate. At the same time a dedicated group from New York, audited by their endocrinologist, was reporting long-term cure rates of 62%. Comparison audits like this make a very strong argument for specialist groups. The Internet and pressure from patient groups will do the rest.

Another major challenge is the aggressive marketing of endoscopic "minimally invasive" pituitary surgery. Responsible surgeons such as Cappabianca are well aware that the argument favoring this form of surgery over traditional transsphenoidal methods has yet to be made. The studies necessary to show improvement in outcome and shortened inpatient stay have yet to be started. For most of us, the event that prolongs inpatient stay is postoperative endocrine testing and, to a certain extent in the UK, tradition. However, it cannot be denied that minimally invasive surgery is less painful, and less likely to produce facial marking.

In 1995, the regular use of growth hormone replacement was hardly considered. Now in the UK it is a contentious issue, currently before the UK government's National Institute for Clinical Excellence (NICE), who will decide on "evidence-based" grounds whether we can prescribe this modestly priced medication to our patients. However, in the US, patients who have been shown to be GH deficient on dynamic testing are usually approved for therapy.

We hope that by broadening our author base we have been able to make *Management of Pituitary Tumors: A Clinician's Practical Guide, Second Edition,* less parochial. Clearly there are significant trans-Atlantic differences—in units of measurement (both of which are used in this edition) and in surgical procedure (in the US a neurosurgeon will often carry out the surgery after an otolaryngologist has made the approach). The trans-Atlantic editorial collaboration has the virtue of bringing out the similarities and differences in our respective approaches.

A number of developments in the use of radiotherapy in the last few years have not yet been shown to be genuine advances. Clearly, fewer patients are being referred for conventional radiotherapy and there is a significant increase in the use of the Gamma Knife. Sadly, despite theoretical advantages in this technique, which has been available for 20 years, there is surprisingly little good data available to assess its advantages and disadvantages. This issue is addressed in the relevant chapters.

A much neglected area in practice is consideration of the patient's experience during investigation, treatment, and followup. With the recent recognition and expansion of patient support groups, we believed it important to provide a patient's viewpoint. Although there may be trans-Atlantic differences in management, the fears and experiences of the patient will be essentially identical wherever they are treated.

***Michael P. Powell**, MB, BS, FRCS*
***Stafford L. Lightman**, MB, BChir, PhD, FRCP, FMedSci*
***Edward R. Laws, Jr.**, MD, FACS*

REFERENCES

1. Ciric I, Ragin A, Baumgartner C, Pierce D. Complications of transsphenoidal surgery: results of a national survey, review of the literature, and personal experience. Neurosurgery 1997;40:225-236; discussion 236-237.
2. Lissett CA, Peacey SR, Laing I, Tetlow L, Davis JR, Shalet SM. The outcome of surgery for acromegaly: the need for a specialist pituitary surgeon for all types of growth hormone secreting adenoma. Clin Endocrinol (Oxf) 1998;49:653-657.

Preface to the First Edition

The pituitary gland is an organ that has fascinated scientists and clinicians for centuries. The ancient Greeks believed that the pituitary drained waste products from the brain and secreted them as nasal mucus from the nose. There was remarkably little advance from this notion until the revolutionary discovery in the early 1930s of the neurosecretion of vasopressin and oxytocin from the posterior pituitary gland, and the demonstration of the primary importance of the anterior gland in the regulation of reproduction. It was a decade later that Geoffrey Harris and John Green suggested that nerve fibers in the hypothalamus secreted substances into the portal capillaries whence they were carried to the pituitary gland to excite or inhibit the activity of specialized secreting cells. After centuries of belief that it was a secretory organ, the pituitary became the "conductor of the endocrine orchestra" and subsequently, and more accurately, an amplifier for messages sent by the real conductor, the hypothalamus.

The first hypothalamic-releasing factor, thyrotropin-releasing hormone, was finally characterized by Roger Guillemin and Andrew Schally in 1971, rapidly followed by the other releasing factors. In 1977, the Nobel Prize for Medicine was awarded to them in recognition of this work. Since then, the identification of many other hypothalamic-releasing and -inhibitory factors has continued and to date almost 30 neuropeptides have been localized in the endocrine hypothalamus with neuroendocrine or neurotransmitter effects on hypothalamohypophyseal regulation. The CIBA Foundation has recently published an up-to-date review on this field, which we would recommend (Functional anatomy of the neuroendocrine hypothalamus, CIBA Foundations symposium 168, 1992, John Wiley).

Harvey Cushing stands as a giant in the history of pituitary disease. The founder of modern neurosurgery (in his surgical work, pioneering one of the transsphenoidal routes to the pituitary fossa) and a brilliant neurophysiologist, he made full and detailed descriptions of acromegaly and, of course, demonstrated the connection between the disease that bears his name and pituitary adenomas. Less well known, he also suggested that the patient with postpartum amenorrhea and persistent lactation might be secreting a lactogenic hormone, which has now been identified as prolactin.

Since Cushing's day, pituitary management has benefited significantly from a number of technological advances in three main fields. First, endocrinology, through radioimmunoassay, has led to the early diagnosis of disease caused by microadenomas and allowed us to assess the therapeutic value of the different treatments of the disease. Second, advances in computer imaging, initially with transmission computed tomography and now magnetic resonance imaging, have allowed anatomical diagnosis of microadenomas at a very early stage. Finally, the operating microscope and microinstruments have allowed surgeons to make enormous improvements in surgical technique.

The history of the surgical management of pituitary disease starts, other than anecdotally, at the turn of the 20th century. The first unsuccessful attempt to remove pituitary tumors was made in 1889 by Sir Victor Horsley, who went on to perform a series of 10 such operations between 1904 and 1906. The first partial removal of pituitary tumor via the transsphenoidal approach was in 1907 by Schloffer. Surgeons such as Hirsch in Vienna and Cushing in Boston experimented with transsphenoidal surgery via the nasal and sublabial routes, although this was largely abandoned. We must admire their bravery in attempting their pioneering approaches with poor anesthesia, poor lighting, and lack of magnification, but we should not be surprised that for a long time radiotherapy held the center ground in terms of useful treatment.

In the UK, the interest in transsphenoidal surgery was rekindled after the World War II and hypophysectomy was used as endocrine control of the spread of hormone-sensitive secondary cancers, such as breast and prostate. As neurosurgery was developing in other directions at that time, otolaryngologists such as Angel-James in Bristol, Richards in Cardiff, and Williams in London developed the transethmoidal technique, gaining enormous experience at a time when endocrinologists were able to measure accurately and to a certain extent control pituitary diseases medically. It was only on the continent and in Canada, through the legacy of Cushing's trainees (Norman Dott, who taught Guiot in Paris, who taught Jules Hardy in Montreal), that transsphenoidal surgery remained in the neurosurgical domain.

The interest in radiation treatment of pituitary gland began after Carl Beck (1905) described positive treatment results with the use of Roentgen rays in "Basedow's syndrome." Two French physicians working separately, Gramagnea and Beclere, extended this work to the management of acromegaly associated with the "acidophil" pituitary tumor in 1909. During the succeeding 20 years, several reports confirmed the value of radiotherapy in the management of pituitary tumors. With the major advances in megavoltage equipment and other developments in medical physics, the superiority of high-energy X-rays and particle radiation compared with the lower-energy orthovoltage modalities, which were used in the early part of the century, have produced significant advances in the field of radiotherapy to the pituitary gland.

Successful medical management of pituitary tumors is a much more recent therapeutic advance. The use of dopamine agonists in the 1970s and more recently the development of somatostatin analogs have opened new noninvasive approaches to the treatment of pituitary tumors. This is clearly only the vanguard of new pharmacological approaches to pituitary disease.

***Michael P. Powell**, MB, BS, FRCS*
***Stafford L. Lightman**, MB, BChir, PhD, FRCP, FMedSci*

CONTENTS

CONTRIBUTORS

PRAKASH ABRAHAM, MB, BS, MD, MRCP • *Consultant Endocrinologist, Aberdeen Royal Infirmary, Foresterhill, Aberdeen, UK*

STEPHANIE BALDEWEG, MD, MRCP • *Department of Endocrinology, University College (London) Hospitals, London, UK*

JOHN S. BEVAN, MD, FRCP (Edin) • *Consultant Endocrinologist, Aberdeen Royal Infirmary, Foresterhill, Aberdeen, UK*

MICHAEL BRADA, MD, FRCP, FRCR • *Neuro-Oncology Unit and Academic Unit of Radiotherapy and Oncology, The Institute of Cancer Research; The Royal Marsden NHS Trust, Sutton, Surrey, UK*

PAOLO CAPPABIANCA, MD • *Associate Professor of Neurosurgery, Department of Neurological Sciences, Università degli Studi di Napoli Federico II, Naples, Italy*

PAUL V. CARROLL, MD, MRCP • *Lecturer in Medicine, Department of Endocrinology, St. Thomas's Hospital, London, UK*

GEORGE P. CHROUSOS, MD, FACP, FAAP, MACE • *Chief, Pediatric and Reproductive Endocrinology Branch, National Institute of Child Health and Human Development, National Institutes of Health, Bethesda, MD*

ENRICO DE DIVITIIS, MD • *Professor of Neurosurgery and Chairman, Department of Neurological Sciences, Università degli Studi di Napoli Federico II, Naples, Italy*

ASHLEY B. GROSSMAN, MD, FRCP, FMedSci • *Professor of Neuroendocrinology, Department of Endocrinology, St. Bartholomew's Hospital, London, UK*

NICHOLAS P. HIRSCH, MB, BS, FRCA • *Consultant Neuroanaesthetist, The National Hospital for Neurology and Neurosurgery, London, UK*

CHRISTIAN A. KOCH, MD, FACP, FACE • *Assistant Professor, Department of Endocrinology and Nephrology, University of Leipzig, Leipzig, Germany*

TOMOHIKO KOHATA, MD • *Neurosurgery Fellow, Division of Neurosurgery, Arthur and Sonia Labatt Brain Tumor Research Center, Hospital for Sick Children; University of Toronto, Toronto, Ontario, Canada*

EDWARD R. LAWS, JR., MD, FACS • *Professor of Neurological Surgery and Medicine, University of Virginia School of Medicine, Charlottesville, VA*

ANDREW LEVY • *Reader in Medicine, University Research Center for Neuroendocrinology, Bristol University; Bristol Royal Infirmary, Bristol, UK*

Stafford L. Lightman, MB, BChir, PhD, FRCP, FMedSci • *Professor of Medicine, University of Bristol; Bristol Royal Infirmary, Bristol, UK*

Ian MacDonald, BMedSc, MB, ChB, PhD, FRCAP, FRCP, FRCOphth • *Emeritus Professor of Neurology, University of London; The Institute of Neurology, Queen Square, London, UK*

Patsy Perrin • *The Pituitary Foundation, Bristol, UK*

Jonathan R. Pollock, BM, BCh, FRCS (S/N) • *Pituitary Fellow, Victor Horsley Department of Neurosurgery, National Hospital for Neurology and Neurosurgery, London, UK*

Michael P. Powell, MB, BS, FRCS • *Consultant Neurosurgeon, The National Hospital for Neurology and Neurosurgery, London, UK*

Mary H. Samuels, MD • *Associate Professor, Division of Endocrinology, Diabetes, and Clinical Nutrition, Oregon Health Sciences University, Portland, OR*

Kamal Thapar, MD, PhD, FRCS (C) • *Division of Neurosurgery, University Health Network (Toronto Western Hospital); Staff Scientist, Arthur and Sonia Labatt Brain Tumor Research Center, Hospital for Sick Children; University of Toronto, Toronto, Ontario, Canada*

Mary Lee Vance, MD • *Professor of Medicine, Division of Endocrinology and Metabolism, Departments of Medicine and Neurological Surgery, University of Virginia, Charlottesville, VA*

1 Pathogenesis of Pituitary Adenomas

Andrew Levy

Contents

INTRODUCTION

The pituitary gland is an extremely well-defined structure that occupies a central place both anatomically and physiologically in the chain of neuroendocrine command from the hypothalamus and higher brain centers to the peripheral endocrine organs. Isolated as it is from ultraviolet radiation and from direct contact with ingested and inhaled irritants and carcinogens, it is remarkable that occult pituitary adenomas can be disclosed by imaging and histologic studies in as many as 11% of people at autopsy *(1)* (Fig. 1). Overt pituitary adenoma formation presenting with symptoms and signs of space occupation, hypopituitarism, and/or one of the classic syndromes of hormone excess is fortunately relatively rare, and true pituitary carcinoma characterized by metastatic spread has been described fewer than 100 times *(2)*.

From: *Management of Pituitary Tumors: The Clinician's Practical Guide, Second Edition*
Edited by: M. P. Powell, S. L. Lightman, and E. R. Laws, Jr. © Humana Press Inc., Totowa, NJ

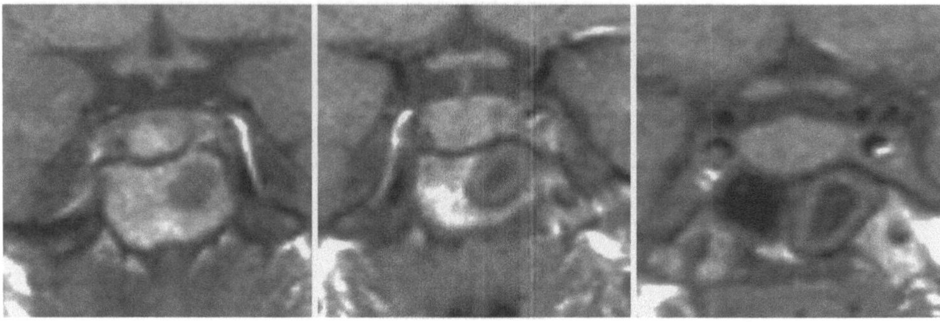

Fig. 1. Coronal MRI reconstructions, 3 mm apart, through the pituitary of a patient with an incidentally discovered, nonfunctional microadenoma.

Much of the literature that addresses the pathogenesis of pituitary adenomas centers on an examination of whether they are likely to arise after the acquisition of an intrinsic pituitary defect, such as chromosomal instability or point mutation, or whether an inappropriate quantity, combination, or pattern of exposure to growth factors from the hypothalamus or elsewhere acting on one or more genetically normal pituitary cells is to blame.

This chapter summarizes current understanding of the pathogenesis of pituitary adenomas. Its brevity is consistent with the fundamental reality that the pathogenesis of pituitary adenomas remains almost entirely obscure. The molecular defects that have been identified do not have the consistency, strength, and biologic plausibility to necessarily be pathogenic, and many of the mechanisms suggested are difficult to verify experimentally because of profound differences between the behavior of spontaneous pituitary adenomas in humans, which tend to have low levels of mitotic activity and in animal models, which tend to have relatively high levels.

ARE PITUITARY ADENOMAS TUMORS?

Currently, pituitary adenomas are a group of related conditions that require a combination of congenital or acquired intracellular abnormalities acting together with a permissive extrapituitary microenvironment to bring about the distinct pathologic processes of tumor induction and subsequent propagation. The temptation is to assume that pituitary adenomas are "true tumors"; in other words, the mechanisms responsible for neoplasia in most other organ systems are responsible for pituitary adenomas. For those who believe this scenario, if pituitary adenomas behave in an atypically benign fashion, the responsible mechanisms merely differ quantitatively rather than qualitatively from those seen in rapidly progressive malignancies.

An alternative opinion might be that in many cases pituitary adenomas are developmentally and behaviorally little different from, for example, thyroid nodules; however, by being more confined anatomically and by having a broader synthetic portfolio at the time of their departure into malignancy, pituitary adenomas appear as true tumors and require treatment as such. The distinction between the latter mechanism, which might be likened to "exuberant normality," and the former mechanism, "benign malignancy," is important because the molecular miscreants are likely to lurk in quite different places.

One of the most useful guides to help evaluate the legitimacy of the various pathogenic mechanisms is to consider how they correspond with the observed behavior of pituitary adenomas. Clearly, if activation of a new powerful oncogene is adduced *(3)*, studies investigating why a tumor harboring such a mutation should behave in such a benign fashion must immediately follow.

PITUITARY ADENOMA BEHAVIOR

When compared with normal tumors, the behavior of pituitary adenomas is extremely unusual. Clinical follow-up of patients with pituitary tumors indicates that the majority of pituitary tumors grow slowly and predictably, with a prolonged and often increasing doubling time. As a consequence, in the majority of cases, pituitary tumors remain trophically stable and show little evidence of overall growth over years. Surgical debulking is a perfectly adequate primary treatment in most cases, and strenuous efforts to remove every vestige of pituitary adenoma for fear that rapid recurrence will negate the benefit of decompression or allow remnant tissue to metastasize is rarely considered or required. For the same reason, the routine use of adjuvant radiotherapy at debulking has become a management strategy of the past.

Perhaps the most unique and unexpected characteristic of pituitary adenomas is the tendency for microprolactinomas to resolve of their own accord *(4–7)*. Whether part of this behavior is the result of epiphenomena such as impaired induction of tumor microvasculature with microhemorrhagic destruction or silent infarction, is not known, but the composite achievement of modest growth through the summation of discrete hemorrhagic or ischemic events superimposed on faster turnover or spontaneous resolution through neat and otherwise asymptomatic infarction is intuitively unlikely. Pituitary adenomas display one further remarkable and mechanistically eloquent feature: in a minority of cases of unequivocal Cushing's disease, removal of histologically entirely normal tissue results in unambiguous cure of the disease *(8)*. Specifically, in a retrospective audit of 57 patients with Cushing's disease, the macroscopically abnormal tissue removed was histologically indistinguishable from normal pituitary gland in 27% of patients, but the cure rate was nevertheless 82% *(8)*.

A central question is how to equate these familiar but nevertheless rather extraordinary behavioral characteristics with mechanisms that, when present in most tumors in most other organ systems, give rise to lesions characterized by inexorable growth, progressive genomic instability, metastatic spread, and, ulti-

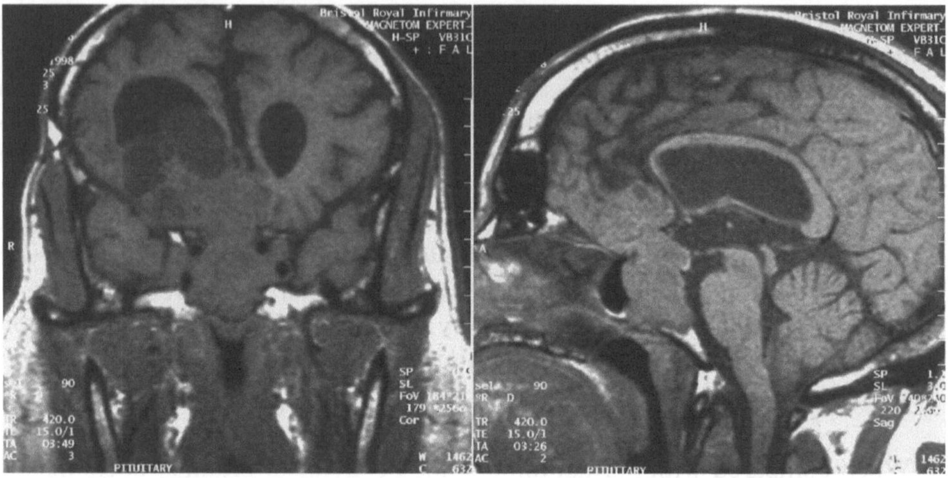

Fig. 2. Coronal and saggital MRI of an acromegalic patient with a somatotroph adenoma that had spread extensively prior to presentation. Modest debulking surgery and radiotherapy prevented further tumor growth and the patient remians well at the time of writing, 5 yr after the MRI.

mately, the death of the patient. In other words, what kind of oncogene implicated in the pathogenesis of pituitary adenomas would be so modest in its malignant aspirations that it would allow for these lesions to remain trophically stable for decades or resolve of their own accord? In the case of the Cushing's disease cases noted, what kind of intrinsic defect in an expansion of pituitary cells would be so affected by removal of adjacent normal pituitary tissue that it would regress or at least resume entirely normal trophic and functional activity?

There are exceptions, of course, and the pituitary adenomas that are most taxing clinically are relatively aggressive lesions, often corticotroph, silent corticotroph, or somatotroph adenomas, that have either infiltrated surrounding structures at the time of initial presentation or rapidly recur after debulking, but these form a minority of tumors that come to clinical attention and a small proportion of pituitary adenomas as a whole (Fig. 2). Thus, using behavior as a guide, classic irreversible mechanisms of tumor formation, such as gene mutation or allelic loss of tumor suppressors, can hardly be the whole story.

PITUITARY ADENOMA DIFFERENTIATION

A further characteristic that distinguishes pituitary adenomas from other tumors is that pituitary adenomas are well differentiated and often remain responsive to normal physiologic stimuli. It is unusual for the secretory identity

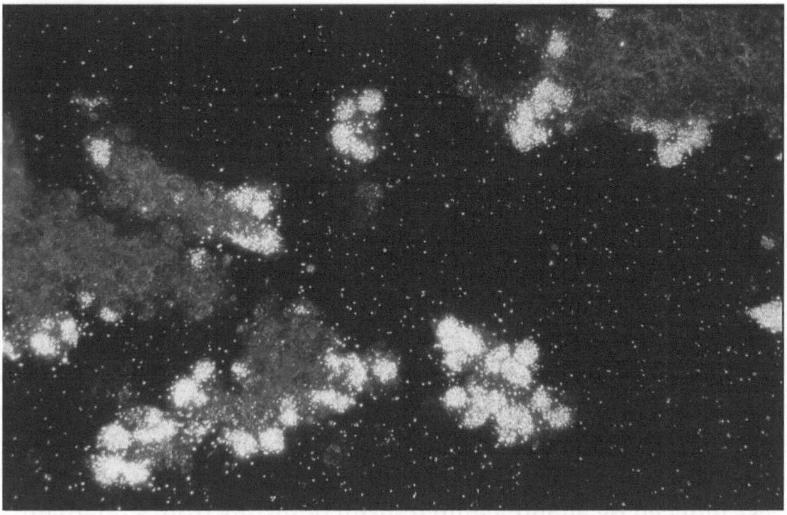

Fig. 3. Dark-field photomicrograph of tissue fragments at the edge of a 12-μm-thick frozen section of a somatotroph adenoma hybridized to an oligonucleotide probe complementary to TRH. A subset of individual cells and small clusters of cells expressing TRH at high level are clearly seen.

of the presumed cells of origin to fluctuate and the efficacy of somatostatin and dopamine analogues in somatotroph and lactotroph adenomas and the effects of changes in levels of circulating glucocorticoids in corticotroph adenomas attest to their continued expression of hormone receptors. Progressive deregulation of pituitary adenoma functional activity during propagation and how colonic neoplasms acquire a sequential series of genetic defects over time and become increasingly malignant is unusual. Indeed, although thyrotroph adenomas, for example, may become more resistant to somatostatin analogs over time, the hormone secretory potential of silent corticotroph adenomas may resume years after the original diagnosis and secreting corticotroph adenomas may alternate between quantitatively normal and abnormal hormone secretion *(9–11)*, findings that are difficult to equate with progressive dedifferentiation.

Despite the belief that they develop from the deregulated division of single cells harboring either point mutations or some degree of chromosomal disruption, pituitary adenomas frequently contain well-defined subsets of cells, with distinct transcriptional activity, expressing not only pituitary but also hypothalamic hormones *(12–14)* (Fig. 3). It is almost as if in these cases differentiation has not just been maintained but new neuroendocrine-differentiated function has been unmasked in subsets of cells. Even when hormone secretion is not continued, the histology of endocrinologically inactive adenomas at light and electron microscopic levels clearly identifies the subset of secretory cells of origin in most cases. In summary, pituitary adenomas are usually well differentiated at diagnosis and retain their differentiation in the long-term.

IS PITUITARY PATHOGENESIS INTRINSIC OR DRIVEN BY EXTERNAL GROWTH SIGNALS?

As mentioned, whether pituitary adenomas arise from intracellular defects or from excessive trophic influences from outside remains central to discussions about pathogenesis. The observation that has been pivotal in guiding opinion resolutely towards intracellular defects—to the extent that pituitary behavior has been all but ignored—is pituitary adenoma clonality. This issue is so important conceptually that it warrants explanation and examination even in such a brief summary as this. The clonality of a cellular expansion is a secure archaeologic tool capable of distinguishing an irreversible and potentially inexorably progressive process induced by an intracellular insult or insults from a relatively excessive but possibly reversible or self-limiting trophic response to stromal or microenvironmental signals *(15,16)*.

The basis of clonality is that during early female embryogenesis, each cell randomly but permanently inactivates genes on either the maternally or the paternally derived X-chromosome by cytosine methylation of promoter regions. Once methylated, the pattern of functional inactivation is stably inherited by the progeny of each cell *(17)*. Thus, all adult female tissues consist of a mosaic of cells, in each of which genes on either the maternal or paternal X-chromosome have been inactivated.

Clonality analysis depends first on being able to obtain the tissue of interest (in this case a pituitary adenoma) from a female patient who happens by chance to be heterozygotic for X-chromosome-linked markers, second on being able to distinguish between different X-chromosome alleles in such a patient (straightforward, given the known X-chromosome-linked markers), and finally, on being able to establish, on the basis of the methylation pattern of the alleles, which of the two X-chromosomes is active. If migration and dispersal of cells between assignment of clonality in utero and postnatal life leads to the formation of a mosaic at a single-cell level and mature tissues do not continue to divide, then, unless motile cells of similar identity and clonality spontaneously cosegregate in differentiated tissue or a polyclonal field spontaneously undergoes differential apoptosis leaving a single clone, a monoclonal cellular expansion in a polyclonal field must represent the progeny of a single cell. Conversely, a tumor that develops through inappropriate exogenous stimulation is likely to be derived from more than one susceptible cell and the resulting mass will be polyclonal.

Thus, the finding of monoclonality in pituitary adenomas is broadly taken to be the most compelling evidence for the neoplastic origin of these lesions, and in published series, approx 90% of the 60 or so pituitary tumors that have been analyzed for clonality have been reported to be monoclonal. The summated findings of studies from five different groups *(18–22)* show that all of the eight endocrinologically inactive adenomas, two gonadotroph adenomas, three somatotroph adenomas, and one mammosomatotroph adenoma analyzed were monoclonal. Two of the six lactotroph adenomas examined and the single plurihormonal adenoma were apparently polyclonal but were contaminated with normal pituitary tissue, and of the 22 corticotrophs examined, 17 were monoclonal, including five of the six tumors recovered from patients with Nelson's syndrome. On the basis of these studies, which were conducted 10 yrs ago, the search for the pathogenesis of pituitary adenomas has focused almost entirely on primary intracellular pituitary defects.

There are several technical and conceptual problems with clonality studies, however, that may have made the decision to abandon studies of the effects of pituitary architecture, hypothalamic stimulation, and feedback effects on pituitary adenoma pathogenesis and propagation premature.

The strategy used to define clonality relies on qualitative assessments of the consistency of deoxyribonucleic acid (DNA) recovery and probe hybridization to membrane-bound DNA that has been subjected to sequential restriction enzyme digestions. Absence of monoclonality could be dismissed as tissue contamination, and arbitrary cut offs, such as a reduction of more than 80% in the optical density of one hybridization band and less than 40% in the other, or decreases of between 70% and 30%, have to be defined as indicative of clonal skewing or polyclonality respectively *(23)*. Publication bias toward a positive result is thus compounded by considerable technical bias in favor of monoclonality.

Despite their presumed monoclonal origin, many pituitary tumors transcribe *(14)* and translate *(24)* multiple pituitary hormones in subsets of cells. The explanations adduced for this observation, if monoclonality is taken at face value, include sample contamination, monoclonal expansion of pleurihormonal precursors, a cell cycle phase effect, or further mutations of the original malignant clone. These interpretations are not supported by the pattern of hormones represented, which include hypothalamic hormones *(12–14,25,26)*, by the lack of evidence of new genomic deletions or mutations appearing with time in the majority of cases *(27,28)*, or by the slow and stable intrinsic rate of cellular turnover, which is too low to allow new subclones to emerge *(29)*.

Aside from these inconsistencies, a further critical possibility may confound the simplistic interpretation of clonality studies, which is that dispersal of cells after trophic assignment during development may not be complete *(15,16)*. There are precedents for exactly this macroscopic monoclonality in the absence of neoplasia in other tissues. Smooth muscle cell proliferation in human myometrium *(30)* normal aortic smooth muscle and atherosclerotic plaques *(31,32)*

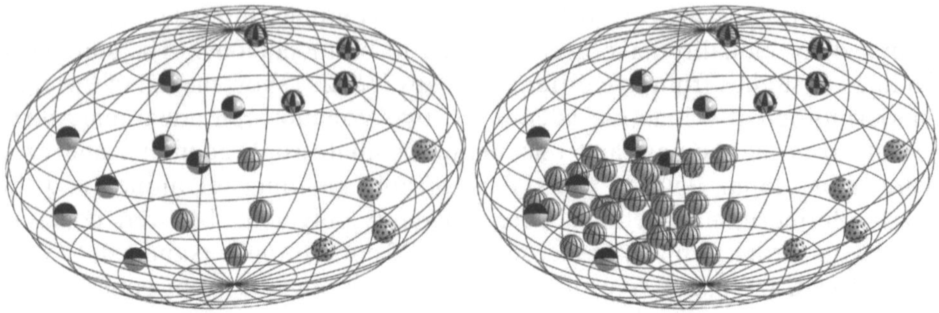

Fig. 4. Cartoon of the appearance of a non-neoplastic monoclonal expansion as an artefact of preexisting clonal topography. The left hand panel shows five different clones of a cellular subtype (depicted as differently shaded spheres), with distinct but overlapping clonal territories distributed within the pituitary (which is represented here as a 'wireframe' ovoid). The remaining pituitary cell types, which under normal circumstances fill the spaces between them (not shown), ensure that despite the nonrandom clonal topography of the particular cellular subtype shown, a random tissue sample will be truly polyclonal. By displacing intervening cells, expansion of a single clone in response to a physiologic stimulus (right hand panel) might lead to the appearance of skewing towards monoclonality in biopsy analysis, yet be derived from a physiologic response of a preexisting clone of normal cells rather than a single mutant.

all exhibit macroscopic monoclonality. The aorta, for example, consists of a patchwork of contiguous 4-mm patches skewed to the same allele *(32)*. The same is true of regenerative nodules in cirrhotic liver, which are monoclonal but entirely benign *(33)*, and in bladder urothelium, where it is estimated that 200–300 founder cells each give rise to approx 2 million cells arranged in macroscopic monoclonal patches approx 120 mm^2 *(34)*. Thus, in several tissues in which relatively pure cellular populations allow clonality to be ascertained, and perhaps in the majority of human tissues, macroscopic monoclonality is the norm.

These observations are extremely pertinent because an unusually strong or prolonged stimulus or a sequence of unusually timed stimuli might induce an excessive but nevertheless physiologic trophic response in one clone of pituitary cells that would lead to its progeny increasingly outnumbering and displacing other interspersed cell subtypes, skewing the clonality pattern in that territory. Depending on the threshold dictated by the techniques used to analyze clonality and the timing and location of pituitary biopsy, it is possible that the responsive cell population would become identifiable in vitro as a monoclonal expansion (Fig. 4).

Unlike a neoplastic monoclonal expansion derived from a single abnormal cell, expansion of a clonal patch might represent an entirely physiologic trophic response that would be expected to be well differentiated and physiologically responsive and demonstrate fluctuations in activity or spontaneous resolution, depending on the nature and duration of the trophic stimulus. This scenario would predict the twin paradoxes of a relatively high long-term failure rate for tumor excision and that partial removal of histologically normal pituitary might produce a functional remission—events that are known to occur in clinical practice *(8,35–38)*. The implication is that monoclonality does not necessarily mean neoplasia in the normal sense of the word.

One further extraordinary recent observation has called simple monoclonality into question. In more than half of recurrent pituitary tumors in which it was possible to repeat examination for loss of heterozygosity after further surgery, the loci originally implicated were heterozygous once again; in other words, the missing chromosomal region had been restored *(28)*. The explanation that the recurrence represented a second entirely independent monoclonal tumor derived from another abnormal clone after complete resection of the first is not consistant with clinical experience because a pituitary adenoma that has been almost entirely resected does not normally recur significantly. Restoration of the original allelic deletion by further mutation is clearly vanishingly improbable. A more likely scenario is that in the cases where the integrity of the genome has been restored in tumor recurrence, the original adenomas were initiated as oligoclonal rather than monoclonal expansions and that clonal interference (i.e., selection pressure) facing the newly established expansion resulted in several of the original clones being suppressed and diluted below detectable levels *(39–42)*. Debulking of the original trophically disinhibited clone allowed another clone to become trophically dominant. A more modest trophic response in a second clone with distinct transcriptional and translational activity, such as cotranscription of pro-opiomelanocortin and growth hormone-releasing hormone or corticotrophin-releasing hormone, could account for the appearance of cellular subpopulations yet be insufficient to mask monoclonality *(16)*.

Conceptual arguments about benign monoclonality aside, the pathogenesis of pituitary adenomas is still widely perceived to be related to relatively benign neoplasia rather than to a qualitatively normal but quantitatively excessive response to physiologic trophic stimuli. Proto-oncogene activation is therefore still a critical prerequisite for pituitary tumor formation.

EXOGENOUS TROPHIC INFLUENCES

Growth hormone-releasing hormone has trophic activity in the human pituitary *(43)* and, in addition to a case report of diffuse somatotroph hyperplasia in a patient with a growth hormone-releasing hormone-producing bronchial carcinoid *(44)*, there are several cases of true somatotroph adenoma formation in patients with growth hormone-releasing hormone-producing hypothalamic gangliocytomas *(45,46)*. Corticotrophin-releasing hormone is trophic to corticotrophs*(47,48)*, and a corticotroph adenoma developing in association with a corticotropin-releasing hormone-containing sellar gangliocytoma *(49)* suggests, as do the observations in growth hormone-releasing hormone-producing transgenic mice *(50)*, that duration, pattern, and local level of exposure to hypothalamic hormone may be critical in defining the stability of the trophic response induced.

For abnormal pituitary trophic responses in the presence of normal levels of hypothalamic hormones, no constitutionally active corticotrophin-releasing hormone receptor mutations in corticotroph adenomas *(51)* or growth hormone-releasing hormone receptor mutations in sporadic *(52)* or familial isolated acromegaly *(53)* have been identified. There is no evidence of somatostatin receptor (SSTR2 or SSTR5) mutations even in the presence of somatostatin analog resistance *(54,55)*, and only isolated cases of Cushing's disease preceded by generalized glucocorticoid resistance resulting from a dominant-negative glucocorticoid receptor mutation *(56)* and of Nelson's syndrome, in which a glucocorticoid receptor frame shift mutation may have modified glucocorticoid sensitivity *(57)*, have been reported.

In practical terms, the rarity with which ectopic hypothalamic hormone secretion has resulted in pituitary adenoma induction is good evidence against a major primary hypothalamic etiology in the majority of pituitary adenomas. When an association is present, it is far from clear how the shift from hyperplasia to stimulus-independent growth in the pituitary is mediated at the molecular level, even though such transitions are familiar in other endocrine tissues. This in no way excludes an important influence of the hypothalamus in tumor propagation.

ENDOGENOUS TROPHIC INFLUENCES

Activation of the gsp *Oncogene*

The strongest pathogenic mechanism yet defined for pituitary adenomas is the association between activation of the *gsp* oncogene and the development of somatotroph adenomas *(58–62)*. The GSα subunit of the heterotrimeric GTPase binds guanosine triphosphate (GTP) when growth hormone-releasing hormone receptors are occupied by ligand. Bound to GTP, the α subunit dissociates from the β and α subunits and associates with adenylyl cyclase, stimulating production of cAMP (cyclic adenosine 3', 5'-monophosphate) until the α subunit-bound GTP is hydrolysis to GDP. At this point, cAMP production stops and the α subunit reassociates with the β and γ subunits attached to the receptor.

One of two single point mutations in the Gs α subunit of GTPase has been identified in approx 40% of somatotrophinomas and results in constitutive activation of adenylyl cyclase by reducing the susceptibility of α subunit-bound GTP to hydrolysis. In tumors in which one of these mutations is present, sella morphology is more often normal than in somatotroph adenomas arising from other causes, suggesting that Gs mutant-containing adenomas tend to be smaller *(61,63)*, but there is little consistent difference in growth hormone (GH) levels in *gsp*-positive tumors compared to *gsp*-negative tumors *(61,63,64)*. Similarly, the patient's age and gender, and the duration and clinical features of the disease are also indistinguishable between groups with and without the *gsp* mutation. Although intuitively the association between the *gsp* mutation and induction of somatotroph adenomas is sensible, it is worth noting that activating mutations of *gsp* have also been reported, albeit at lower frequency, in endocrinologically inactive adenomas where the immediate consequences of the metabolic association is more obscure *(65,66)*.

Multiple Endocrine Neoplasia Type I and Menin

Multiple endocrine neoplasia type 1 (MEN-1) is a dominantly inherited condition characterized by the association of pancreatic (75%), parathyroid (80%) and pituitary (65%) adenomas. The gene responsible on chromosome 11q13 codes for a 610-amino acid predominantly nuclear protein named menin, the structure of which has no apparent similarities to any previously known proteins *(67)* and the functions of which are still being defined *(68–71)*. Whether loss of heterozygosity at the menin locus or mutations in the menin coding region are responsible for sporadic pituitary adenomas has been addressed in several reports. In 14 studies examining sporadic pituitary adenomas, loss of heterozygosity on 11q13 was identified in 57 out of 415 cases (13.7%), with results varying from 0% *(72–74)* to 28% *(75)*. Nine studies found inactivating mutations in the coding region of the menin gene to be relatively rare: 5 out of 368 cases (1.4%) ranging from 0% *(72,76–78)* to 5% *(79)*. Menin mutations have also been examined in 15 cases of isolated familial acromegaly, none of which was found to harbor a mutation *(53,80,81)*. So far there is an association between loss of heterozygosity at this locus and pituitary tumor formation, but until the portfolio of functions of menin are defined and the specificity of the finding clarified, the location of menin deletion in sporadic pituitary adenomas remains unclear.

Pituitary Tumor Transforming Gene

Successful cell cycle phase transition, such as the progression from G1 to S phase, depends on timed degradation of cyclin-dependent kinases. One of the key proteins in controlling timed degradation is securin, which is expressed in proliferating cells and in several kinds of tumors in a cell cycle-dependent manner *(82)*—increasing throughout S phase from low levels at the end of G1 to maximum prevalence at the junction of G2 and M phase *(83)*. The same protein (securin) was subsequently isolated by comparing differences in transcriptional activity between normal and neoplastic rat pituitary and called pituitary tumor-transforming gene (PTTG) *(3)*. More than 50% increases in PTTG have been observed in 23 of 30 endocrinologically inactive pituitary tumors, 13 of 13 GH-producing tumors, 9 of 10 prolactinomas, and 1 adrenocorticotropic hormone (ACTH)-secreting tumor, with more than 10-fold increases evident in some tumors *(84)*. Although this may imply a role for PTTG in pituitary tumorigenesis, the findings might also be expected of any marker of cell division measured semiquantitatively in comparison to a control tissue containing low levels (i.e., normal pituitary). Its place in pituitary tumor formation is still being assessed.

Other Oncogenes

As discussed, an oncogene implicated in the pathogenesis of pituitary adenomas would have to allow for these lesions to remain trophically stable for decades or resolve of their own accord. It is not too surprising, therefore, that there is little evidence for classic oncogene activation, except in the less than 1% of pituitary adenomas that also adopt the aggressive behavior typical of malignant tumors seen in other organ systems *(85–90)*. This is also true for the tumor suppressor genes p53, Rb, and DCC, which are strongly associated with human tumor formation *(91–96)*. The p53 gene codes for a protein that under normal circumstances prevents replication until the integrity of the genome has been assured *(97,98)*, or, failing that, activates apoptosis *(99)*. Inactivation of p53 is the most common genetic alteration found in human tumors, yet the 600-bp region within which 98% of all substitution mutations occur in other tumors shows no evidence of mutation in pituitary adenomas *(100)*. Despite the association of pituitary tumors with p27 and retinoblastoma gene inactivation in mice, no consistent point mutations of p21 and p27 have been found in human pituitary tumors *(101,102)*.

Abnormalities of tumor suppressor's on the short arm of chromosome 9 (p16INK4A and p15INK4B genes encoding the cyclin inhibitors p15 and p16), N-*ras*, H-*ras*, K-*ras*, mycL1, N-*myc*, *myc*, bcl1, H-stf1, sea, kraS2, p53, and fos are rarely or at least inconsistently implicated *(86,100,103–114)*. In the absence of known proto-oncogene mutations, perplexed investigators have adduced hypermethylation, dose effects *(112,115)*, and co-induction of tumor suppressors, such as nm23 *(116)* to explain pituitary adenoma behavior.

GENOMIC INTEGRITY

Although specific mutations leading to activation of proto-oncogenes or loss of tumor suppressors are rare in pituitary adenoma pathogenesis, loss or duplication of chromosomal regions is more common. No particular loci examined in pituitary adenomas are free of allelic deletions, and the impression that some regions or chromosomes are more involved than others (such as 11 *(107)*, 11q13, 13q12–14, 10q, and 1p *(117)*, 9p, 10, 11 and 13 *(118)*, 1, 3 and 12 *(115)*, 1, 4, 7, and 19 *(119)* or 7, 9, 12, 20 and X *(120–123)*), or that there is a direct relationship between the frequency or characteristics of deletions and the aggressiveness of the adenoma *(107)* may be artifacts of the probe batteries used rather than genuine associations. Nevertheless, the rate of gross aneuploidy in pituitary adenomas is at least 40% to 55% *(115,119,124,125)* and studies of specific loci find a similar high rate of one or more allelic deletions *(87,126)*.

The immediate assumption is that the appearance of aneuploidy implicates chromosomal instability in pituitary adenoma pathogenesis. However, in the same way that the significance of monoclonality in a pituitary tumor is quite different if the normal pituitary tissue from which it originated is clonally skewed by the presence of large clonal patches, the significance of chromosomal defects is different if normal pituitary tissue is not uniformly diploid. Is it possible, in other words, that rather than each cell in the normal pituitary being diploid, different pituitary clones normally have some degree of aneuploidy and that the pituitary, although diploid as a whole, has some degree of chromosomal tattiness? The answer to this question is unknown, but there are precedents for aneuploidy in normal human tissue. Trisomy 7, for example, which has been implicated in the pathogenesis of many tumors, including those of the thyroid, kidney, ovary, prostate, lung, and brain, has been found in macroscopically normal tissue away from obvious neoplastic involvement. This suggest that the clones with trisomy 7 detected in tumor may not represent the tumor parenchyma *(127)*. Trisomy 7 and other chromosomal aberrations have also been found in synovial tissue, cartilage, and bone of patients with osteoarthritis *(128,129)* and in addition to increasing with age in normal tissue *(130)*, trisomy 7 and trisomy 12 have been found in benign follicular thyroid nodules *(131)*.

So far, the significance of the finding of a high prevalence of aneuploidy remains obscure, but because different cancers exhibit either instability at the sequence level (i.e., point mutations) or chromosomal instability, but not usually both *(132,133)*, this issue needs more concerted examination.

CONCLUSION

With the exception of the *gsp* oncogene, which is implicated in the induction of a minority of somatotroph adenomas, the pathogenesis of pituitary adenomas remains unknown. Because removal of normal tissue from an adjacent corticotroph adenoma is sometimes curative and because pituitary adenomas may resolve without treatment, exogenous factors must be implicated in tumor propagation and are likely to be required for tumor initiation as well. Without clear information about trophic activity and clonal architecture in the normal pituitary, the presence of monoclonality cannot necessarily be taken to imply proto-oncogene activation and inexorable clonal expansion from a single cell. Equally, apparent loss of heterozygosity at various chromosomal regions cannot necessarily be implicated in pituitary adenoma formation without information about the ploidy of normal pituitary parenchymal cell clones.

It remains to be seen whether loss of heterozygosity or clonal expansion causes quantitative rather than qualitative abnormalities of gene products and somehow affects the ability of pituitary cells to correctly interpret their identities and functions, leading them to excessively exuberant trophic responses to recurrent physiologic stimuli and the development of the typical pituitary adenoma phenotype. In any case, given the strange and sometimes paradoxical behavior of these fascinating lesions, whichever mechanisms are adduced for pituitary adenoma induction and propagation must include an assessment of biologic plausibility in their evaluations of their causality.

REFERENCES

1. Molitch M. Meta-analytical data from 19 published series of pituitary incidentalomas totalling 12,300 autopsy examinations. Paper presented at: Ann. Meeting of the American Endocrine Society; June 11–14, 1997; Minneapolis, MN.
2. Lubke D, Saeger W. Carcinomas of the pituitary: definition and review of the literature. Gen Diagn Pathol 1995;141:81–92.
3. Pei L, Melmed S. Isolation and characterization of a pituitary tumor-transforming gene (PTTG). Mol Endocrinol 1997;11:433–441.
4. Jeffcoate WJ, Pound N, Sturrock NDC, Lambourne J. Long-term follow-up of patients with hyperprolactinaemia. Clin. Endocrinol. 1996;45:299–303.
5. Buchfelder M, Nomikos P, Schott W, Fahlbusch R. Persistent suppression of prolactin following surgery and dopamine-agonist treatment in a patient with a large macroprolactinoma. Paper presented at: 81st Ann. Meeting of the American Endocrine Society; June 12–15, 1999; San Diego: P576.
6. Robinson DB, Michaels RD. Empty sella resulting from the spontaneous resolution of a pituitary macroadenoma. Arch Intern Med 1992;152:1920–1923.
7. Van Zandijcke M, Casselman J. The vanishing pituitary adenoma. Acta Neurol Belg 1994;94:256–258.
8. Burke CW, Adams CB, Esiri MM, Morris C, Bevan JS. Transsphenoidal surgery for Cushing's disease: does what is removed determine the endocrine outcome? Clin Endocrinol (Oxf) 1990;33:525–537.
9. Atkinson AB, Chestnutt A, Crothers E, et al. Cyclical Cushing's disease: two distinct rhythms in a patient with a basophil adenoma. J Clin Endocrinol Metab 1985;60:328–332.
10. Atkinson AB, Kennedy AL, Carson DJ, Hadden DR, Weaver JA, Sheridan B. Five cases of cyclical Cushing's syndrome. Br Med J 1985;291:1453–1457.
11. Popovic V, Micic D, Nesovic M, et al. Cushing's disease cycling over ten years. Exp Clin Endocrinol 1990;92:143–148.
12. Levy A, Lightman SL. Local production of hypothalamic trophic peptides in human pituitary tumors. Clin Chem Enz Comm 1992;5:265–273.
13. Levy A, Powell M, Lightman SL. Colocalization of corticotrophin-releasing hormone and oxytocin transcripts in human pituitary adenomas. Endocr J 1993;1:117–122.
14. Levy A, Lightman SL. Quantitative in-situ hybridization histochemistry of anterior pituitary hormone mRNA species in human pituitary adenomas. Acta Endocrinal (Copen) 1988;119:397–404.
15. Levy A. Monoclonality of endocrine tumors: what does it mean? Trends Endocrinol Metab 2001;12:301–307.
16. Levy A. Is monoclonality in pituitary adenomas synonymous with neoplasia? Clin Endocrinol (Oxf) 2000;52:393–397.
17. Gartler SM, Riggs AD. Mammalian X-chromosome inactivation. Annu Rev Genet 1983;17:155–190

18. Alexander JM, Biller BM, Bikkal H, Zervas NT, Arnold A, Klibanski A. Clinically nonfunctioning pituitary tumors are monoclonal in origin. J Clin Invest 1990;86:336–340.
19. Herman V, Fagin J, Gonsky E, Kovacs K, Melmed S. Clonal origins of pituitary adenomas. J Clin Endocrinol Metab 1990;71:1427–1433.
20. Jacoby LB, Hedley-Whyte ET, Pulaski K, Seizinger BR, Martuza RL. Clonal origin of pituitary adenomas. J Neurosurg 1990;73:731–735.
21. Schulte HM, Oldfield EH, Allolio B, Katz DA, Berkman RA, Ali IU. Clonal composition of pituitary adenomas in patients with Cushing's disease: determination by X-chromosome inactivation analysis. J Clin Endocrinol Metab 1991;73:1302–1308.
22. Gicquel C, LeBouc Y, Craig I, Luton JP, Girard F, Bertagna X. Pituitary corticotroph adenomas are monoclonal. Paper presented at: Endocrine Society 73rd Annual Meeting; 1991; Atlanta, GA: 439.
23. Vogelstein B, Fearon ER, Hamilton SR, et al. Clonal analysis using recombinant DNA probes from the X-chromosome. Cancer Res 1987;47:4806–4813.
24. Laws E, Jr., Scheithauer BW, Carpenter S, Randall RV, Abbound CF. The pathogenesis of acromegaly. Clinical and immunocytochemical analysis in 75 patients. J Neurosurg 1985;63:35–38.
25. Levy A, Lightman SL. Growth hormone-releasing hormone transcripts in human pituitary adenomas. J Clin Endocrinol Metab 1992;74:1474–1476.
26. Wakabayashi I, Inokuchi K, Hasegawa O, Sugihara H, Minami S. Expression of growth hormone(GH)-releasing factor gene in GH-producing pituitary adenoma. J Clin Endocrinol Metab 1992;74:357–361.
27. Clayton RN, Pfeifer M, Wass JAH, et al. Human pituitary tumors have multiclonal origins. Paper produced at: The Endocrine Society's 81st Annual Meeting; 1999, San Diego, California: P121.
28. Clayton RN, Pfeifer M, Atkinson AB, et al. Different patterns of allelic loss (loss of heterozygosity) in recurrent human pituitary tumors provide evidence for multiclonal origins. Clin Cancer Res 2000;6:3973–3982.
29. Nolan LA, Lunness HR, Lightman SL, Levy A. The effects of age and spontaneous adenoma formation on trophic activity in the rat pituitary gland: a comparison with trophic activity in the human pituitary and in human pituitary adenomas. J Neuroendocrinol 1999; 11:393–401.
30. Tiltman AJ. Smooth muscle neoplasms of the uterus. Curr Opin Obstet Gynecol 1997;9:48–51.
31. Murry CE, Gipaya CT, Bartosek T, Benditt EP, Schwartz SM. Monoclonality of smooth muscle cells in human atherosclerosis. Am J Pathol 1997;151:697–705.
32. Chung IM, Schwartz SM, Murry CE. Clonal architecture of normal and atherosclerotic aorta: implications for atherogenesis and vascular development. Am J Pathol 1998;152:913–923.
33. Aihara T, Noguchi S, Sasaki Y, Imaoka S. Does monoclonality mean malignancy. Hepatology 1996;24:1550.
34. Tsai YC, Simoneau AR, Spruck CHr, et al. Mosaicism in human epithelium: macroscopic monoclonal patches cover the urothelium. J Urol 1995;153:1698–1700.
35. Schnall AM, Kovacs K, Brodkey JS, Pearson OH. Pituitary Cushing's disease without adenoma. Acta Endocrinol (Copen) 1980;94:297–303.
36. Kruse A, Klinken L, Holck S, Lindholm J. Pituitary histology in Cushing's disease. Clin Endocrinol (Oxf) 1992;37:254–259.
37. Bochicchio D, Losa M, Buchfelder M. Factors influencing the immediate and late outcome of Cushing's disease treated by transsphenoidal surgery: a retrospective study by the European Cushing's Disease Survey Group. J Clin Endocrinol Metab 1995;80:3114–3120.
38. Lissett CA, Peacey SR, Laing I, Tetlow L, Davis JR, Shalet SM. The outcome of surgery for acromegaly: the need for a specialist pituitary surgeon for all types of growth hormone (GH) secreting adenoma. Clin Endocrinol (Oxf) 1998;49:653–657.

39. Nowell PC, Croce CM. Chromosomal approaches to oncogenes and oncogenesis. FASEB J. 1988;2:3054–3060.
40. Migeon BR, Axelman J, Stetten G. Clonal evolution in human lymphoblast cultures. Am J Hum Genet 1988;42:742–747.
41. Heim S, Caron M, Jin Y, Mandahl N, Mitelman F. Genetic convergence during serial in vitro passage of a polyclonal squamous cell carcinoma. Cytogenet Cell Genet 1989;52:133–135.
42. Jiang X, Yao KT. The clonal progression in the neoplastic process of nasopharyngeal carcinoma. Biochem Biophys Res Commun 1996;221:122–128.
43. Thorner MO, Perryman RL, Cronin MJ, et al. Somatotroph hyperplasia: successful treatment of acromegaly by removal of a pancreatic islet tumor secreting a growth hormone releasing factor. J Clin Invest 1982;70:965–977.
44. Ezzat S, Asa SL, Stefaneanu L, et al. Somatotroph hyperplasia without pituitary adenoma associated with a long standing growth hormone-releasing hormone-producing bronchial carcinoid. J Clin Endocrinol Metab 1994;78:555–560.
45. Asa SL, Scheithauer BW, Bilbao JM, et al. A case for hypothalamic acromegaly: a clinicopathological study of six patients with hypothalamic gangliocytomas producing growth hormone-releasing hormone. J Clin Endocrinol Metab 1984;58:796–803.
46. Bevan JS, Asa SL, Rossi ML, Esiri MM, Adams CB, Burke CW. Intrasellar gangliocytoma containing gastrin and growth hormone-releasing hormone associated with a growth hormone-secreting pituitary adenoma. Clin Endocrinol (Oxf) 1989;30:213–234.
47. Carey RM, Varma SK, Drake JCR, et al. Ectopic secretion of corticotropin-releasing factor as a cause of Cushing's syndrome; a clinical, morphologic and biochemical study. N Engl J Med 1984;311:381–388.
48. Childs GV, Rougeau D, Unabia G. Corticotropin-releasing hormone and epidermal growth factor: mitogens for anterior pituitary corticotropes. Endocrinology 1995;136:1595–1602.
49. Saeger W, Puchner MJA, Ludecke DK. Combined sellar gangliocytoma and pituitary adenoma in acromegaly or Cushing's disease: a report of 3 cases. Virchows Arch 1994;425:93–99.
50. Asa SL, Kovacs K, Stefaneanu L, et al. Pituitary adenomas in mice transgenic for growth hormone-releasing hormone. Endocrinology 1992;131:2083–2089.
51 Asa SL, Ezzat S. The cytogenesis and pathogenesis of pituitary adenomas. Endocr Rev 1998;19:798–827.
52. Salvatori R, Thakker RV, Lopes MB, et al. Absence of mutations in the growth hormone (GH)-releasing hormone receptor gene in GH-secreting pituitary adenomas. Clin Endocrinol (Oxf) 2001;54:301–307.
53. Jorge BH, Agarwal SK, Lando VS, et al. Study of the multiple endocrine neoplasia type 1, growth hormone-releasing hormone receptor, Gs alpha, and Gi2 alpha genes in isolated familial acromegaly. J Clin Endocrinol Metab 2001;86:542–544.
54. Petersenn S, Heyens M, Ludecke DK, Beil FU, Schulte HM. Absence of somatostatin receptor type 2 A mutations and gip oncogene in pituitary somatotroph adenomas. Clin Endocrinol (Oxf) 2000;52:35–42.
55. Corbetta S, Ballare E, Mantovani G, et al. Somatostatin receptor subtype 2 and 5 in human GH-secreting pituitary adenomas: analysis of gene sequence and mRNA expression. Eur J Clin Invest 2001;31:208–214.
56. Karl M, Lamberts SW, Koper JW, et al. Cushing's disease preceded by generalized glucocorticoid resistance: clinical consequences of a novel, dominant-negative glucocorticoid receptor mutation. Proc Assoc Am Physicians 1996;108:296–307.
57. Karl M, Von Wichert G, Kempter E, et al. Nelson's syndrome associated with a somatic frame shift mutation in the glucocorticoid receptor gene. J Clin Endocrinol Metab 1996;81:124–129.
58. Vallar L, Spada A, Giannattasio G. Altered Gs and adenylate cyclase activity in human growth hormone-secreting pituitary adenomas. Nature 1987;330:566–568.

59. Landis CA, Masters SB, Spada A, Pace AM, Bourne HR, Vallar L. GTPase inhibiting mutations activate the a chain of Gs and stimulate adenylyl cyclase in human pituitary tumors. Nature 1989;340:692–696.
60. Lyons J, Landis CA, Harsh G, et al. Two G protein oncogenes in human endocrine tumors. Science 1990;249:655–659.
61. Spada A, Arosio M, Bochicchio D, et al. Clinical, biochemical, and morphological correlates in patients bearing growth hormone-secreting pituitary tumors with or without constitutively active adenylyl cyclase. J Clin Endocrinol Metab 1990;71:1421–1426.
62. Johnson MC, Codner E, Eggers M, Mosso L, Rodriguez JA, Cassorla F. Gsp mutations in Chilean patients harboring growth hormone-secreting pituitary tumors. J Pediatr Endocrinol Metab 1999;12:381–387.
63. Landis CA, Harsh G, Lyons J, Davis RL, McCormick F, Bourne HR. Clinical characteristics of acromegalic patients whose pituitary tumors contain mutant Gs protein. J Clin Endocrinol Metab 1990;71:1089–1095.
64. Harris PE, Alexander JM, Bikkal HA, et al. Glycoprotein hormone alpha-subunit production in somatotroph adenomas with and without Gs alpha mutations. J Clin Endocrinol Metab 1992;75:918–923.
65. Williamson EA, Daniels M, Foster S, Kelly WF, Kendall-Taylor P, Harris PE. Gs alpha and Gi2 alpha mutations in clinically non-functioning pituitary tumors. Clin Endocrinol (Oxf) 1994;41:815–520.
66. Williamson EA, Ince PG, Harrison D, Kendall-Taylor P, Harris PE. G-protein mutations in human pituitary adrenocorticotrophic hormone-secreting adenomas. Eur J Clin Invest 1995;25:128–131.
67. Chandrasekharappa SC, Guru SC, Manickam P, et al. Positional cloning of the gene for multiple endocrine neoplasia-type 1. Science 1997;276:404–407.
68. Marx SJ, Agarwal SK, Heppner C, et al. The gene for multiple endocrine neoplasia type 1: recent findings. Bone 1999;25:119–122.
69. Yazgan O, Pfarr CM. Differential binding of the Menin tumor suppressor protein to JunD isoforms. Cancer Res 2001;61:916–920.
70. Ohkura N, Kishi M, Tsukada T, Yamaguchi K. Menin, a gene product responsible for multiple endocrine neoplasia type 1, interacts with the putative tumor metastasis suppressor nm23. Biochem Biophys Res Commun 2001;282:1206–1210.
71. Kaji H, Canaff L, Lebrun JJ, Goltzman D, Hendy GN. Inactivation of menin, a Smad3-interacting protein, blocks transforming growth factor type beta signaling. Proc Natl Acad Sci USA 2001;98:3837–3842.
72. Fukino K, Kitamura Y, Sanno N, Teramoto A, Emi M. Analysis of the MEN1 gene in sporadic pituitary adenomas from Japanese patients. Cancer Lett 1999;144:85–92.
73. Bergman L, Boothroyd C, Palmer J, et al. Identification of somatic mutations of the MEN1 gene in sporadic endocrine tumors. Br J Cancer 2000;83:1003–1008.
74. Friedman E, Adams EF, Höög A, et al. Normal structural dopamine type 2 receptor gene in prolactin-secreting and other pituitary tumors. J Clin Endocrinol Metab 1994;78:568–574.
75. Eubanks PJ, Sawicki MP, Samara GJ, et al. Putative tumor-suppressor gene on chromosome 11 is important in sporadic endocrine tumor formation. Am J Surg 1994;167:180–185.
76. Evans CO, Brown MR, Parks JS, Oyesiku NM. Screening for MEN1 tumor suppressor gene mutations in sporadic pituitary tumors. J Endocrinol Invest 2000;23:304–309.
77. Prezant TR, Levine J, Melmed S. Molecular characterization of the men1 tumor suppressor gene in sporadic pituitary tumors. J Clin Endocrinol Metab 1998;83:1388–1391.
78. Farrell WE, Simpson DJ, Bicknell J, et al. Sequence analysis and transcript expression of the MEN1 gene in sporadic pituitary tumors. Br J Cancer 1999;80:44–50.
79. Zhuang Z, Ezzat SZ, Vortmeyer AO, et al. Mutations of the MEN1 tumor suppressor gene in pituitary tumors. Cancer Res 1997;57:5446–5451.

80. Teh BT, Kytola S, Farnebo F, et al. Mutation analysis of the MEN1 gene in multiple endocrine neoplasia type 1, familial acromegaly and familial isolated hyperparathyroidism. J Clin Endocrinol Metab 1998;83:2621–2626.
81. Gadelha MR, Prezant TR, Une KN, et al. Loss of heterozygosity on chromosome 11q13 in two families with acromegaly/gigantism is independent of mutations of the multiple endocrine neoplasia type I gene. J Clin Endocrinol Metab 2000;85:4920–4921.
82. Romero F, Multon MC, Ramos-Morales F, et al. Human securin, hPTTG, is associated with Ku heterodimer, the regulatory subunit of the DNA-dependent protein kinase. Nucleic Acids Res 2001;29:1300–1307.
83. Yu R, Ren SG, Horwitz GA, Wang Z, Melmed S. Pituitary tumor transforming gene (PTTG) regulates placental JEG-3 cell division and survival: evidence from live cell imaging. Mol Endocrinol 2000;14:1137–1146.
84 Zhang X, Horwitz GA, Heaney AP, et al. Pituitary tumor transforming gene (PTTG) expression in pituitary adenomas. J Clin Endocrinol Metab 1999;84:761–767.
85. Barbacid M. *Ras* genes. Annu Rev Biochem 1987;56:779–827.
86. Karga HJ, Alexander JM, Hedley-Whyte ET, Klibanski A, Jameson JL. *Ras* mutations in human pituitary tumors. J Clin Endocrinol Metab 1992;74:914–919.
87. Bates AS, Buckley N, Boggild MD, et al. Clinical and genetic changes in a case of a Cushing's carcinoma. Clin Endocrinol (Oxf) 1995;42:663–670.
88. Pei L, Melmed S, Scheithauer BW, Kovacs K, Benedict WF, Prager D. Frequent loss of heterozygosity at the retinoblastoma susceptibility gene (RB) locus in aggressive pituitary tumors: evidence for a chromosome 13 tumor suppressor gene other than RB. Cancer Res 1995;55:1613–1616.
89. Kulig E, Jin L, Qian X, et al. Apoptosis in nontumorous and neoplastic human pituitaries: expression of the Bcl-2 family of proteins. Am J Pathol 1999;154:767–774.
90. Harada K, Aria K, Kurisu K, Tahara H. Telomerase activity and the expression of telomerase components in pituitary adenoma with malignant transformation. Surg Neurol 2000;53: 267–274.
91. Wu SQ, Storer BE, Bookland EA, et al. Nonrandom chromosome losses in stepwise neoplastic transformation in vitro of human uroepithelial cells. Cancer Res 1991;51:3323–3326.
92. Tanaka K, Oshimura M, Kikuchi R, Seki M, Hayashi T, Miyaki M. Suppression of tumorigenicity in human colon carcinoma cells by introduction of normal chromosome 5 or 18. Nature 1991;349:340–342.
93. Hollstein M, Sidransky D, Vogelstein B, Harris CC. p53 mutations in human cancers. Science 1991;253:49–53
94. Malkin D, Li FP, Strong LC, et al. Germ line p53 mutations in a familial syndrome of breast cancer, sarcomas, and other neoplasms. Science 1990;250:1223–1238.
95. Oliner JD, Kinzler KW, Meltzer PS, George DL, Vogelstein B. Amplification of a gene encoding a p53-associated protein in human sarcomas. Nature 1992;358:80–83.
96. Michalovitz D, Halevy O, Oren M. p53 mutations: gains or losses? J Cell Biochem 1991;45:22–29.
97. Farmer G, Bargonetti J, Zhu H, Friedman P, Prywes R, Prives C. Wild-type p53 activates transcription in vitro. Nature 1992;358:83–86.
98. Lane DP. p53, guardian of the genome. Nature 1992;358:15–16.
99. Yonish RE, Resnitzky D, Lotem J, Sachs L, Kimchi A, Oren M. Wild-type p53 induces apoptosis of myeloid leukaemic cells that is inhibited by interleukin-6. Nature 1991;353:345–347.
100. Levy A, Hall L, Yeudall WA, Lightman SL. P53 gene mutations in pituitary adenomas: a rare event. Clin Endocrinol 1994;41:809–814.
101. Ikeda H, Yoshimoto T, Shida N. Molecular analysis of p21 and p27 genes in human pituitary adenomas. Br J Cancer 1997;76:1119–1123.

102. Dahia PL, Aguiar RC, Honegger J, et al. Mutation and expression analysis of the p27/kip1 gene in corticotrophin-secreting tumors. Oncogene 1998;16:69–76.
103. Byström C, Larsson C, Blomberg C, et al. Localization of the MEN 1 gene to a small region within chromosome 11q13 by deletion mapping in tumors. Proc Natl Acad Sci USA 1990;87:1968–1972.
104. Herman V, Drazin NZ, Gonsky R, Melmed S. Molecular screening of pituitary adenomas for gene mutations and rearrangements. J Clin Endocrinol Metab 1993;77:50–55.
105. Cai WY, Alexander JM, Hedley-Whyte ET, et al. *Ras* mutations in human prolactinomas and pituitary carcinomas. J Clin Endocrinol Metab 1994;78:89–93.
106. Pei L, Melmed S, Scheithauer B, Kovacs K, Prager D. H-*ras* mutations in human pituitary carcinoma metastases. J Clin Endocrinol Metab 1994;78:842–846.
107. Boggild MD, Jenkinson S, Pistorello M, et al. Molecular genetic studies of sporadic pituitary adenomas. J Clin Endocrinol Metab 1994;78:387–392.
108. Woloschak M, Roberts JL, Post K. *c-Myc*, *c-fos*, and *c-myb* gene expression in human pituitary adenomas. J Clin Endocrinol Metab 1994;79:253–257.
109. Cryns VL, Alexander JM, Klibanski A, Arnold A. The retinoblastoma gene in human pituitary tumors. J Clin Endocrinol Metab 1993;77:644–646.
110. Farrell WE, Simpson DJ, Bicknell JE, Talbot AJ, Bates AS, Clayton RN. Chromosome 9p deletions in invasive and noninvasive nonfunctional pituitary adenomas: the deleted region involves markers outside of the MTS1 and MTS2 genes. Cancer Res 1997;57:2703–2709.
111. Yoshimoto K, Tanaka C, Yamada S, et al. Infrequent mutations of p16INK4A and p15INK4B genes in human pituitary adenomas. Eur J Endocrinol 1997;136:74–80.
112. Jaffrain-Rea ML, Ferretti E, Toniato E, et al. p16 (INK4a, MTS-1) gene polymorphism and methylation status in human pituitary tumors. Clin Endocrinol (Oxf) 1999;51:317–325.
113. Wenbin C, Asai A, Teramoto A, Sanno N, Kirino T. Mutations of the MEN1 tumor suppressor gene in sporadic pituitary tumors. Cancer Lett 1999;142:43–47.
114. Poncin J, Stevenaert A, Beckers A. Somatic MEN1 gene mutation does not contribute significantly to sporadic pituitary tumorigenesis. Eur J Endocrinol 1999;140:573–576.
115. Finelli P, Giardino D, Rizzi N, et al. Non-random trisomies of chromosomes 5, 8 and 12 in the prolactinoma sub-type of pituitary adenomas: conventional cytogenetics and interphase FISH study. Int J Cancer 2000;86:344–350.
116. Takino H, Herman V, Weiss M, Melmed S. Purine-binding factor (nm23) gene expression in pituitary tumors: marker of adenoma invasiveness. J Clin Endocrinol Metab 1995;80: 1733–1738.
117. Clayton RN, Boggild M, Bates AS, Bicknell J, Simpson D, Farrell W. Tumor suppressor genes in the pathogenesis of human pituitary tumors. Horm Res 1997;47:185–193.
118. Farrell WE, Clayton RN. Tumor suppressor genes in pituitary tumor formation. Baillieres Best Pract Res Clin Endocrinol Metab 1999;13:381–393.
119. Rock JP, Babu VR, Drumheller T, Chason J. Cytogenetic findings in pituitary adenoma: results of a pilot study. Surg Neurol 1993;40:224–229.
120. Rey JA, Bello MJ, de Campos JM, Kusak ME, Martinez-Castro P, Benitez J. A case of pituitary adenoma with 58 chromosomes. Cancer Genet Cytogenet 1986;23:171–174.
121. Dietrich CU, Pandis N, Bjerre P, Schroder HD, Heim S. Simple numerical chromosome aberrations in two pituitary adenomas. Cancer Genet Cytogenet 1993;69:118–121.
122 Larsen JB, Schroder HD, Sorensen AG, Bjerre P, Heim S. Simple numerical chromosome aberrations characterize pituitary adenomas. Cancer Genet Cytogenet 1999;114:144–149.
123. Mertens F, Johansson B, Hoglund M, Mitelman F. Chromosomal imbalance maps of malignant solid tumors: a cytogenetic survey of 3185 neoplasms. Cancer Res 1997;57: 2765–2780.
124. Anniko M, Tribukait B, Wersall J. DNA ploidy and cell phase in human pituitary tumors. Cancer 1984;53:1708–1713.

125. Anniko M, Tribukait B. DNA pattern of human pituitary tumors. Am J Otolaryngol 1985;6:103–110.
126. Bates AS, Farrell WE, Bicknell EJ, et al. Allelic deletion in pituitary adenomas reflects aggressive biological activity and has potential value as a prognostic marker. J Clin Endocrinol Metab 1997;82:818–824.
127. Johansson B, Heim S, Mandahl N, Mertens F, Mitelman F. Trisomy 7 in nonneoplastic cells. Genes Chromosomes Cancer 1993;6:199–205.
128. Mertens F, Palsson E, Lindstrand A, et al. Evidence of somatic mutations in osteoarthritis. Hum Genet 1996;98:651–656.
129. Broberg K, Hoglund M, Lindstrand A, Toksvig-Larsen S, Mandahl N, Mertens F. Polyclonal expansion of cells with trisomy 7 in synovia from patients with osteoarthritis. Cytogenet Cell Genet 1998;83:30–34.
130. Broberg K, Toksvig-Larsen S, Lindstrand A, Mertens F. Trisomy 7 accumulates with age in solid tumors and non-neoplastic synovia. Genes Chromosomes Cancer 2001;30:310–315.
131. Roque L, Serpa A, Clode A, Castedo S, Soares J. Significance of trisomy 7 and 12 in thyroid lesions with follicular differentiation: a cytogenetic and in situ hybridization study. Lab Invest 1999;79:369–378.
132. Aaltonen LA, Peltomaki P, Leach FS, et al. Clues to the pathogenesis of familial colorectal cancer. Science 1993;260:812–816.
133. Cahill DP, Kinzler KW, Vogelstein B, Lengauer C. Genetic instability and darwinian selection in tumors. Trends Cell Biol 1999;9:M57–60.

2 Prolactinoma

Prakash Abraham, MB, BS, MD, MRCP,
and John S. Bevan, MD, FRCP (Edin)

CONTENTS

INTRODUCTION

Prolactin (PRL) was characterized as a hormone distinct from growth hormone, which also has lactogenic activity, as recently as 1971. In humans, the predominant PRL species is a 23 kDa, 199-amino-acid, polypeptide synthesized and secreted by lactotroph cells in the anterior pituitary gland. Pituitary PRL production is under tonic inhibitory control by hypothalamic dopamine, such that pituitary stalk interruption produces hyperprolactinemia. The neuropeptides thyrotropin-releasing hormone (TRH) and vasoactive intestinal peptide (VIP) exert less important stimulatory effects on pituitary PRL release *(1)*. Prolactin is essential for postpartum milk production and lactation. During pregnancy, increasing estrogen production stimulates the pituitary lactotrophs and causes increased PRL secretion. However, high estrogen levels inhibit PRL stimulation of the breasts, and, as a result, lactation does not occur until the estrogen levels decline postpartum.

Prolactinomas are the most common hormonally active pituitary tumors. There is a marked female preponderance, and prolactinoma is relatively rare in men. Several studies have revealed small prolactinomas in approx 5% of autopsy pituitaries, most of which are undiagnosed during life. From a clinical stand-

From: *Management of Pituitary Tumors: The Clinician's Practical Guide, Second Edition*
Edited by: M. P. Powell, S. L. Lightman, and E. R. Laws, Jr.

point, prolactinomas may be divided arbitrarily into *micro*prolactinomas (<10-mm diameter) and *macro*prolactinomas (>10-mm diameter). This is a useful distinction that predicts tumor behavior and indicates appropriate management strategies. Generally, microprolactinomas run a benign course. Some regress spontaneously, most stay unchanged for many years, and few expand to cause local pressure effects. Pooled data from seven studies, including 139 patients with untreated microprolactinomas, show documented tumor expansion in only 9 patients (7%) *(2)*. In contrast, macroprolactinomas may present with pressure symptoms, often increase in size if untreated, and rarely disappear.

Prolactinomas are usually sporadic tumors. Molecular genetics have shown nearly all to be monoclonal, suggesting that an intrinsic pituitary defect is likely to be responsible for pituitary tumorigenesis. Occasionally, prolactinoma may be part of a multiple endocrine neoplasia syndrome (MEN-1), but this occurs too infrequently to justify MEN-1 screening in every patient with a prolactinoma. Mixed growth hormone (GH)- and PRL-secreting tumors are well recognized and give rise to acromegaly in association with hyperprolactinemia. Malignant prolactinomas are rare. A few cases have been described that have proved resistant to aggressive treatment with surgery, radiotherapy, dopamine agonists, and, occasionally, chemotherapy. In a small proportion, extracranial metastases in liver, lungs, bone, and lymph nodes have been documented.

CLINICAL FEATURES OF PROLACTINOMA

The clinical features of prolactinoma are attributable to three main factors: hyperprolactinemia, space occupation by the tumor, and varying degrees of hypopituitarism (Table 1). The individual clinical picture will be determined by the gender and age of the patient and the tumor size. In brief, hyperprolactinemia stimulates milk production, particularly from the estrogen-primed breast, and inhibits hypothalamic gonadotropin-releasing hormone (GnRH) release, which leads to hypogonadotropic hypogonadism.

Premenopausal women, most of whom have microprolactinomas, usually have oligomenorrhea or amenorrhea (90%) and/or galactorrhea (up to 80%). Anovulatory infertility is common. Excluding pregnancy, hyperprolactinemia accounts for 10–20% of cases of secondary amenorrhea. In passing, it is worth remembering that most women with galactorrhea do not have menstrual disturbance, hyperprolactinemia, or a pituitary tumor.

Postmenopausal women are, by definition, already hypogonadal and markedly hypoestrogenemic. Hyperprolactinemia in this age group does not, therefore, present with classic symptoms and may be recognized only when a large pituitary adenoma produces headache and/or visual disturbance.

The men with hyperprolactinemia experience reduced libido, impotence (75%), and infertility associated with a reduced sperm count. Such symptoms

Table 1
Clinical Features of Prolactinoma

A. Caused by prolactin excess
- Women
  - Oligomenorrhea/amenorrhea
  - Galactorrhea
  - Infertility
  - Hirsutism/acne[a]
- Men
  - Reduced libido
  - Impotence
  - Infertility
  - Galactorrhea[a]

B. Caused by tumor size (usually in men)
  - Headache
  - Visual failure, classically bitemporal hemianopia
  - Cranial nerve palsies

C. Caused by other pituitary hormone deficiency
  - *Microprolactinoma*—other pituitary function usually normal
  - *Macroprolactinoma*—varying degrees of hypopituitarism may be present

[a]Less common features.

are often concealed or ignored, particularly by older men, so men tend to present later with larger tumors causing pressure symptoms (Table 1). Galactorrhea is uncommon in men but does occur occasionally. Weight gain is noted frequently by men with hyperprolactinemia. Prolactinoma is an unusual cause of delayed puberty in both sexes, and some advocate the routine measurement of serum PRL in this situation.

Reduced bone mineral density (BMD) is a well-recognized long-term effect of untreated hyperprolactinemia. Studies of women with hyperprolactinemia and amenorrheia women have shown reductions in trabecular BMD of approx 20% (range 10%–26%) and cortical BMD of 6% (range 2.5%–11%) *(3)*. Reduced estrogen levels, as well as the direct effect of hyperprolactinemia, play a role in osteopenia. A longitudinal follow-up study of untreated women with amenorrheia suggested that BMD loss is progressive in some but not all cases, patients who are overweight and those with higher androgen levels being afforded some protection *(4)*. Restoration of menses after therapy results in an increase in bone density, although it may not return to normal *(4,5)*. Men with hypogonadism secondary to hyperprolactinemia also have significant BMD reductions. In one study of 20 men, 16 had osteopenia at the spine and 6 at the hip *(6)*. Adolescents had lower bone densities at the time of diagnosis, and less improvement was observed after two yr of dopamine agonist therapy, compared with adults with prolactinomas *(7)*.

Table 2
Causes of Hyperprolactinemia

A. Physiologic
- Stress (venipuncture?)
- Pregnancy
- Lactation

B. Pharmacologic
- Anti-emetics (e.g., metoclopramide, domperidone, prochlorperazine)
- Phenothiazines (e.g., chlorpromazine, thioridazine)
- Many others[1]

C. Pathologic
- Primary hypothyroidism
- Pituitary tumors
  - Prolactinoma
  - GH secreting (30% of people with acromegaly)
  - Nonfunctioning (stalk pressure or disconnection hyperprolactinemia)
- Polycystic ovarian syndrome (10% of people with polycystic ovary syndrome)
- Hypothalamic lesions (rare)
  - Sarcoidosis
  - Langerhan's cell histiocytosis
  - Hypothalamic tumors
- Chest wall stimulation
  - Repeated breast self-examination
  - Post-herpes zoster
- Liver or renal failure

GH, growth hormone.

DIAGNOSTIC INVESTIGATIONS

Causes of Hyperprolactinemia

The causes of hyperprolactinemia can be divided simply into physiologic, pharmacologic, and pathologic (Table 2). The normal PRL range for nonpregnant women is <500 mU/L (20 μg/L) and for men <300 mU/L (12 μg/L). Pregnancy is the most common cause of hyperprolactinemic amenorrhea, and serum PRL concentrations may rise as high as 8000 mU/L (320 μg/L) during the third trimester. Normal lactation is also associated with quite marked elevation of serum PRL. As predicted from the physiologic dopaminergic inhibition of PRL secretion, treatment with dopamine receptor antagonist drugs commonly induces hyperprolactinemia. Serum PRL levels may rise as high as 5000 mU/L (200 μg/L). This is a particular problem with the major tranquilizers (e.g., chlorpromazine) and anti-emetics (e.g., metoclopramide). A source of potential confusion may arise if a patient does not reveal that he or she is taking an over-the-counter preparation, such as a combined medication for the treatment of migraine, which contains both an analgesic and an anti-emetic. Similarly, some nonprescribed herbal or alternative remedies contain constituents that cause PRL elevation. Thus, a comprehensive drug history is essential. With regard to pathologic causes of hyperprolactinemia, it is important to exclude primary hypothyroidism. Modest hyperprolactinemia is present in 40% of patients, although only 10% have levels > 600 mU/L (24 μg/L). Nevertheless, some young women with hypothyroidism may present with menstrual disturbance and galactorrhea, together with few typical hypothyroid symptoms. Once venipuncture stress, pregnancy, interfering drugs, and primary hypothyroidism are excluded, significant hyperprolactinemia is usually associated with a pituitary adenoma (Table 2).

Interpretation of Prolactin Immunoassay Results

Macroprolactin

PRL in human serum exists in multiple molecular forms, with three dominant species identified by gel filtration chromatography: monomeric PRL (23 kDa), big PRL (50–60 kDa), and big-big PRL (macroprolactin, 150–170 kDa). Macroprolactin is a complex of PRL, with an IgG antibody that is detected by most, but not all, PRL immunoassays. The clinical significance and biologic activity of macroprolactin remain contentious. Recent studies have indicated that this PRL species is present in significant amounts in up to 20% of hyperprolactinemic sera. However, many patients with macroprolactinemia do not exhibit typical hyperprolactinemic symptoms, and preliminary data suggest that this prolactin variant is virtually never associated with macroprolactinoma. The presence of macroprolactin can be confirmed by a simple polyethylene glycol precipitation method *(8)*. Presently, there is little justification for detailed pituitary investigation after the finding of macroprolactinemia in an essentially asymptomatic individual.

Prolactin Hook Effect

If serum PRL concentrations are extremely high (as in some men with giant prolactinomas), the amount of PRL antigen may cause antibody saturation in PRL immunoradiometric assays (IRMAs), leading to artifactually low PRL results. This is known as the high-dose hook effect and has been occasionally recognized in other immunoassays (e.g., β-human chorionic gonadotropin [hCG]). This artifact may lead to misdiagnosis and inappropriate surgery for some patients with macroprolactinoma. If an IRMA is employed, serum PRL should always be assayed *in dilution* in any patient with a large pituitary lesion that might be a prolactinoma *(9)*.

Dynamic Prolactin Function Tests

Several dynamic tests have been proposed for the evaluation of hyperprolactinemia. However, a recent survey showed that only 15% of UK clinical endocrinologists routinely use dynamic PRL function tests, with most using thyrotropin-releasing hormone (TRH) rather than a dopamine antagonist. In our experience, the intravenous (iv) administration of a dopamine antagonist (such as 10 mg metoclopramide) is a simple well-tolerated procedure that provides clinically useful information, particularly for patients with modest serum PRL elevations. Dopamine antagonist administration to normal individuals results in a marked rise in serum PRL concentration (to at least three times basal) together with little or no change in serum thyroid-stimulating hormone (TSH) (<2 mU/L rise). In contrast, patients with pituitary microlesions and macrolesions have blunted PRL responses. Patients with microprolactinomas may, in addition, show exaggerated TSH responses owing to enhanced dopaminergic tone on the anterior pituitary thyrotrophs (via short-loop hypothalamic feedback).

Sawers and coworkers reviewed 84 patients with hyperprolactinemia whose screening had included a domperidone test and high-resolution magnetic resonance imaging (MRI) *(10)*. They found that 18 of 20 patients with normal PRL responses to domperidone had normal MRI scans, and the other 2 had only microadenomas. In contrast, 18 of the remaining 64 patients with abnormal PRL responses had lesions greater than 10 mm in diameter. Of the rest, 63% had microadenomas. Dopamine antagonist testing can therefore identify a subset of hyperprolactinemic patients for whom detailed pituitary imaging is mandatory. Conversely, a normal PRL response to domperidone obviates the need for pituitary imaging and can reduce usage of this limited resource.

Dopamine antagonist testing can also be useful before and after surgery for microprolactinoma. Webster and colleagues described a series of 82 patients with hyperprolactinemia submitted to surgery for suspected prolactinoma *(11)*. No tumor was found in three cases, including the only two patients with normal PRL and TSH responses to domperidone. Overall, 79% of patients had early postoperative normalization of serum PRL, but there were three relapses during long-term follow-up. Two of these had persistently abnormal PRL and TSH responses to domperidone, even when basal PRL levels remained normal.

Thus, although few patients with microprolactinoma are now treated surgically, these data are important because they indicate that dopamine antagonist testing can confirm (or refute) the presence of a microprolactinoma with reasonable certainty. Clinicians may regard this confirmatory biochemical evidence to be helpful in the medical management of such patients when histologic proof of the diagnosis will not be forthcoming.

TRH testing is less discriminatory and generally not helpful in hyperprolactinemia investigation. However, the test may have limited use in the evaluation of patients with GH- or gonadotrophin-secreting tumors, a proportion of whom will show paradoxical stimulation of hormone release.

Diagnostic Value of the Basal Serum Prolactin Concentration

Most patients with microprolactinomas have basal serum PRL concentrations less than 5000 mU/L (200 μg/L). In patients with pituitary macrolesions, the basal serum PRL is of considerable diagnostic value. A value greater than 5000 mU/L is virtually diagnostic of a macroprolactinoma and with a level greater than 10,000 mU/L (400 μg/L), there is no other possible diagnosis. A serum PRL concentration lower than 2000 mU/L (18 μg/L) in a patient with a pituitary macrolesion usually indicates disconnection hyperprolactinemia rather than tumoral secretion of the hormone. This is due most commonly to a nonfunctioning pituitary macroadenoma, although intrasellar craniopharyngioma and numerous other neoplastic and inflammatory pathologies may masquerade as pseudopituitary adenomas *(12)*. An intermediate serum PRL level (2000–5000 mU/L or 80–200 μg/L) in a patient with a large pituitary lesion produces an area of diagnostic uncertainty that dynamic PRL function tests cannot resolve; approx 50% of such patients will have true prolactinomas and the remainder disconnection hyperprolactinemia *(12,13)*.

Pituitary Imaging and Ophthalmological Assessment

This is similar to the assessment of patients with other pituitary and parapituitary lesions and is described in Chapters 5 and 6.

General Pituitary Function

Larger pituitary masses may cause hypopituitarism by either direct pituitary compression or disruption of hypothalamic control mechanisms. Patients with microprolactinomas usually have normal GH, adenocorticotropic hormone (ACTH), and TSH function. However, with macroprolactinomas, the degree of hypopituitarism is likely to be proportional to the size of the tumor. With the largest tumors, ACTH and TSH deficits may be present at diagnosis in approx 20% of patients, and GH deficiency is almost invariable. All patients with macroprolactinomas should have full pituitary function testing, using the methods described in Chapter 12.

TREATMENT OF PROLACTINOMA

An algorithm for the management of prolactinoma is given in Fig. 1.

Treatment Indications

Most patients with prolactinoma require active treatment. Infertility, menstrual disturbance with long-standing hypogonadism (risk of secondary osteoporosis), troublesome galactorrhea, an enlarging pituitary tumor and tumor

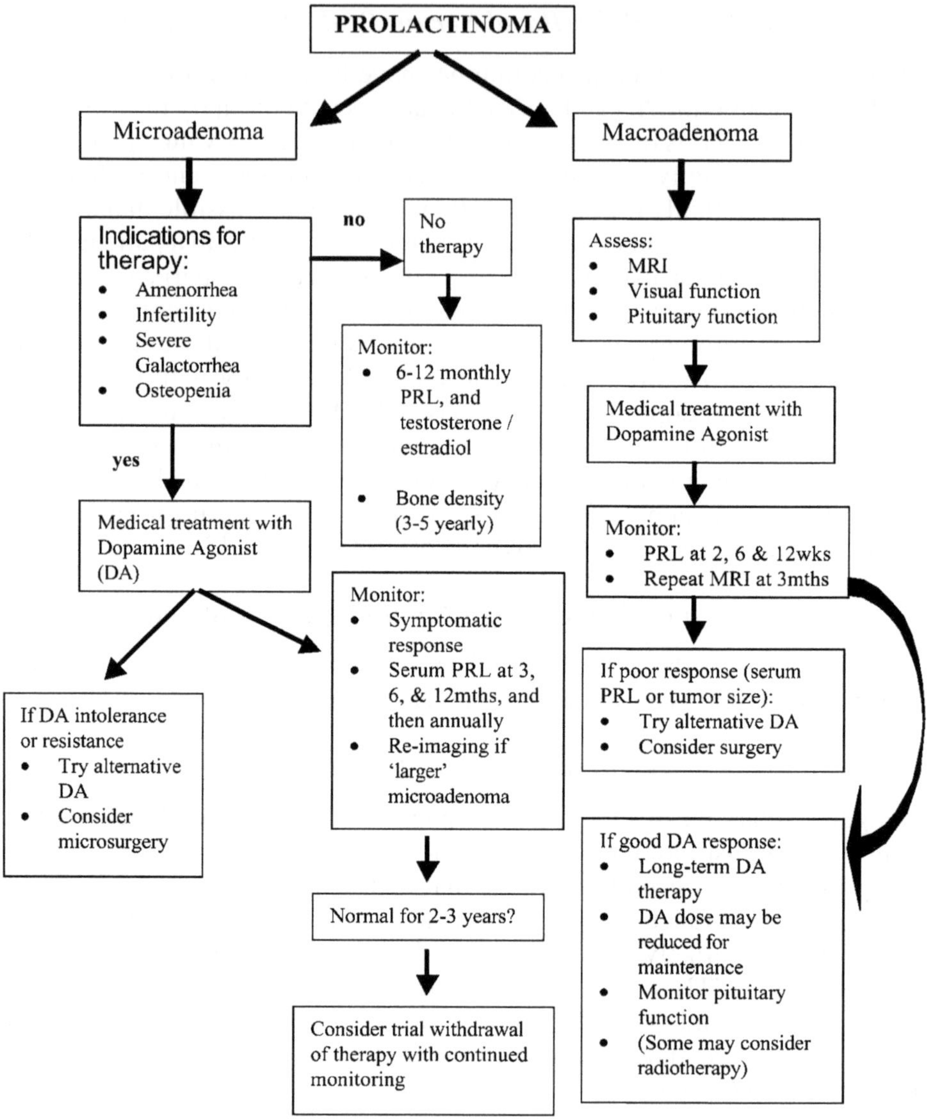

Fig. 1. Management algorithm for prolactinoma.

pressure effects (particularly visual failure) are all indications for treatment. As will be seen, dopamine agonist drugs are now indicated as primary medical therapy for patients with prolactinomas of *all* sizes. However, an important exception is the patient with a pituitary macrolesion and minor PRL elevation, who is most likely to have a nonfunctioning pituitary adenoma requiring surgery for decompression and histologic diagnosis. It may be reasonable to simply observe some patients with microprolactinomas, particularly if circulating sex steroid concentrations are judged to be adequate and BMD is normal.

Dopamine Agonists

The introduction of medical therapy with dopamine agonists revolutionized the treatment of patients with prolactinoma. The first such drug was bromocriptine, a semisynthetic ergopeptine derivative, introduced in 1971. On a global basis, this probably remains the most widely used dopamine agonist, but the introduction of other longer acting and better tolerated drugs, such as cabergoline and quinagolide, is altering this pattern, at least in the Western world. Many UK endocrine units now use cabergoline as first-choice dopamine agonist after a large comparative study with bromocriptine, which convincingly demonstrated its superiority in terms of tolerability, patient convenience, and possibly also efficacy *(14)*. All dopamine agonists may produce unwanted side effects, including, in decreasing order of importance, upper gastrointestinal disturbance (especially nausea), postural hypotension, constipation, nasal stuffiness, and Raynaud's phenomenon. These can be minimized by using an incremental dosage schedule and taking tablets during meals.

Cabergoline and quinagolide are newer dopamine agonists, which have been licensed in the UK during the last decade. Table 3 summarizes the recent prospective comparative studies of these agents, both with each other and with bromocriptine. Bromocriptine normalized PRL in 57% of patients, compared with 85% taking cabergoline and 78% taking quinagolide. Cabergoline was better tolerated, with mild adverse effects reported in only 37% and fewer than 3% of patients withdrawing from therapy. Bromocriptine caused mild adverse effects in 67%, with 13% of patients needing to cease therapy. Table 4 provides an overview of recent publications addressing cabergoline efficacy and tolerability. In pooled data from 1485 patients (972 with microadenomas and 513 with macroadenomas), PRL was normalized in 87% of patients. Adverse effects were noted in 26% of patients, but only 1.7% of patients had to discontinue therapy. It is notable that cabergoline was effective (approx 80%) and well tolerated (>90%) in the majority of patients with bromocriptine resistance (164 patients) and bromocriptine intolerance (267 patients). Colao and colleagues reported that 17 of 20 patients resistant to quinagolide achieved normoprolactinemia during cabergoline therapy, although a proportion may have been poorly compliant with quinagolide *(29)*.

Bromocriptine is used in a dose of 2.5 mg two or three times daily. It is now clear that the doses of 20–40 mg/d used in early studies are no more efficacious and produce more side-effects. Cabergoline is usually effective in a dose of 0.5–1.0 mg once or twice *weekly* and quinagolide in a *once-daily* dose of 75–150 μg. To minimize side effects, patients should be advised to take these two newer

Table 3
Prospective Comparative Studies of Bromocriptine, Cabergoline, and Quinagolide

Study author (year) (ref)	*Drugs*[a]	*Total patients*	*Study design and duration*	*Prolactin normalization (PRL n)*	*Return of menses or normal gonadal function (G) (%)*	*Mild adverse effects (AD) (%)*	*Drug withdrawal (WD)*
Webster	BCR	236	MC,R	138 (58%)	84	78	27 (12%)
(1994) *(14)*	CBG	223	DB (8 wk)	186 (83%)	93	68	7 (3%)
Van der Heijden	BCR	24	R, DB,	14 (70%)	79	66	4 (16%)
(1991) *(15)*	QUI	23	24 wk	17 (81%)	80	78	1 (14%)
Verhelst	BCR	5	R, DB,	2 (40%)	70	60	0
(1991) *(16)*	QUI	7	24 wk	3 (43%)	82	57	1 (14%)
Homburgh	BCR	11	R, DB,	3 (27%)	82	64	4 (36%)
(1990) *(17)*	QUI	11	24 wk	10 (91%)	91	82	0
Giusti	CBG	12	R, NB	10 (83%)	82	50	1 (8%)
(1994) *(18)*	QUI		CO, 12 wk	6 (50%)	80	90	2 (16%)
Di Sarno (2000) *(19)*	CBG	39[b] (23 mic and 16 mac)	NB, CO 52 wk	22 (95%) mic 14 (87%) mac	100% (mic)	0	0
	QUI			23 (100%) mic 14 (87%) mac	100% mic 62% mac	30	0
De Luis DA	CBG	20	R, NB,	18 (90%)	95	30	0
(2000) *(20)*	QUI		CO, 12 wk	15 (75%)	90	55	0

[a]Bromocriptine: Total 276, PRL n: 157 (57%), G: 79%, AD: 67%, WD: 35 (13%); Cabergoline: Total 294, PRL n: 256 (85%), G: 91%, AD: 37%, WD: 8 (2.5%); Quinagolide: Total 112, PRL n: 88 (78%), G: 84%, AD: 65%, WD: 4 (3.5%)

[b]All other studies had few macroadenomas (only 6 out of 643 patients).

BCR, bromocriptine; CBG, cabergoline; QUI, quinagolide; R, Randomized; MC, multicenter; DB, double blind; NB, nonblinded; CO, crossover; PRL n, PRL normalization; G, gonadal function; AD, adverse effects; WD, drug withdrawal; mic, microadenoma; mac, macroadenoma.

Table 4
Overview of Cabergoline Efficacy and Tolerability in Patients With Hyperprolactinemic Disorders

Year	*Author (reference)*	*Microa/ macro adenoma*	*% Patients with PRL normalization*	*% Side effects*	*% Dropouts*	*% Patients with tumor reductionb*	*BCR-resistant/ intolerant*
1989	Ciccarelli *(21)*	27/3	81	48	11	71	0/7
1989	Ferrari *(22)*	38/8	85	15	0	83	
1992	Ferrari *(23)*	108/19	90	23	0	79	10/1
1993	Webster *(24)*	161/1	92	40	3		0/27
1994	Webster *(14)*	223/0	83	68	3		
1995	Pascal-Vigneron *(25)*	60/0	93	52	3.3		
1996	Biller *(26)*	0/15	73	Minimal	0	73	5/5
1997	Ferrari *(27)*	0/85	61	25	4.7	66	16/32
1997	Muratori *(28)*	26/0	96	24	0	68	
1997	Colao *(29)*	8/19	85	22	0	48	27/0
1997	Colao *(30)*	0/23	83	4	0	61	6/2
1999	Verhelst *(31)*	249/181	86	13	3.9	67	58/140
1999	Cannavo *(32)*	26/11	92	12	0	96	
2000	Pontikides *(33)*	0/12	100	15	0	100	
2000	Pinzone *(34)*	3/10	92				
2000	Di Sarno *(19)*	23/16	92	0	0	30	23/16
2000	De Luis *(20)*	20/0	90	30	0		
2000	Colao *(35)*	0/110	99*c*	5	0	47*d*	19/37
Totals or means		972/513	87	26	1.7	66	164/267

[a] Includes idiopathic hyperprolactinemia and empty sella.
[b] Criteria differ between studies and imaging was performed on only subgroups of patients.
[c] 74% after 6 mo, the remainder after higher doses (up to 3.5 mg/wk) *for 18 to 24 mo.*
[d] 92% in patients who had no previous exposure to dopamine agonists, with complete disappearance in 61%.

drugs, together with a snack, just before retiring to bed. It is worth noting that acute psychotic reactions have been described with quinagolide, albeit rarely. It is unclear whether this important side effect is drug specific because acute psychosis was encountered occasionally in previous patients treated with large bromocriptine doses.

Microprolactinomas

Dopamine Agonists

Medical therapy is remarkably effective in the treatment of microprolactinoma. In the early studies of patients treated with bromocriptine, normoprolactinemia or ovulatory cycles were restored in 80%–90% of patients. Fertility returned within 2 mo in 70% of women. Galactorrhea disappeared or was greatly reduced in the majority of patients, usually within a few days or weeks. In the more recent comparative study of cabergoline and bromocriptine, resumption of ovulatory cycles or occurrence of pregnancy was documented in 72% of cabergoline patients (up to 1.0 mg twice weekly) compared with 52% in the bromocriptine group (up to 5.0 mg twice daily) *(14)*. The number of women with stable normoprolactinemia was also higher in the cabergoline group (83% vs 58%).

Tumor shrinkage occurs during long-term treatment, although this is less critical than for patients with macroprolactinomas. Importantly, a minority of patients may be cured after a period of dopamine agonist treatment. The mechanism is unknown. The probability of cure remains unclear but perhaps between 10% and 20% of microprolactinomas remit with time. It has been suggested that a dopamine agonist-induced pregnancy increases the chances of remission *(36)*. For these reasons, most endocrinologists interrupt dopamine agonist treatment every 2–3 yr, for further clinical assessment and PRL testing. In doing so, one should remember that women may continue to have ovulatory cycles for 3–6 mo after withdrawal of the long-acting drug cabergoline *(23)*.

Transsphenoidal Surgery

In some centers, transsphenoidal surgery may be offered as an alternative to medical therapy. Indeed, surgery may be essential if the patient is intolerant of or resistant to dopamine receptor agonists. Surgical success is critically dependent on surgical experience and tumor size. In most large centers, normoprolactinemia is achieved postoperatively in 60% to 90% of patients, with results for larger microprolactinomas (4–9 mm diameter) being significantly better than for smaller ones *(11)*. Previous dopamine agonist therapy may hamper surgery but this is less troublesome for microprolactinomas than it is for macroprolactinomas. Recurrence of hyperprolactinemia, usually without radiologically evident tumor, is well recognized. Early reports suggested this might occur in up to 50% of microprolactinoma patients, but a recent meta-analysis of 1224 surgically treated microprolactinomas gave a recurrence figure of 17% *(2)*. However, it should be stressed that long-term follow-up is still quite short. Using normoprolactinemia as the main criterion of cure, it is probably reasonable to speak of a *long-term surgical cure rate* of between 50% and 70% when counseling patients with respect to choice of therapy. It is, of course, important also to mention the small but measurable morbidity of transsphenoidal surgery (*see* Chapter 8), together with the small risk of loss of normal pituitary function. The latter would be particularly important if the patient wished fertility.

Owing to the excellent therapeutic responses to either dopamine agonists or transsphenoidal surgery, radiotherapy is no longer considered acceptable primary therapy for microprolactinoma.

Observation (Including Oral Contraception)

Longitudinal studies suggest that only 7% of microprolactinomas progress to larger lesions. Hence, in a woman with a microprolactinoma who has normal menses and libido and nontroublesome galactorrhoea and who does not wish to become pregnant, there may be no clear indication for antiprolactinoma therapy. Before recommending simple observation of a microprolactinoma, most endocrinologists would wish to confirm adequate circulating sex steroid concentrations (mean estradiol >200 pmol/L [55 pg/mL]) in a woman and testosterone >7 nmol/L (2 ng/mL) in a man), together with BMD within one standard deviation of age-related mean values. In this situation it would be reasonable to monitor the patient with 6–12 monthly serum PRL and estradiol/testosterone estimations, supplemented with bone densitometry every 3–5 yr, thus enabling individualized timing of any intervention. The question of oral contraceptive safety often arises. There are good data confirming the safety of oral contraceptive in combination with a dopamine agonist in women with microprolactinomas but no satisfactory prospective studies of treatment with an oral contraceptive alone. If the latter course of action is taken, serum PRL should be checked every 3–6 mo, with the addition of dopamine agonist therapy should the serum PRL level rise above an arbitrary target level (e.g., twice the basal level).

Macroprolactinomas

Dopamine Agonists

These drugs directly activate pituitary D2 dopamine receptors, mimicking the action of endogenous hypothalamic dopamine. In addition to reducing PRL secretion, D2 receptor stimulation results in rapid involution of the cellular protein synthetic machinery and thus marked reduction in lactotroph cell size. This effect, together with an antimitotic action, accounts for the rapid and sustained tumor shrinkage, which enables these drugs to be used as *primary therapy* for patients with larger prolactinomas, even those with pressure effects.

Dopamine agonist treatment is followed typically by a rapid fall in serum PRL (within hours) and tumor shrinkage (within days or weeks). Tumor regression is often followed by an improvement in visual function over a (short) time course that rivals that seen after surgical decompression of the chiasm. Thus, patients with macroprolactinomas with visual failure are no longer the neurosurgical emergency they were previously regarded to be. Nevertheless, it is important that all patients with a pituitary macrolesion producing chiasmal compression should have serum PRL measured urgently (and checked in dilution—*see* "Interpretation of Prolactin Immunoassay Result," earlier). An illustrative patient is shown in Fig. 2.

Shrinkage rates. A meta-analysis of 271 well-characterized macroprolactinomas treated with dopamine agonists showed that 79% of tumors shrank by more than a quarter and 89% shrank to some degree *(37)*. The pretreatment PRL level is not a reliable predictor of tumor shrinkage, because 83% of tumors showed significant tumor shrinkage in both the >100,000 mU/L (4000 μg/L) and 5000–10,000 mU/L (200–400 μg/L) groups. Of the macroprolactinomas large enough to produce chiasmal compression, 85% showed significant tumor shrinkage.

Time course of shrinkage. Tumor shrinkage can be demonstrated with a week or two of starting dopamine agonist therapy, and most shrinkage takes place during the first 3 mo of treatment *(37,38)*. However, in many patients, shrinkage continues at a slower rate during many months. It is recommended to repeat MRI 2–3 mo after commencing dopamine agonist therapy and, if there has been an acceptable response, at longer intervals thereafter.

Amount of shrinkage and visual recovery. Approx 40% of macroprolactinomas treated with dopamine agonists for between 1 and 3 mo show tumor-size reduction of at least one half. Of those treated for 1 yr or longer, almost 90% show such shrinkage *(37)*. Colao and colleagues in a recent prospective study of 110 patients with macroprolactinoma have suggested that tumor shrinkage is greater in previously untreated (*de novo*) patients *(35)*. Tumor shrinkage (>80% of pretreatment volume) was noted, with standard doses of cabergoline in 92% of *de novo* patients, compared with 42% of dopamine-agonist-intolerant and 30% of dopamine-agonist-resistant patients. Tumor shrinkage was only 38% in patients with previously responsive tumors switched to cabergoline because of poor compliance with or nonavailability of a previous dopamine agonist.

Visual field defects improve in approx 90% with these abnormalities. It is important to stress that although early visual improvement occurs frequently, it may be several months before maximum benefit accrues. Thus, persistence of a visual field defect is not an absolute indication to proceed to surgery.

Serum PRL responses. Suppression of serum PRL usually accompanies successful tumor shrinkage. Indeed, all of the responsive patients in the meta-analysis showed a fall in serum PRL of at least 50%, and in 58% of patients serum PRL became entirely normal *(37)*.

Effects on pituitary function. Several investigators have demonstrated recovery of impaired anterior pituitary function in association with tumor shrinkage. Importantly, these data have been extended recently to include recovery of GH

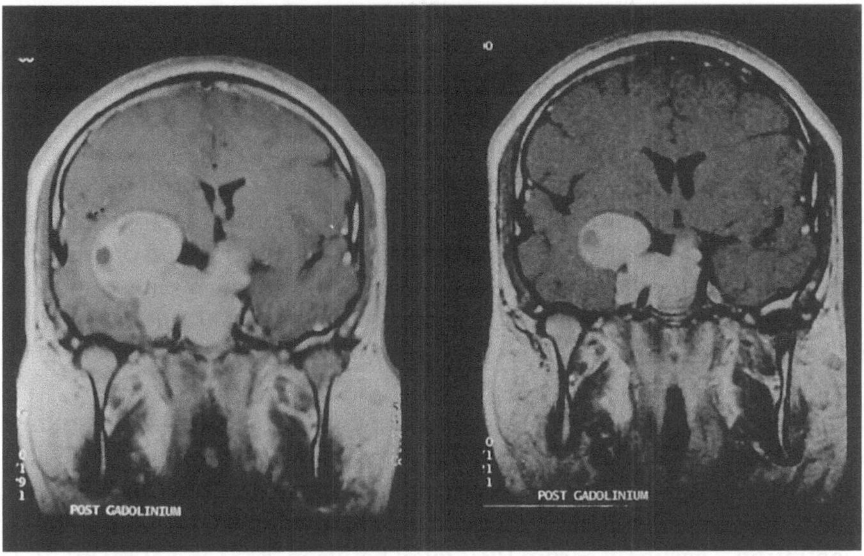

Fig. 2. This 26-yr-old-man presented via the ophthalmology clinic with a 6-mo history of headache and decreased color vision and a 1-mo history of bitemporal visual field loss. He also described episodes suggestive of temporal lobe epilepsy. Initial serum prolactin level was enormously raised at 821,000 mU/L (normal <300) and MRI showed a 7.4-cm invasive macroadenoma, extending into the right temporal lobe (left hand panel). Serum testosterone was reduced at 4 nmol/L and gonadotropin concentrations were low. Thyroid and adrenal functions were normal. He commenced cabergoline 0.5 mg twice weekly, and the dose was incremented to 1 mg twice weekly after 4 mo. His headaches subsided within 1 mo, visual fields were normal after 4 mo and the TLE episodes disappeared. Serum prolactin fell to 84,060 mU/L after 4 d and to 12,790 mU/L after 9 mo. MRI showed a considerable reduction in tumor size after 3 mo of medical therapy (right hand panel).

reserve, which may obviate the need for expensive GH replacement in a proportion of patients *(39,40)*. In contrast, it is worth noting that at least two thirds of men with successfully treated prolactinomas have persistently subnormal testosterone levels and require androgen supplementation *(37)*. Details of gonadal function in women with medically treated macroprolactinomas are difficult to glean from the literature. Cyclical menses return in more than 90% of premenopausal women. The effects on pregnancy are discussed in "Pregnancy and Prolactinomas," following.

Dopamine agonist resistance. Overall, the acquisition of dopamine agonist resistance during therapy is rare, even with treatment periods of 10 or more years. A handful of cases have been described, however *(37)*.

Dopamine agonist withdrawal. Although prolactinomas usually remain sensitive to dopamine agonists, the drugs do not appear to provide a definitive cure for macroprolactinoma and most patients have to remain on long-term therapy.

Immediate tumor re-expansion may occur after drug withdrawal following medium-term therapy (up to 1 yr). Such re-expansion is less common after long-term treatment (several years), but the return of hyperprolactinemia in most patients suggests that tumor regrowth would occur over time. In practice, the dose of dopamine agonist can often be reduced considerably once initial tumor regression has been achieved, with ongoing satisfactory control of tumor size.

Nonshrinking prolactinomas. Approx 10% of genuine macroprolactinomas fail to regress during dopamine agonist therapy. The mechanism of this primary resistance is obscure because most patients with nonshrinking tumors have marked suppression of serum PRL levels. Some resistant tumors have large cystic components, some have atypical histology, and some have a deficiency of membrane-bound D2 dopamine receptors *(37)*.

Management strategies. Macroprolactinoma is virtually certain if serum PRL is greater than 5000 mU/L (200 μg/L) in a patient with a pituitary macrolesion, and primary treatment with a dopamine agonist has an excellent chance of tumor volume reduction. As noted in"Diagnostic Value of the Basal Serum Prolactin Concentration," earlier, a serum PRL level between 2000 and 5000 mU/L (80–200 μg/L) presents some diagnostic uncertainty. The choice between dopamine agonists and surgery will depend on several factors, including local surgical expertise, the severity of any visual failure, patient preference, and clinical judgment. A closely supervised dopamine agonist therapy trial is perfectly reasonable, provided surgery is performed in the event of visual deterioration or failure of the lesion to shrink after, at most, 3 mo of therapy. Using dopamine agonists, visual failure will persist for longer if the lesion is not a prolactinoma, but up to 50% of patients will avoid surgery. It is important to note that dopamine agonists reduce PRL secretion from both normal and tumorous lactotrophs; therefore, serum PRL is likely to fall, irrespective of the cause of the hyperprolactinemia. Pituitary macrolesions associated with PRL levels less than 2000 mU/L (80 μg/L) are rarely prolactinoma, and surgery should be undertaken to decompress the lesion and provide a histologic diagnosis.

The Present Role of Radiotherapy and Surgery

Medical treatment alone is an acceptable option for most patients with macroprolactinoma, particularly those with fertility needs in whom adjunctive therapy might compromise gonadotropin function. Physicians should be aware of the infrequent complication of cerebrospinal fluid (CSF) rhinorrhea, which may occur after shrinkage of inferiorly invasive tumors and may be difficult to correct surgically.

Some endocrinologists consider that dopamine agonist therapy alone is unsuitable for long-term management of macroprolactinoma and recommend external beam radiotherapy. Although PRL levels fall during a several-year period after radiotherapy, enabling dopamine agonist withdrawal in a proportion of patients, this treatment is likely to be followed by varying degrees of hypopituitarism.

A meta-analysis of 1256 macroprolactinomas treated with primary surgery showed PRL normalization in only 32% of patients *(2)*. Consequently, in view of the effectiveness of medical treatment, only a minority of patients with large tumors should now require surgical intervention. There are three situations in which some clinicians might consider surgery, and a cautionary note on the effect of dopamine agonists on prolactinoma fibrosis is necessary.

First, some macroprolactinomas have considerable suprasellar tissue, even after prolonged dopamine agonist therapy, and some clinicians may be inclined to debulk these tumors before radiotherapy. However, there is a direct relationship between tumor fibrosis and duration of medical treatment such that surgery is made much more difficult and may even be hazardous if dopamine agonists have been given for more than 3 mo *(38,41)*. Furthermore, it is now clear that external radiotherapy can be given safely to patients with persistent suprasellar disease, and anecdotal reports of tumor swelling and visual deterioration have assumed undeserved prominence. Second, up to 10% of macroprolactinomas may require surgery after failure of dopamine agonist shrinkage, most of which are likely to be treated surgically within a few months of presentation, particularly if vision is compromised. Third, it is possible that if short-term dopamine agonist therapy produces a compact intrasellar tumor, which will be uncommon with large adenomas, some may be curable by subsequent surgery. This remains unproven. Overall, it would seem prudent to limit pre-operative medical treatment to a maximum of 3 mo, if surgery is to be undertaken. Gamma Knife radiosurgery is offered in few specialized centers, especially in situations where PRL cannot be normalized with dopamine agonists or microsurgery *(42)*.

Pregnancy and Prolactinomas

Management Recommendations

Estrogens have a marked effect on PRL synthesis and secretion, and the hormonal changes of normal pregnancy cause marked lactotroph hyperplasia. MRI studies have confirmed a gradual doubling in pituitary volume during gestation. In view of these effects of pregnancy on normal lactotrophs, it is not surprising that prolactinomas may also increase in size.

The potential risk to the patient depends on the prepregnancy size of the prolactinoma. For women with microprolactinomas, the risk of clinically relevant tumor expansion is small indeed—less than 2%. Dopamine agonists can be safely stopped in such patients as soon as pregnancy is confirmed. Nevertheless, they should be advised to report for urgent assessment in the event of severe headache or any visual disturbance. Routine endocrine review may be arranged on two or three occasions during the pregnancy, but formal charting of visual fields is unnecessary and measurement of serum PRL provides no useful information, given the considerable PRL rise during normal gestation. Patients can safely breast-feed their infants.

There has been some controversy concerning the risk of pregnancy for women with larger prolactinomas. In early reviews, macroprolactinoma expansion was reported to occur in nearly 40%, but many of these women received ovulation induction with gonadotrophins and not dopamine agonists. More recent reviews suggest that symptomatic macroprolactinoma expansion occurs in well under 20% of women. The figure is probably 5% or lower in women, given a several-month course of dopamine agonist before conception *(43)*.

Some clinicians continue to recommend conservative debulking surgery or even radiotherapy before pregnancy in women with macroprolactinomas to reduce the likelihood of major tumor expansion. However, dopamine agonists may be safely employed as sole therapy, using the following strategy. Medical treatment should be used for a minimum of 6 mo preferably 12 mo, together with follow-up MRI to assess residual suprasellar extension, *before* conception is attempted. If the tumor has shrunk to within the fossa, the dopamine agonist can be withdrawn once pregnancy is confirmed, with a less than 10% chance of re-expansion problems. If neurologic problems do occur, *bromocriptine* should be started during the pregnancy and this will restore tumor control in nearly all cases *(38)*. If there is significant suprasellar tumor before conception, the choice is between debulking surgery or continuing bromocriptine throughout the pregnancy. The latter is effective but present experience is limited to slightly more than 100 women.

Dopamine Agonist Safety

There is no evidence of teratogenicity in the offspring of women treated with simple bromocriptine-induced ovulation or those treated throughout pregnancy with the drug. Nevertheless, the oldest bromocriptine child is still only 25 years old, and it is prudent not to use the drug during pregnancy unless absolutely necessary.

Safety data for the newer dopamine agonists, cabergoline and quinagolide, are limited to a few hundred pregnancies, compared with several thousand for bromocriptine. Nevertheless, no new problems have yet emerged. As of May 1999, the manufacturer of cabergoline had data on 334 pregnancies in 301 women treated with the drug. The spontaneous abortion rate in 294 pregnancies with known outcome was 9.5%, well within the expected range. The fetal malformation rate also falls within reported ranges for the general population, and no malformation has occurred more than once. Because clinical experience is limited in relation to pregnancy and because the drug has a long half-life, it is still recommended that cabergoline be stopped 1 mo before intended conception. However, this is clinically inconvenient and requires repeated monitoring of prolactin and ovarian status. Ultimately, it is hoped that sufficient safety data will be gathered to enable the drug to be used in the same way as bromocriptine. As of March 1999, the manufacturer of quinagolide had data on 178 pregnancies in 159 women treated with the drug, 14.6% of whom ended in spontaneous abortion. Nine fetal malformations were diagnosed, including two infants with Down syndrome. These figures also fall within the expected normal ranges. Quinagolide has an intermediate duration of action and, in acknowledgment of the limited pregnancy experience, the data sheet recommends that the drug be withdrawn as soon as pregnancy is confirmed.

REFERENCES

1. Molitch ME. Prolactin. In: Melmed M, ed. *The Pituitary*. Cambridge, MA: Blackwell Science; 1995:164–166.
2. Molitch ME. Prolactinoma. In: Melmed M, ed. *The Pituitary*. Cambridge, MA: Blackwell Science; 1995:443–477.
3. Webster J. Clinical management of prolactinomas. Baillieres Best Pract Res Clin Endocrinol Metab 1999;13(3):395–408.
4. Biller BMK, Baum HBA, Rosenthal DI, et al. Progressive trabecular osteopenia in women with hyperprolactinemic amenorrhea. J Clin Endocrinol Metab 1992;75:692.
5. Schlechte J, Walkner L, Kathol M. A longitudinal analysis of premenopausal bone loss in healthy women and women with hyperprolactinemia. J Clin Endocrinol Metab 1992;75:698.
6. Di Somma C, Colao A, Di Sarno A, et al. Bone marker and bone density responses to dopamine agonist therapy in hyperprolactinemic males. J Clin Endocrinol Metab 1998;83:807.
7. Colao A, Di Somma C, Loche S, et al. Prolactinomas in adolescents: persistent bone loss after 2 years of prolactin normalization. Clin Endocrinol 2000;52:319.
8. Fahie-Wilson MN, Soule SG. Macroprolactinemia: contribution to hyperprolactinemia in a district general hospital and evaluation of a screening test based on precipitation with polyethylene glycol. Ann Clin Biochem 1997;34:252–258.
9. St-Jean E, Blain F, Comtois R. High prolactin levels may be missed by immunoradiometric assay in patients with macroprolactinomas. Clin Endocrinol 1996;44:305–309.
10. Sawers HA, Robb OJ, Walmsley D, Strachan FM, Shaw J, Bevan JS. An audit of the diagnostic usefulness of PRL and TSH responses to domperidone and high resolution magnetic resonance imaging of the pituitary in the evaluation of hyperprolactinemia. Clin Endocrinol 1997;46:321–326.
11. Webster J, Page MD, Bevan JS, Richards SH, Douglas-John AG, Scanlon MF. Low recurrence rate after partial hypophysectomy for prolactinoma; the predictive value of dynamic prolactin function tests. Clin Endocrinol 1992; 36:35–44.
12. Bevan JS, Burke CW, Esiri MM, Adams CBT. Misinterpretation of prolactin levels leading to management errors in patients with sellar enlargement. Am J Med 1987;82:29–32.
13. Ross RJM, Grossman A, Bouloux P, Rees LH, Doniach I, Besser GM. The relationship between serum prolactin and immunocytochemical staining for prolactin in patients with pituitary macroadenomas. Clin Endocrinol 1985;23:227–235.
14. Webster J, Piscitelli G, Polli A, et al. A comparison of cabergoline and bromocriptine in the treatment of hyperprolactinemic amenorrhea. N Engl J Med 1994;331:904–909.
15. van der Heijden PFM., de Wit W., Brownell J., Schoemaker J., Rolland, R. CV205-502, a new dopamine agonist, versus bromocriptine in the treatment of hyperprolactinemia. Eur J Obstet Gynecol Reprod Biol 1991;40:111–118.
16. Verhelst JA, Froud AL, Touzel R, Wass JA, Besser GM, Grossman AB. Acute and long-term effects of once-daily oral bromocriptine and a new long-acting non-ergot dopamine agonist,

quinagolide, in the treatment of hyperprolactinemia: a double blind study. Acta Endocrinol 1991;125:385–391.

17. Homburg R, West C, Brownell J, Jacobs HS. A double-blind study comparing a new non-ergot, long-acting dopamine agonist, CV 205±502, with bromocriptine in women with hyperpro-lactinemia. Clin Endocrinol (Oxf) 1990;32:565–571.
18. Giusti M, Porcella E, Carraro A, Cuttica M, Valenti S, Giordano G. A cross-over study with the two novel dopaminergic drugs cabergoline and quinagolide in hyperprolactinemic patients. J Endocrinol Investig 1994; 17:51–57.
19. Di Sarno A, Landi ML, Marzullo P, et al. The effect of quinagolide and cabergoline, two selective dopamine receptor type 2 agonists, in the treatment of prolactinomas. Clin Endocrinol (Oxf) 2000;53(1):53–60.
20. De Luis DA, Becerra A, Lahera M, Botella JI, Valero, Varela C. A randomized cross-over study comparing cabergoline and quinagolide in the treatment of hyperprolactinemic patients. J Endocrinol Invest 2000;23(7):428–434.
21. Ciccarelli E, Giusti M, Miola C, et al. Effectiveness and tolerability of long-term treatment with cabergoline, a new long-lasting ergoline derivative, in hyperprolactinemic patients. J Clin Endocrinol Metab 1989;69:725–728.
22. Ferrari C, Mattei A, Melis GB, et al. Cabergoline: long-acting oral treatment of hyperprolactinemic disorders. J Clin Endocrinol Metab 1989;68:1201–1206.
23. Ferrari C, Paracchi A, Mattei AM, de Vincentiis S, D'Alberton A, Crosignani P. Cabergoline in the long-term therapy of hyperprolactinemic disorders. Acta Endocrinol (Copen) 1992;126:489–494.
24. Webster J, Piscitelli G, Polli A, et al. The efficacy and tolerability of long-term cabergoline therapy in hyperprolactinaemic disorders: an open, uncontrolled, multicentre study. Clin Endocrinol (Oxf) 1993;39:323–329.
25. Pascal-Vigneron V, Weryha G, Bosc M, Leclere J. Hyperprolactinemic amenorrhea: treatment with cabergoline vs. bromocriptine. Results of a national multicenter randomized double-blind study. Presse Med. 1995;24:753–757.
26. Biller BMK, Molitch ME, Vance ML, et al. Treatment of prolactin-secreting macroadenomas with the once-weekly dopamine agonist cabergoline. J Clin Endocrinol Metab 1996;81:2338–2343.
27. Ferrari CI, Abs R, Bevan JS, et al. Treatment of macroprolactinoma with cabergoline: a study of 85 patients. Clin Endocrinol (Oxf) 1997;46:409–413.
28. Muratori M, Arosio M, Gambino G, Romano C, Biella O, Faglia G. Use of cabergoline in the long-term treatment of hyperprolactinemic and acromegalic patients. J Endocrinol Invest 1997;20:537–546.
29. Colao A, Di Sarno A, Sarnacchiaro F, et al. Prolactinomas resistant to standard dopamine agonists respond to chronic cabergoline treatment. J Clin Endocrinol Metab 1997;82:876–883.
30. Colao A, Di Sarno A, Landi ML, et al. Long-term and low-dose treatment with cabergoline induces macroprolactinoma shrinkage. J Clin Endocrinol Metab 1997;82:3574–3579.
31. Verhelst J, Abs R, Maiter D, et al. Cabergoline in the treatment of hyperprolactinemia: a study in 455 patients. J Clin Endocrinol Metab 1999;84:2518-2522.
32. Cannavo S, Curto L, Squadrito S, Almoto B, Vieni A, Trimarchi F. Cabergoline: a first-choice treatment in patients with previously untreated prolactin-secreting pituitary adenoma. J Endocrinol Invest 1999;22(5):354–359.
33. Pontikides N, Krassas GE, Nikopoulou E, Kaltsas T. Cabergoline as a first-line treatment in newly diagnosed macroprolactinomas. Pituitary 2000;2(4):277–281.
34. Pinzone JJ, Katznelson L, Danila DC, Pauler DK, Miller CS, Klibanski A. Primary medical therapy of micro and macroprolactinomas in men. J Clin Endocrinol Metab 2000; 85(9):3053–3057.
35. Colao A, Di Sarno A, Landi ML, et al. Macroprolactinoma shrinkage during cabergoline treatment is greater in naive patients than in patients pretreated with other dopamine agonists: a prospective study in 110 patients. J Clin Endocrinol Metab 2000;85(6):2247–2252.

36. Jeffcoate WJ, Pound N, Sturrock NDC, Lambourne J. Long-term follow-up of patients with hyperprolactinemia. Clin Endocrinol 1997;45:299–303.
37. Bevan JS, Webster J, Burke CW, Scanlon MF. Dopamine agonists and pituitary tumor shrinkage. Endocr Rev 1992;13:220–240.
38. Bevan JS, Adams CBT, Burke CW, et al. Factors in the outcome of trans-sphenoidal surgery for prolactinoma and non-functioning pituitary tumor, including pre-operative bromocriptine therapy. Clin Endocrinol 1987;26:541–556.
39. Popovic V, Simic M, Ilic LJ, et al. Growth hormone secretion elicited by GHRH, GHRP-6 or GHRH plus GHRP-6 in patients with microprolactinoma and macroprolactinoma before and after bromocriptine therapy. Clin Endocrinol 1998;48:103–108.
40. George LD, Nicolau N, Scanlon MF, Davies JS. Recovery of growth hormone secretion following cabergoline treatment of macroprolactinomas. Clin Endocrinol (Oxf) 2000;53(5):595–599.
41. Esiri MM, Bevan JS, Burke CW, Adams CBT. Effect of bromocriptine treatment on the fibrous tissue content of prolactin-secreting and non-functioning macroadenomas of the pituitary gland. J Clin Endocrinol Metab 1986; 63:383–388.
42. Landolt AM, Lomax N. Gamma knife radiosurgery for prolactinomas. J Neurosurg 2000;93 (Suppl 3):14–18.
43. Molitch ME. Management of prolactinomas during pregnancy. J Reprod Med 1999;44(12 Suppl):1121–1126.

3 Acromegaly

Mary Lee Vance, MD

Contents

INTRODUCTION

The diagnosis of acromegaly is clinical, biochemical, and anatomic. The clinical diagnosis involves a suspicion of excessive growth hormone (GH) production when the patient has symptoms such as changes in facial features, enlargement of hands and feet, excessive sweating, dental malocclusion, sleep apnea, hypertension, diabetes mellitus, colon polyps, and skin tags. Unfortunately, the majority of patients with acromegaly have symptoms of the disease for 7 to 8 yr before the diagnosis is ascertained. Untreated acromegaly results in premature mortality, most commonly from cardiovascular disease *(1–6)*. Thus, prompt diagnosis and treatment are essential to reduce the risk of morbidity and premature mortality; reduction in GH production to normal reduces this risk of premature death *(7)*.

DIAGNOSIS OF ACROMEGALY

Excessive GH production is chacterized by an elevated serum insulin-like growth hormone factor-1 (IGF-1) and the lack of adequate GH reduction after oral glucose ingestion. Serum IGF-1 concentrations are age and gender dependent. GH secretion and serum IGF-1 concentrations decline with increasing age,

From: *Management of Pituitary Tumors: The Clinician's Practical Guide, Second Edition*
Edited by: M. P. Powell, S. L. Lightman, and E. R. Laws, Jr.

and women have higher levels than men. An accurate IGF-1 assay with a suitable database reflecting normal age- and gender-matched values is the keystone in screening patients with possible acromegaly. An important consideration is the young woman with galactorrhea, menstrual disturbance, and hyperprolactinemia. In this setting, the patient may not have the classic features of acromegaly. Patients with early acromegaly may not have the suggestive features of facial changes, hyperhidrosis, and acral enlargement. Thus, any patient with hyperprolactinemia should be screened for acromegaly by measurement of serum IGF-1. GH-producing pituitary adenomas may also produce excessive prolactin (PRL) (bihormonal tumor or mammosomatotrope tumor). This distinction is essential because the treatment of a prolactinoma and a GH plus prolactin-producing tumor is different, with medical therapy the first choice for a prolactinoma and surgery for a GH and prolactin-producing tumor. The diagnosis of acromegaly is ascertained by the presence of an elevated serum IGF-1 concentration and the failure of GH to decline to <1 ng/mL (µg/L) (2.5 mU/L) after ingestion of 75 or 100 g of glucose. With the refinement of GH assays with increased sensitivity, this criterion of a GH of <1 ng/mL (µg/L) (2.5 mU/L) has replaced the value of a GH of <2 ng/mL (µg/L) (5 mU/L)*(8)*. It is important that the oral glucose test be performed properly with measurement of GH levels before and every 30 min after glucose ingestion during 120 min (2 h, a total of five blood samples).

TREATMENT OF ACROMEGALY

After the biochemical diagnosis is determined, the patient should have magnetic resonance imaging (MRI) of the pituitary gland. The majority of patients with acromegaly have a pituitary macroadenoma (>10 mm), and some patients have a smaller tumor which is more amenable to complete surgical resection. First-line treatment is surgical removal of the adenoma by an experienced pituitary neurosurgeon; results of pituitary surgery are dependent on the experience and expertise of the neurosurgeon *(9)*. A pituitary macroadenoma, particularly with invasion into the cavernous sinus or bone, is less likely to be cured surgically but does require removal to alleviate or prevent visual loss and to allow for optimal additional treatment with focused radiation (stereotactic radiation) or conventional fractionated radiation to treat the residual tumor. Surgical treatment of acromegaly results in remission or cure in approx 66% of patients, thus a substantial number of patients require additional treatment, including medical therapy and pituitary radiation.

RESULTS OF TREATMENT OF ACROMEGALY

Surgery

The results of transsphenoidal removal of a GH adenoma vary according to the experience and expertise of the neurosurgeon. Results from medical centers in

Table 1
Results of Transsphenoidal Removal of GH Adenoma from Medical Centers Performing a Large Number of Pituitary Surgeries

Location	*No. of patients*	*Nl. IGF-1*	*OGTT GH <2 ng/mL 5.0 mU/mL*	*OGTT GH <1 ng/mL 2.5 mU/mL*	*Random GH <2.5 ng/mL 6.5 mU/mL*	*Random GH <5 ng/mL <13 mU/mL*
Boston	162	70%	58%	......	0%	......
New York	115	61%	53%	—	—	71%
San Francisco	254	......	......	......	......	76%
Charlottesville	57	67%	—	52%	49%	—

OGGT, oral glucose tolerance test; GH, growth hormone.

which a large number of pituitary surgeries are performed by an experienced neurosurgeon report that achievement of a normal serum IGF-1 concentration ranges from 61% to 70%. Using the strict criterion of a postglucose GH of <1 ng/mL (μg/L) (2.5 mU/L), one study reported a 52% success rate. Table 1 summarizes the results from centers in which pituitary surgery is frequently performed.

In contrast, surgery in 73 patients performed by nine neurosurgeons in one community, (Manchester, England) resulted in an overall remission rate of 18% (39% for patients with a microadenoma, 12% for patients with a macroadenoma) *(9)*. In comparing these results with those of dedicated pituitary neurosurgeons, the authors concluded that pituitary surgery should be performed by those with experience and expertise. Despite considerable surgical expertise, many patients are not cured, which relates to the size of the adenoma and invasion of adjoining structures (dura, bone, cavernous sinuses). Thus, additional treatment or treatments are necessary for symptomatic improvement and to reduce the risk of premature mortality.

Postoperative Evaluation

After pituitary surgery the patient should undergo measurement of serum IGF-1 (6 wk to 3 or more mo after surgery, delayed clearance of IGF-1) and an oral glucose test (can be performed within a week of surgery, short half-life of GH, approx 19 min) The definition of cure or remission is a serum GH of <1 ng/mL (μg/L) (2.5 mU/L) after glucose ingestion *(8)*. A normal age- and gender-matched serum IGF-1 concentration is also the optimal outcome, if there is a discrepancy between the serum IGF-1 and glucose-suppressed GH value, the GH value should be used and the IGF-1 level measured 2 to 3 mo later. Persistent acromegaly requires additional treatment.

Table 2
Short-Acting Somatostatin Analog (Octreotide)

Author, year (ref.)	*No. of patients*	*Duration Rx (mo)*	*Serum GH <2.5 µg/L (6.5 mU/L) (%)*	*Normal IGF-1 (%)*
Ho, 1990 *(17)*	19	3–6	42[a]	42
Vance, 1990 *(18)*	189	6[b]	NR[c]	46
Ezzat, 1992 *(19)*	98	6	NR	61
Newman, 1995 *(20)*	84	24	NR	64

[a]Mean GH compared with age-matched normal subjects.
[b]Median duration of treatment.
[c]NR: not reported.

Table 3
Long-Acting Somatostatin Analogs

Medication author, year (ref.)	*No. of patients*	*Duration Rx (mo)*	*Normal IGF-1 (%)*
Octreotide LAR			
Stewart, 1995 *(22)*	8	11–17	88
Octreotide LAR			
Flogstad, 1997 *(23)*	14	18	64
Lanreotide			
Marek, 1994 *(24)*	13	9	23
Lanreotide			
Giusti, 1996 *(25)*	50	6	38
Lanreotide			
Al-Maskari, 1996 *(26)*	10	6	50
Lanreotide			
Caron, 1997 *(27)*	22	12	63

Medical Treatment

Currently available medical therapies include dopamine agonist drugs and somatostatin analogs. Dopamine agonist drugs (bromocriptine, pergolide, cabergoline), provide symptomatic relief in approx 90% of patients, but reduction in serum IGF-1 to normal occurs in less than 20% *(14)*. Somatostatin, the naturally occurring hypothalamic hormone that suppresses GH secretion, is effective only when given by continuous intravenous (iv) infusion. Analogs of somatostatin are effective when given by subcutaneous or intramuscular injection. Currently available analogs include octreotide, lanreotide and octreotide LAR (Sandostatin LAR®). This class of drugs reduces GH and IGF-1 concentrations to normal in 50% to 60% of patients and improves symptoms in more than

90% *(15–27)*. Tables 2 and 3 summarize the results of short-acting (octreotide) and long-acting (lanreotide, octreotide LAR) somatostatin analogs in patients with acromegaly

Side effects of somatostatin analog drugs include transient abdominal discomfort, acholic stools, and diarrhea. These symptoms usually resolve within a few days to a week. Development of gall bladder sludge or gallstones occurs in approx 18% of patients *(19)*.

A recent development in the medical treatment of acromegaly is a modification of the GH molecule, a 9-amino-acid substitution and pegylation to reduce immunogenicity, resulting in a GH antagonist. This antagonist, pegvisomant, prevents dimerization of the GH receptor and thus reduces IGF-1 generation. A consequence of reducing circulating IGF-1 concentrations is an increase in serum GH concentrations. Pegvisomant reduced serum IGF-1 concentrations in a dose-dependent fashion in a study of 112 patients with acromegaly, with suppression of IGF-1 to normal in 89% of patients treated with 20 mg/d *(28)*. This medication is self- administered as a daily sc injection. A long-term study of pegvisomant of patients treated up to 18 mo (n=131) found that in the 90 patients treated for 12 mo or more, 97% achieved a normal serum IGF-1 concentration. Serum GH increased and achieved a plateau after 6 mo of treatment. In this study two patients developed abnormal liver enzymes and two patients had enlargement of the residual pituitary adenoma. The remaining patients had no change in pituitary size *(29)*. This experimental medication is the most effective medical therapy for acromegaly and is currently under review by government regulatory agencies regarding approval for clinical use.

Radiation Therapy

Pituitary radiation has been used for more than 50 yr, usually as adjunctive therapy after surgery. Conventional or fractionated radiation given during 4 to 5 wk requires 10 to 20 yr to be effective. Stereotactic or focused radiation allows for precise delivery of radiation to a circumscribed area, with reduction in the amount of radiation to the brain; more focused methods of radiation delivery include the Gamma Knife, LINEAC, and proton beam. The widely quoted study in 1979 from the National Institutes of Health (NIH) reported on 47 patients treated with fractionated radiotherapy as primary treatment found that serum GH levels were reduced to <5 ng/mL (μg/L) (13 mU/L) in 67% of patients within 10 yr of treatment *(30)*. Considering what is now known about the importance of lowering GH (and presumably IGF-1) levels to normal to reduce the risk of premature death, all efforts should be made to recommend treatment that has the best chance of accomplishing this goal. Thus, pituitary radiation should be reserved for patients who have residual disease after surgery. Because it usually requires months to years for radiation to be effective in lowering GH and IGF-1 to normal, patients should be given medical therapy when awaiting the therapeutic effect of radiation. The conventional method of administering pituitary radiation is delivery through 3 ports (bitemporal and frontal) in fractions during 4 to 5 wk. Other methods include particle beam (protons, deuterons, helium ions), usually administered in 4 fractions during 5 d, or the more recently developed stereotactic methods, Gamma Knife, and LINEAC. Particle beam radiotherapy in 220 patients with acromegaly lowered the median GH level to 5 ng/mL (μg/L) (13 mU/L) or less 4 yr after treatment in 169 patients (77%). Another study of 114 patients treated with helium ion radiotherapy resulted in lowered fasting GH to 5 ng/mL (μg/L) (13 mUu/L) or less 7 yr after treatment in 26 patients (23%) *(31)*. Stereotactic radiation with the Gamma Knife involves delivery of focused radiation through 201 ports, usually in one treatment. The theoretical advantage of this method is minimal exposure of brain tissue to radiation, the ability to treat a very circumscribed area and with minimal exposure to the hypothalamus and optic chiasm. This method is best reserved for patients with a small amount of residual tumor that is not close to the optic chiasm. Gamma Knife radiotherapy in 20 patients resulted in reduction in fasting GH to <2.5 ng/mL (μg/L) in 7 (35%) 6 mo to 7 yr after treatment *(32)*. Using MRI planning, 56 patients with acromegaly were given postoperative Gamma Knife radiotherapy; 36 were followed for >6 mo of whom 25% (9 out of 36) achieved a normal serum IGF-1 5 to 43 mo after treatment (average 20 mo) *(33)*. It is important to note that the technique of planning the radiation field for the Gamma Knife has advanced throughout the years, from the less precise use of pneumoencephalography to the computer tomography (CT) scan to the current use of MRI planning. Comparison of results among studies using different techniques is difficult given radiation delivery methods and the evolution of the criterion for cure.

Anticipated complications of radiation include development of hypopituitarism. Deficiency of some or all of the pituitary hormones usually occurs in a progressive fashion, the earliest and most common deficiency is that of the gonadotropins (luteinizing hormone [LH], follicle-stimulating hormone [FSH]) with consequent gonadal failure *(34)*. Development of GH deficiency in these patients has not been studied systematically. In 35 patients treated with conventional radiotherapy, adenocortictropic hormone (ACTH) deficiency developed in 67%, thyroid-stimulating hormone (TSH) deficiency in 55%, and gonadotropin deficiency in 67% after a mean follow-up of 4.2 yr *(35)*.

Patients who receive pituitary radiation should be followed regularly (at least every 6 mo) with appropriate hormone measurements and prompt institution of replacement therapy as indicated. The risk of developing a CNS malignancy is low but is a consideration. Prospective studies detailing intellectual function before and after radiotherapy are not available. The incidence of pituitary failure after stereotactic radiation (Gamma Knife, LINEAC, proton beam) is not as well established. Prospective follow up of these patients is necessary.

SUMMARY

The diagnosis and treatment of acromegaly is straightforward once the possibility of this disorder is entertained. Because many patients have a tumor too large for complete resection, multiple treatments are necessary. A combined approach of surgery, medical therapy to control residual disease, and pituitary radiation to effect permanent control is a suitable approach. The ultimate goal is to lower GH production to normal and reduce morbidity and the risk of premature mortality.

REFERENCES

1. Wright AD, Hill DM, Lowery C, et al. mortality in acromegaly. Quart J Med 1970;39:1–16.
2. Alexander L, Appleton D, Hall R, et al. Epidemiology of acromegaly in the Newcastle region. Clin Endocrinol 1980;12:71–79.
3. Ritchie CM, Atkinson AB, Kennedy AL, et al. Ascertainment and natural history of treated acromegaly in Northern Ireland. Ulster Med J 1990;59:55–62.
4. Etxabe J, Gaztambide S, Latorre P, et al. Acromegaly: An epidemiologic study. J Endocrinol Invest 1993;16:181–187.
5. Rajasoorya C, Holdaway IM, Wrightson P, Scott DJ, Ibbertson HK. Determinants of clinical outcome and survival in acromegaly. Clin Endocrinol 1994;41:95–102.
6. Orme SM, McNally RJQ, Cartwright RA, Belchetz PE. Mortality and cancer incidence in acromegaly: a retrospective cohort study. J Clin Endocrinol Metab 1998;83:2730–2734.
7. Bates AS, Van't Hoff, W, Jones JM, Clayton RN. An audit of outcome of treatment in acromegaly. Quart J Med 1993;86:293–299.
8. Giustina A, Barkan A, Casanueva FF, et al. Criteria for cure of acromegaly: A consensus statement. J Clin Endocrinol Metab 2000;85:526–529.
9. Lissett CA, Peacey SR, Laing I, Tetlow L, Davis JRE, Shalet SM. The outcome of surgery for acromegaly: the need for a specialist pituitary surgeon for all types of growth hormone secreting adenomas. Clin Endocrinol 1998;45:517–522.
10. Swearingen B, Barker FG, Katznelson L, et al. Long-term mortality after transsphenoidal surgery and adjunctive therapy for acromegaly. J Clin Endocrinol Metab 1998;83:3419–3426.
11. Freda PU, Wardlaw SL, Post KD. Long-term endocrinological follow-up in 115 patients who underwent transsphenoidal surgery for acromegaly. J Neurosurg 1998;89:353–358.
12. Abosch A, Tyrrell JB, Lamborn KR, Hannegan LT, Applebury CB, Wilson CB. J Clin Endocrinol Metab 1998;83:3411–3418.
13. Kreutzer J, Vance ML, Lopes MBS, Laws ER. Surgical management of growth hormone secreting pituitary adenomas. An outcome study using modern remission criteria. J Clin Endocrinol Metab 2001;86:4072–4077.
14. Barkan AL. Acromegaly: diagnosis and therapy. Endocrinol Metab Clin North Am 1989;18:277–310.
15. Quabbe HJ, Plockinger U Dose-response study and long-term effects of the somatostatin analog octreotide in patients with therapy-resistant acromegaly. J Clin Endocrinol Metab 1989;68:873–881.
16. McKnight JA, McCance DR, Sheridan B, et al. A long-term dose-response study of somatostatin analogue (SMS 201-995, octreotide) in resistant acromegaly. Clin Endocrinol 1991;34:119–125
17. Ho KY, Weissberger AJ, Marbach P, Lazarus L. Therapeutic efficacy of the somatostatin analog SMS 201–995 (octreotide) in acromegaly—effects of dose and frequency and long-term safety. Ann Inter Med 1990;112:173–181.

18. Vance ML, Harris AG. Long-term treatment of 189 acromegalic patients with the somatostatin analog octreotide. Arch Intern Med 1991;151:1573–1578.
19. Ezzat S, Snyder PJ, Yourn WF, et al. Octreotide treatment of acromegaly: a randomized multicenter trial. Ann Intern Med 1992;117:711–718.
20. Newman CB, Melmed S, Snyder PJ et al. Safety and efficacy of long-term octreotide therapy of acromegaly: results of a multicenter trial in 103 patients. J Clin Endocrinol Metab 1995;80:2768–2775.
21. Lucas-Morante T, Garcia-Urda J, Estada J, et al. Treatment of invasive growth hormone pituitary adenomas with long-acting somatostatin analog SMS 201-995 before transsphenoidal surgery. J Neurosurg 1994;81:10–14.
22. Stewart PM, Kane KF, Stewart SE, Lancranjan I, Sheppard MC. Depot long-acting somatostatin analog (Sandostatin-LAR) is an effective treatment for acromegaly. J Clin Endocrinol Metab 1995;80:3267–3272.
23. Flogstad AK, Halse J, Bakke S, et al. Sandostatin LAR in acromegalic patients: long-term treatment. J Clin Endocrinol Metab 1997;82:23–28.
24. Marek J, Hana V, Krsek M, Justova V, Catus F, Thomas F. Long-term treatment of acromegaly with the slow-release somatostatin analogue Lanreotide. Eur J Endocrinol 1994;131:20–26.
25. Giusti M, Gussoni G, Cuttica CM, Giordano G, and the Italian Multicenter Slow Release Lanreotide Study Group. Effectiveness and tolerability of slow release lanreotide treatment in active acromegaly: six-month report on an Italian Multicenter Study. J Clin Endocrinol Metab 1996;81:2089–2097
26. Al-Maskari M, Gebbie J, Kendall-Taylor P. The effect of a new slow-release, long-acting somatostatin analogue, lanreotide, in acromegaly. Clin Endocrinol 1996;45:415–421.
27. Caron P, Morange-Ramos I, Cogne M, Jaquet P. Three year follow-up of acromegalic patients treated with intramuscular slow-release lanreotide. J Clin Endocrinol Metab 1997;82:18–22.
28. Trainer PJ, Drake WM, Katznelson L, et al. Treatment of acromegaly with the growth hormone-receptor antagonist pegvisomant. N Engl J Med 2000;342:1171–1177.
29. van der Lely AJ, Hutson RK, Trainer PJ, et al. Long-term treatment of acromegaly with pegvisomant, a growth hormone receptor antagonist. Lancet 2001;358:1754–1759.
30. Eastman RC, Gorden P, Roth J. Conventional supervoltage irradiation is an effective treatment for acromegaly. J Clin Endocrinol Metab 1979;48:931–940.
31. Levy RP, Fabrikant JI, Frankel KA. Particle-beam irradiation of the pituitary gland. E Alexander, JS Woffler, CD Lunsford, eds. In: *Stereotactic Radiosurgery*. 1993;157–165.
32. Thoren M, Rahn T, Gou WY, Werner S. Stereotactic radiosurgery with the cobalt-60 gamma unit in the treatment of growth hormone-producing pituitary tumors. Neurosurgery 1991;29:663–668.
33. Laws ER, Vance ML. Radiosurgery for pituitary tumors and craniopharyngiomas. Neurosurg Clin North Am 1999;10:327–336.
34. Vance ML. Medical progress: hypopituitarism. New Engl J Med 1994;330:1651–1662.
35. Synder PJ, Fowble BF, Shatz NJ. Hypopituitarism following radiation therapy for pituitary adenomas. Am J Med 1986;81:457–462.

4 Cushing's Disease

Christian A. Koch, MD, FACP, FACE
and George P. Chrousos, MD, FACP, FAAP, MACE

Contents

Cushing's syndrome (CS) results from prolonged exposure of tissues to excess of glucocorticoids. After Harvey Cushing's initial report in the early 20th century *(1)*, CS has been etiologically subdivided into adenocorticotropin hormone (ACTH)-independent (nonpituitary) or ACTH-dependent *(2–4)*. Endogenous CS is rare, with an overall incidence of approx two to four new cases per million of population per year. ACTH-dependent CS accounts for approx 85% of endogenous cases. In the majority of these cases (80%), the cause is autonomous pituitary ACTH secretion and is referred to as Cushing's disease (CD). In the remaining 20%, the ACTH secretion source is ectopic. CD has a female to male preponderance (8/1), whereas the ectopic ACTH syndrome is more common in men (3/1). Ectopic corticotropin-releasing hormone (CRH) production causing CS has also been described in approx 11 cases *(5–7)*. In this chapter, we focus on the diagnosis and treatment of CD which generally presents between the second and sixth decades of life, with a peak incidence at age 35 yr *(2)*.

From: *Management of Pituitary Tumors: The Clinician's Practical Guide, Second Edition*
Edited by: M. P. Powell, S. L. Lightman, and E. R. Laws, Jr.

CLINICAL PRESENTATION

CS is a multisystem disorder *(8)*. The typical clinical presentation of CS results primarily from excess glucocorticoids (hypercortisolism) and, to a lesser extent, from excess mineralocorticoids (hypermineralocorticoidism) and/or adrenal androgens (hyperandrogenism).

One of the earliest signs in most all patients with CS (including CD) is obesity; in growing children this is combined with growth deceleration or arrest *(9–12)*. The accumulation of visceral fat in patients with CS, a result of excess cortisol and insulin secretion, is associated with the full expression of the metabolic syndrome X (hypertension, hyperlipidemia, hypercoagulation, insulin resistance) and its long-term (cardiovascular) sequelae. Typical signs of glucocorticoid excess are fat accumulation in the face (especially temple area and cheeks), neck (buffalo hump, supraclavicular fossae), trunk, abdomen, and epidural fat, with sparing of the limbs *(8,13,14)*. Connective tissue atrophy leads to thin fragile skin, violaceous striae, and easy bruising. Hirsutism and a variable degree of acne (depending on the individual sensitivity to glucocortioids and androgens) can also be seen. Although mild to moderate hypertension often are present in patients with CD, hypokalemia and hyperpigmentation occur less frequently, because the ACTH and cortisol levels are usually less elevated than in patients with ectopic ACTH-secreting tumors.

Hypercalciuria with subsequent renal calculi, glucocorticoid-induced osteopenia/osteoporosis, menstrual irregularities (e.g., amenorrhea), loss of libido in both genders (hypogonadism secondary to hypercortisolism), and muscle weakness in association with proximal muscle atrophy are common features of CD/CS. Avascular necrosis of the hip can be the presenting manifestation of an ACTH-secreting pituitary adenoma and requires immediate attention to save the femoral head and avoid subsequent disability *(15)*. Cataracts (classically posterior subcapsular) and glaucoma frequently occur in patients with exogenous CS but not in those with endogenous hypercortisolism *(16)*. Psychiatric manifestations in CD include cognitive deficits with memory loss and poor concentration, anxiety with insomnia, irritability, atypical depression, acute psychosis, and mania *(17–19)*.

Some patients with CS may experience alternating episodes of mania and depression, pointing to the diagnosis of so-called periodic or cyclic glucocorticoid excess with intermittent hypersecretion of cortisol *(20–32)*. Children with CS often are often compulsive and high performers in school.

Increased awareness of the possible diagnosis of CS, for instance, by improved contemporary imaging modalities ("incidentaloma") and biochemical testing, led to the term "subclinical" CS, a state of glucocorticoid excess without the full-blown clinical features *(33)*.

PATHOGENESIS AND ETIOLOGY

An important question is whether CS from excessive ACTH-producing pituitary glands develops by a defect in the pituitary gland or through secondary factors that stimulate the pituitary corticotrophs. Although some past observations suggested that hypothalamic stimulation of the corticotrophs might be responsible for pituitary adenoma formation *(34–37)*, it is now clear that CD arises in the pituitary gland by corticotroph hyperplasia, an adenoma, or extremely rarely a carcinoma *(38–41)*. Transgenic mice with overproduction of CRH show features of CS without concomitant corticotroph proliferation *(42)*. More importantly, most patients (depending on the neurosurgeon; in our institution approx 95%) with CD are in complete remission after adenomectomy (if the adenoma does not infiltrate the cavernous sinus or other structures).

The molecular pathogenesis of pituitary adenomas, including ACTH-producing ones, is the subject of intense investigation *(43)* (Chapter 2). Corticotropinomas are monoclonal, but the exact pathways of tumor formation remain unknown, although some genes, such as *c-myc*, *c-erbB2*, and *ras*, have been associated with more aggressive tumor behavior *(44–48)*. Abnormalities in many other tumor-suppressor genes and oncogenes are found in corticotropinomas, although their exact role in tumorigenesis is not understood *(43, 49)*. Also, abnormalities of the glucocorticoid receptor and its gene have been described in these tumors *(50, 51)*.

DIAGNOSIS AND TUMOR LOCALIZATION

Accurate diagnosis and differential CS diagnosis is crucial for selection of appropriate therapy. Despite major recent advances, the diagnosis of CS continues to challenge the diagnostic skills of physicians. The goal of the clinician should be to identify individuals with CS as early in the course of the disease as possible to maximize the chance for cure and to avoid the chronic complications of hypercortisolism *(8)*.

Once there is clinical suspicion of CS, the first step is the biochemical documentation of endogenous hypercortisolism *(7,14)*. This step can usually be accomplished by outpatient tests. Measurement of 24-h urinary-free cortisol (UFC) and/or 17-hydroxysteroid excretion and the 1-mg overnight dexamethasone suppression test are frequently employed as the first step. Contemporary diagnostic assays (e.g., immunoradiometric plasma ACTH concentrations before and after CRH) and imaging modalities (high-resolution magnetic resonance imaging [MRI]) have dramatically improved the diagnosis of ACTH-dependent CS.

After confirmation of ACTH-dependent CS, the challenge is to localize the ACTH-secreting source by MRI, inferior petrosal or cavernous sinus sampling,

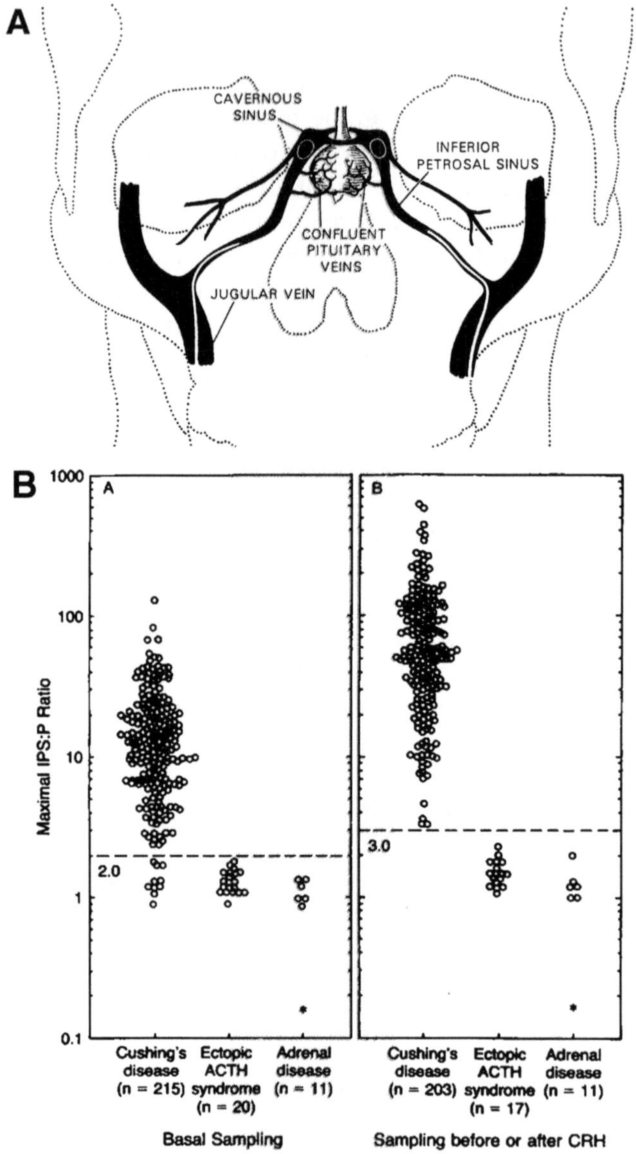

Fig. 1. (A) Catheter placement for bilateral simultaneous blood sampling of the inferior petrosal sinuses. (From Oldfield EH, Chrousos GP, and Schulte HM. Preoperative lateralization of ACTH-secreting pituitary microadenomas by bilateral and simultaneous inferior petrosal venous sinus sampling. N Eng J Med 1985;312:100.) (B) The maximal ratio of ACTH concentration in plasma from either petrosal sinuses and a peripheral vein at baseline (panel A) and after administration of oCRH (panel B). The asterisks represent five patients with primary adrenal disease in whom adrenocorticotropin was undetectable in peripheral-blood plasma before and after CRH administration.

computed tomography, octreoscan, or positron emission tomography (Fig. 1). If ACTH dependency has been established and the pretest probability of CD is high, the next step should be a pituitary MRI. If the pituitary MRI is normal, inferior petrosal or cavernous sinus sampling should be performed. Only rarely in a patient with ACTH-dependent CS does pituitary MRI show a pituitary adenoma that is *not* ACTH producing (incidentaloma), as demonstrated by the lack of a central-to-peripheral ACTH gradient on inferior petrosal sinus sampling.

Diagnosis of Cushing's Syndrome

Determination of 24-h UFC excretion is the best screening test available for documentation of endogenous hypercortisolism *(52,53)*. Values consistently in excess of 200 μg/d (550 nmol) are virtually diagnostic of CS (Fig. 2). Medications or synthetic steroids other than cortisol do not interfere with the performance of high-performance liquid chromatography (HPLC) in measuring urinary cortisol. Assuming complete collections have been performed, there are virtually no false-negative results. In patients with episodic CD *(22–25,27,29,30)*, repeated intermittent UFC collections are necessary, usually in 3-monthly intervals. False-positive results, however, may be obtained in several non-Cushing's hypercortisolemic states (Table 1). Generally, in these states, the UFC levels rarely are higher than 200 μg/d (552 nmol). UFC remains constant throughout life when normalized per square meter of body surface area, obviating the need of using age-specific normal values in children or subjects who are obese *(53)*.

When assays for UFC excretion are not available, measurement of urinary 24-h 17-hydroxysteroids can be helpful. These compounds include all cortisol metabolites with a 17-dihydroxyacetone side chain and, thus, give an indirect measure of cortisol secretion rate. Correction is required, however, for urinary creatinine excretion because size and adiposity influence their daily production.

The overnight 1-mg dexamethasone suppression test is a simple screening procedure for hypercortisolism *(14,54,55)*. The test has a low incidence of false normal suppression (less than 3%). However, the incidence of false-positive results is significantly high (approx 20% to 30%). In children, the dose of dexamethasone that should be employed is 15 μg/kg body weight. In the United States, dexamethasone (in adults, 1 mg) is administered orally at 11 PM and plasma cortisol measured the next morning at 8 AM. The typical plasma cortisol cutoff level (from 5 μg to 2.5 μg/dL; 69 nmol) has been readjusted over the years to improve sensitivity. With these more stringent cortisol cutoff criteria, the

---

Fig. 1. (continued) (From Oldfield EH, Doppman JL, Nieman, LK, et al. Petrosal sinus sampling with and without corticotropin releasing hormone for the differential diagnosis of Cushing's syndrome. N Engl J Med 1991;325:897.)

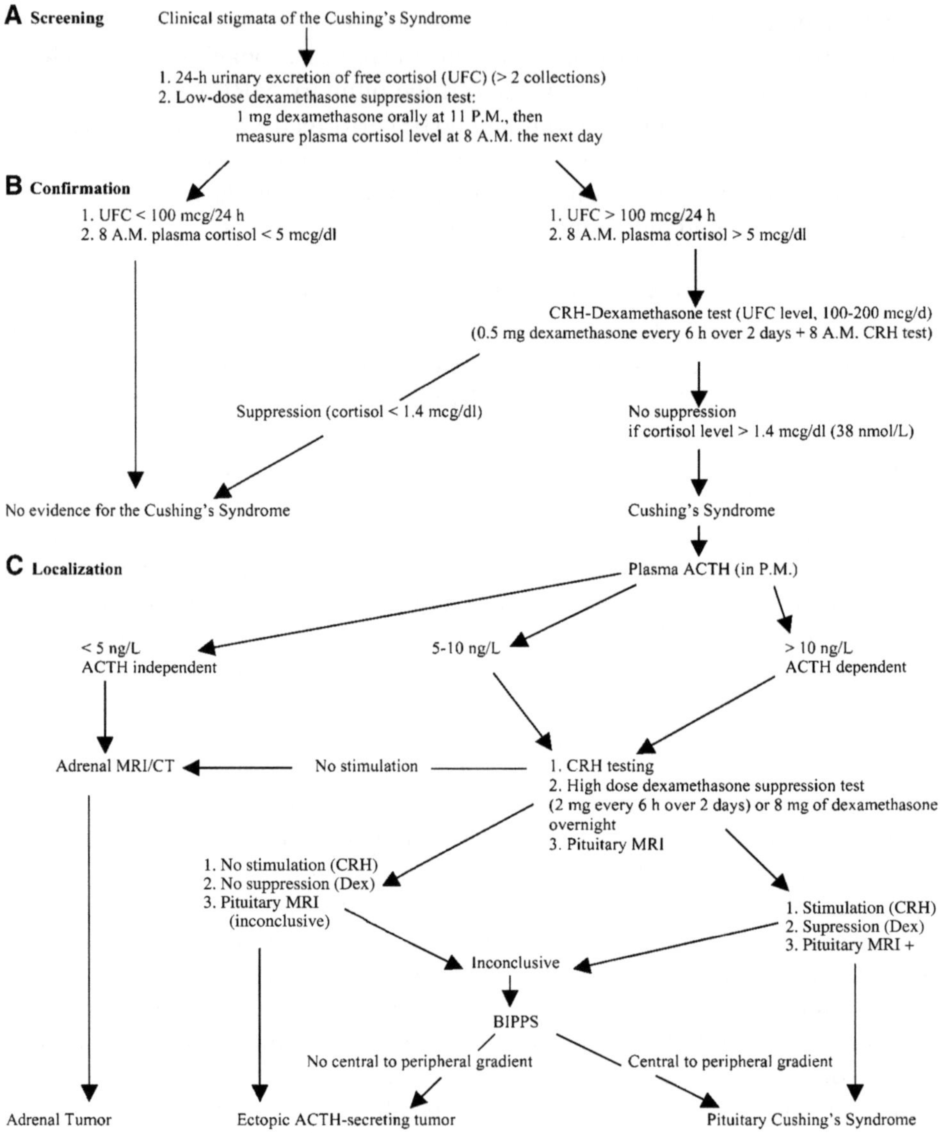

Fig. 2. Algorithm for the diagnosis of Cushing's disease. To convert serum cortisol values to nmol/L and to convert UFC values to nmol/d, multiply by 27.59 (serum) and 2.759 (urine). ACTH, 5 ng/L = 1.1 nmol/L; BIPPS, bilateral inferior petrosal sinus sampling; CRH, corticotropin-releasing hormone; CT, computed tomography; MRI, magnetic resonance imaging.

sensitivity of the overnight low-dose dexamethasone suppression test in CS diagnosis is greater than 95%, whereas the specificity can be as low as 88%.

False-positive results are seen in stress conditions, such as acute illness, extreme obesity, alcoholism, and depression; in high estrogen states; and with medications that accelerate dexamethasone catabolism, such as primidon, phenobarbital, phenytoin, and rifampin.

CS is generally excluded if the response to the single-dose dexamethasone suppression test and the 24-h UFC or 17-hydroxysteroid excretion are normal. One should bear in mind, however, that cortisol hypersecretion may be intermittent and/or periodic in approx 10% of patients with CS of any etiology. Documenting loss of diurnal variation of plasma cortisol (taking into account time zones of travel or shift work) would support the CS diagnosis and vice versa. Multiple blood samples taken in both morning and evening increase the value of the test, because a significant variability of cortisol levels may be present *(7,56)*. Similarly, isolated plasma ACTH determinations are of limited value especially because there is significant overlap between the ACTH levels in patients with Cushing's disease and normal subjects.

On the other hand, plasma ACTH measurements can be useful in providing an early distinction between ACTH-dependent and ACTH-independent sources, because ACTH concentrations higher than 200 pg/mL (44 pmol/L) strongly suggest ectopic (nonpituitary) production. In borderline cases (those with only mild elevation of UFC and/or positive dexamethasone suppression test), the 2-d Liddle test can be conducted *(57)*. In this test, patients receive dexamethasone 0.5 mg orally every 6 h for 48 h, with measurement of UFC and 17-hydroxycorticosteroids (levels of > 25 μg/d [69 nmol] or 4 mg/d [11 μmol], respectively, are abnormal). In addition, a plasma cortisol level 6 h after the last dexamethasone dose can be measured: a level > 1.8 μg/dL (50 nmol) is abnormal, and when using this criterion, the Liddle test has a sensitivity and specificity of 95% *(7)*.

Salivary cortisol is in equilibrium with free plasma cortisol and has been recently used in the diagnosis of CS *(58)*. Measurement of a single midnight plasma cortisol under nonstressed conditions (abnormal if >1.8 μg/dL) is highly sensitive (99%) but not practical for outpatients *(56,59)*.

Distinguishing Mild Cushing's Syndrome From Pseudo-Cushing States

The clinical and biochemical presentation of mild hypercortisolism in CS is often indistinguishable from that seen in pseudo-Cushing states, such as depression or chronic active alcoholism (Table 1) *(60)*. A hyperactive/hyper-responsive hypothalamic CRH neuron is central to the hypercortisolism of pseudo-Cushing states in the context of a pituitary-adrenal axis that is otherwise appropriately, albeit not fully, restrained by negative cortisol feedback *(61)*. In contrast, the hypercortisolism of CS, regardless of the classification, feeds back negatively and completely suppresses hypothalamic CRH secretion. These concepts form the basis for the tests employed in the differential diagnosis of mild hypercortisolism. Thus, most patients with CS (80%–90%) show inadequate suppression to low-dose

Table 1
Classification of Hypercortisolism

Physiologic states
Stress
Pregnancy
Chronic strenuous excercise
Malnutrition
Pathophysiologic states
Cushing's syndrome
ACTH-dependent (85%)
Pituitary adenoma (80%)
Ectopic ACTH (20%)
Ectopic CRH (rare)
ACTH-independent (15%)
Adrenal adenoma
Adrenal carcinoma
Micronodular adrenal disease (rare)
Macronodular adrenal disease (rare)
Psychiatric states
Melancholic depression
Obsessive-compulsive disorder
Chronic active alcoholism
Panic disorder
Anorexia nervosa
Narcotic withdrawal
Glucocorticoid resistance

ACTH, adenocorticotropic hormone; CRH, corticotropin-releasing hormone

(0.5 mg every 6 h for 2 d) dexamethasone and do not respond to insulin-induced hypoglycemia, contrasting the normal responses of depressed and other pseudo-Cushing patients. In addition, patients with CD (85%) have a "normal" or exaggerated ACTH response to CRH, whereas patients with depression (75%) show a blunted response. Whether these three tests, however, are considered individually or evaluated in combination, their diagnostic accuracy in the differential diagnosis of mild hypercortisolism does not exceed 80%.

The combined dexamethasone suppression (0.5 mg every 6 h for 2 d) and ovine CRH stimulation test optimize the ability of oCRH to distinguish between the hypercortisolism of pseudo-Cushing's states and CD *(62)*. In the former, the pituitary corticotroph is appropriately restrained by glucocorticoid feedback and does not respond to CRH, whereas in the latter, the corticotroph tumor is generally resistant to this dose of dexamethasone and responds to CRH. Thus, the dexamethasone/CRH test achieves nearly 100% specificity, sensitivity, and diagnostic accuracy. This test should be reserved, however, for those patients who are borderline/mildly hypercortisolemic who have already failed to suppress to 1 mg of overnight dexamethasone and in whom the clinician suspects CD. The criterion used for the diagnosis of CD is a 15-min cortisol level of >38 nmol per liter (1.4 μg/dL) after the CRH injection.

Another strategy, which is always helpful in diagnosing or ruling out CS, is closely monitoring the patient for a few months. Although true hypercortisolism will persist and cause further symptomatology, the hypercortisolism of pseudo-Cushing's states will frequently subside spontaneously, with effective antidepressant treatment or abstinence from alcohol.

Differential Diagnosis of Cushing's Syndrome

Once the diagnosis of endogenous CS has been established, the next challenge is to establish its specific cause *(7,14)*. Generally, a relatively acute onset of symptoms with rapid progression and associated hypokalemic alkalosis point toward an ectopic ACTH source. Accurate differential diagnosis, however, can only be achieved by the combination of dynamic endocrine testing of the integrity of the feedback regulation of the hypothalamic-pituitary-adrenal (HPA) axis, and imaging techniques used mainly to examine the size and shape of the pituitary and adrenal glands and to localize ectopic ACTH- or CRH-secreting tumors (Fig. 2). It is essential that dynamic adrenal testing is performed when the patient is clearly hypercortisolemic. Hypercortisolemia needs to be documented always at the time of testing to avoid mistakes. To that purpose, all adrenal blocking agents should be discontinued for at least 4 wk before testing.

Basal Plasma Adenocorticotropin Hormone and Corticotropin-Releasing Hormone Concentrations

Morning measurement of plasma ACTH concentrations simultaneously with plasma cortisol would distinguish ACTH-dependent from ACTH-independent CS. Circulating ACTH is typically suppressed/undetectable (<1.1 pmol/L; 5 pg/mL measured by immunoradiometric assay [IRMA]) in adrenal cortisol-secreting tumors, micronodular adrenal disease, and autonomously functioning massive macronodular adrenals. In contrast, plasma ACTH concentrations are normal or elevated in CD and ectopic ACTH and CRH syndrome. Patients with ectopic ACTH syndrome frequently have greater plasma ACTH levels than do those with CD. Interestingly, in many of these patients, ACTH immunoreactivity consists primarily of larger precursor molecules *(63)*. Thus, specific measurement of ACTH precursors, if available, may provide a better marker of ectopic ACTH syndrome.

If ectopic CRH secretion is suspected to be the cause of CS, detection of elevated CRH concentrations in the circulation (>50 pg/mL; 11 pmol/L) is helpful.

CRH Stimulation Test

Most patients (80–90%) with CD respond to CRH with increases in plasma ACTH and cortisol, whereas patients with ectopic ACTH production usually do not *(64)*. New criteria were developed for the interpretation of the morning CRH test that maximize simplicity and cost-effectiveness without compromising diagnostic accuracy *(65)*. The diagnostic accuracy of the CRH test is approx 80–90%. Approximately 10–20% of patients with CD do not respond to CRH stimulation, whereas a few patients with ectopic ACTH syndrome might respond. The best cortisol criterion suggestive of CD is a mean increase at 30 and 45 min of greater than 20% above mean basal values at –5 and 0 min (91% sensitivity and 88% specificity). Similarly, an increase of mean ACTH concentrations at 15 and 30 min after CRH by at least 35% above the mean basal values achieves sensitivity of 91% and specificity of nearly 100%. Indeed, although all patients with ectopic ACTH secretion have less than a 35% increase in ACTH, the probability of CD remains high at all levels of responses, suggesting that in the absence of a discrete lesion on pituitary imaging, it is prudent to perform a second test (e.g., the high-dose dexamethasone suppression test or bilateral inferior petrosal or cavernous sinus sampling) to confirm the diagnosis.

Liddle Dexamethasone Suppression Test

The standard low-dose, high-dose dexamethasone suppression test, developed by Grant Liddle *(57)* has been used extensively for differentiating CD from ectopic ACTH syndrome. In patients with CD, the abnormal corticotrophs are sensitive to glucocorticoid inhibition only at the high dose of dexamethasone (2.0 mg every 6 h for 2 d). In contrast, patients with ectopic ACTH syndrome or cortisol-secreting adrenal tumors usually fail to respond to the dose of 8 mg/d. The classic Liddle criterion for a positive response consistent with CD is a greater than 50% drop in 17-hydroxysteroid excretion on d 2 of high-dose dexamethasone (80% diagnostic accuracy). The diagnostic accuracy of the test, however, increases to 86% by measuring both UFC and 17-hydroxysteroid excretion and by requiring greater suppression of both steroids (greater than 64% and 90%, respectively, for 100% specificity) *(66)*.

Overnight 8-mg Dexamethasone Suppression Test

A simple, reliable, and inexpensive alternative to the Liddle dexamethasone suppression test is the overnight 8-mg dexamethasone suppression test. The advantages are its outpatient administration and the avoidance of errors attributable to incomplete urine collections. The diagnostic accuracy of this overnight test may be similar to that of the standard Liddle dexamethasone suppression test *(67,68)*. Dexamethasone 8 mg orally is administered at 11 PM with measurement of plasma cortisol the next morning at 8 AM. Patients with CD usually show plasma cortisol suppression to <50% (88% sensitivity, 57% specificity but 71% sensitivity, 100% specificity if cutoff <69%) of baseline values *(68)*. Approximately 15% of patients with CD do not show suppression with oral high-dose dexamethasone, whereas approx 30% of patients with ectopic ACTH secretion do show suppression with an iv infusion of dexamethasone for 7 h *(69)*.

Metyrapone Testing

Metyrapone inhibits 11-β-hydroxylase and subsequent cortisol production, thereby stimulating endogenous CRH. This is a relatively simple test but not as reliable as the dexamethasone suppression test. Its overall accuracy ranges from 40% to 70% *(70)*.

Tumor Localization

Imaging Evaluation

Imaging techniques can help to clarify the etiology of hypercortisolism. These usually include MRI of the pituitary and computed tomography (CT) scanning of the adrenal glands. CT and MRI scans of the chest and abdomen and isotope scans are also employed when searching for ectopic ACTH-secreting tumors.

Bilateral enlargement of the adrenal glands with preservation of a relatively normal overall glandular configuration is observed in both CD and ectopic ACTH production *(71,72)*. Approximately 10% to 15% of patients with ACTH-dependent CS demonstrate bilateral adrenocortical nodules (macronodular hyperplasia).

Pituitary adenomas are arbitrarily subdivided into microadenomas and macroadenomas, defined respectively as having a diameter smaller or larger than 10 mm. A more important criterion than size is the topographic location of pituitary adenomas. For instance, adenomas (even when they are small) near the cavernous sinus or posterior pituitary (containing, for instance, vasopressin) can have a greater effect on endocrine function, remission rates, and vision (if near the optic chiasm), than more centrally located adenomas. The majority of pituitary ACTH-secreting tumors are microadenomas with a diameter <10 mm. Currently, MRI scanning is the imaging procedure of choice to visualize pituitary adenomas. Pituitary adenomas are usually best demonstrated on coronal postcontrast T1-weighted images with diminished gadolinium enhancement (hypoenhancing) where they appear as foci of reduced signal intensity (hypointense) within the pituitary gland *(73,74)*. On unenhanced scans, however, ACTH-producing adenomas are detected in only 40% of patients with CD *(75)*. Current MRI techniques have a sensitivity of approx 70% and specificity of approx 85% in detecting ACTH-secreting microadenomas as small as 3 mm *(73)*.

The incidence of pituitary incidentalomas detected by MRI is approx 10% in the general population compared with <27% in autopsy series *(74)*. Most incidentalomas are <5 mm in size and can be mistaken for ACTH-secreting adenomas, which can also occur at this size. Differential diagnosis can be achieved with inferior petrosal or cavernous sinus sampling, which should be employed before any transsphenoidal surgery in patients with Cushing's syndrome whose tumor is not visible or equivocal.

CT scanning with contrast infusion demonstrates microadenomas in less than 20% of patients with bona fide lesions on subsequent surgery. Thus, pituitary CT should be performed only if necessary to demonstrate bone anatomy before transsphenoidal surgery.

Catheterization Studies

Distinguishing CD from ectopic ACTH syndrome frequently presents a major diagnostic challenge. Both pituitary microadenomas and ectopic ACTH-secreting tumors may be radiologically occult and may have similar clinical and laboratory features. Bilateral inferior petrosal venous sinus and peripheral vein catheterization with simultaneous collection of samples for ACTH measurement is one of the most specific tests available to localize the source of ACTH production *(76,77)*.

Venous blood from the anterior pituitary drains into the cavernous sinuses and subsequently into the superior and inferior petrosal sinuses. From there, blood exits the jugular foramen and joins the internal jugular vein (Fig. 1, upper panel). Catheters are led into each inferior petrosal sinus via the ipsilateral femoral vein. Samples for measurement of plasma ACTH are collected from each inferior petrosal sinus and a peripheral vein both before and after injection of 1 μg/kg body weight of oCRH in the United States and 100 μg hCRH in Europe. Patients with ectopic ACTH syndrome have no ACTH concentration gradient between either inferior petrosal sinus and the peripheral sample (Fig. 1, lower panel) *(76)*. A ratio ≥2.0 in basal ACTH samples between either or both of the inferior petrosal sinuses and a peripheral vein is highly suggestive of CD (95% sensitivity, 100% specificity). Patients with ectopic ACTH secretion have a gradient of less than 1.6/1. Stimulation with CRH during the procedure with the resulting ACTH outpouring increases the bilateral inferior petrosal sinus sampling (BIPSS) sensitivity for detecting corticotroph adenomas to 100% when peak ACTH central to peripheral ratio is ≥3.0 (Fig. 1, lower panel). Petrosal sinus sampling must be performed bilaterally and simultaneously, because the sensitivity of the test drops to less than 70% with unilateral catheterization. A false-negative test result with bilateral inferior petrosal sinus sampling (BIPSS) may ensue from a hypoplastic inferior petrosal sinus (<2% of patients with surgically proven CD) *(78)*.

BIPSS is technically difficult and, as with all invasive procedures, can never be risk free even in the most experienced hands *(79,80)*. It should be reserved only for patients with classic CS and negative or equivocal MRI of the pituitary and patients with positive pituitary MRI but equivocal suppression and stimulation tests. In the former group, BIPSS unequivocally distinguishes ACTH-secreting pituitary adenomas from lung and thymic carcinoid tumors and provides lateralization data of potential value to the surgeon. In the latter group, BIPSS will exclude the possibility of a pituitary incidentaloma, which can be visualized on MRI in as many as 10% of young women. The most common complication is a groin hematoma at the site of the venipuncture. Major neurologic complications occur in less than 1% of patients *(79,80)*. In more than 100 patients, the overall complication rate was 13%, including permanent diabetes insipidus, deep venous thrombosis, and pneumonia *(80)*. The diagnostic accuracy of BIPSS in identifying pituitary ACTH hypersecretion is >95%, whereas it is only 60% in lateralizing the adenoma, owing to variable patterns of venous drainage. Routine presampling venography may allow more accurate interpretation of lateralizing ACTH gradients during BIPSS *(81)*. Catheterization of the cavernous sinuses and jugular veins has also been performed in the diagnosis of CD, with high sensitivity and specificity. Although cavernous sinus sampling may be more accurate than BIPPS in predicting the side of the pituitary in which the tumor resides, it can also be more risky than BIPSS *(82)* (John Doppman, personal experience).

Cushing's Syndrome With Unusual Laboratory Behavior

Periodic Cushing's Syndrome

Occasionally, cortisol production in CS may not be constantly increased but may fluctuate in a "periodic" pattern, ranging in length from days to months. This relatively rare phenomenon of periodic, cyclic, or episodic hormonogenesis has been described in patients with CD, ectopic ACTH syndrome (bronchial carcinoids were involved in 50% of the reported cases), and cortisol-secreting adrenal tumors or micronodular adrenal disease *(20–32)*.

Biochemically, patients with periodic hormonogenesis may have consistently normal 24-h UFC and paradoxically "normal" responses to dexamethasone (stimulation of cortisol) in the presence of CS clinical stigmata. In such patients, several weekly 24-h UFC determinations for a period of 3 to 6 mo may be necessary to establish the diagnosis.

Cushing's Syndrome in Pregnancy

In normal pregnancy, a small progressive rise in plasma ACTH and a twofold to threefold increase in plasma total and free cortisol occur. UFC is also elevated above normal, especially between the 34th and 40th wk of gestation (90 to 350 μg/d; 248–966 nmol/d). In the latter part of pregnancy, immunoreactive CRH (irCRH) IR-CRH of placental origin is detected in plasma, with levels reaching up to 10,000 pg/mL (2200 pmol/L) *(83)*. Because plasma cortisol is poorly suppressed in response to dexamethasone in normal pregnancy, the diagnosis of mild or early CS may be difficult to ascertain *(84)*. Transient pregnancy-related and pregnancy-limited CS has been described. Its etiology is unknown.

Primary Cortisol Resistance

Glucocorticoid resistance in humans is characterized by spontaneous hypercortisolism without CS features, owing to an apparent end-organ insensitivity to cortisol usually as a result of genomic defects of the glucocorticoid receptor *(85)*. In addition to increased plasma ACTH and serum and urinary cortisol and decreased cortisol suppression by dexamethasone administration, these patients frequently have elevated plasma and urinary adrenal androgens and mineralocorticoids. Plasma cortisol has a circadian rhythm similar to that of normal subjects, albeit at elevated concentrations, and responds normally to stress tests such as insulin-induced hypoglycemia. The most frequent manifestation of glucocorticoid resistance is adrenal hyperandrogenism in women and children and mild hypertension in both genders.

TREATMENT

Surgery

Selective transsphenoidal microadenomectomy, a procedure with a complete remission rate of nearly 95% on the first exploration (depending on the institution/neurosurgeon) and the added advantage of producing eventually normal anterior pituitary function, is the initial therapy of choice for CD *(4,86)* (*see* Chapter 8).

Less than 10% of ACTH-secreting pituitary adenomas are macroadenomas. Only if these adenomas extend into the lateral parasellar and/or suprasellar regions is the transcranial approach used.

The neurosurgeon should always explore the entire pituitary gland to find the microadenoma responsible for the disease. If the adenoma is <5 mm, it may not be visible on the surface of the gland, but a vertical incision often will reveal it *(87)*. If pituitary MRI did not identify an adenoma, cavernous sinus or inferior petrosal sinus sampling data (if presampling venography confirmed symmetric venous drainage and the lateralizing ACTH gradient is >2) may assist the neurosurgeon in lateralizing the adenoma during transsphenoidal exploration *(88)*. The entire sellar region should be explored before any anterior pituitary tissue is removed. In patients with no identifiable tumor *in situ* at first sight, intraoperative ultrasound may be helpful *(89)*. If an adenoma cannot be found during transsphenoidal exploration, the surgeon may perform a hemihypophysectomy on the site of a lateral IPS ACTH gradient >2. This approach has proved successful in approx 80% of cases *(88,90)*. Few patients have extrapituitary parasellar microadenomas that probably arose from remnants of Rathke's pouch *(88)*. Total hypophysectomy should not be performed in patients without identifiable adenoma during exploration, even if these patients do not insist on reproductive function. Failure of surgery at the first exploration may be followed by a repeat procedure with a 50–60% chance of complete remission *(91)*. Success is defined as a drop of serum cortisol (8 AM) and/or urinary free cortisol to an undetectable level in the postoperative period (after d 2 postoperatively, off glucocorticoid administration) *(92–94)*. A successful outcome can also be predicted by lack of cortisol or ACTH response to oCRH or desmopressin, when the test is performed 7–10 d after surgery *(95,96)*.

In patients without histologically confirmed tumor (an abnormality/tissue that was removed in the belief it was the adenoma), complete remission occurs in 66% on an average follow-up of 38 mo *(97)*.

Criteria to predict long-term remission are controversial and include undetectable serum cortisol, UFC, and ACTH levels in the (immediate) postoperative period and low-dose dexamethasone suppressibility and deficient responses with CRH and/or desmopressin stimulation 7–10 d after surgery *(92–96,98,99)*. However, there are patients with long-term remission who had normal cortisol levels in the immediate postsurgical period *(86,100)*. The lowest risk of relapse has been observed in patients who require prolonged glucocorticoid therapy after adenomectomy *(101)*. A plasma cortisol <6μg/dL (166 nmol) and UFC <15μg/d (41 nmol) between postoperative d 3 and 5 can predict long-term remission *(98)*. At our institution, patients are started on hydrocortisone replacement therapy on d 5 after surgery to treat secondary hypoadrenalism. Cosyntropin (Synacthen) stimulation testing is performed at three monthly intervals to assess recovery of the HPA axis.

The most common reason for residual disease is local invasion of the dura, especially of the lateral sellar wall, possibly with perforation of the sellar floor. The other major cause for surgical failure is the inability to localize the adenoma surgically *(4,91)*.

Overall long-term remission rates for ACTH-secreting microadenomas range from 75% to 95%, depending on the institution and neurosurgeon *(91,102)*. For macroadenomas, surgical long-term success is less than 70% because of frequent invasion of the dura, cavernous sinus, and adjacent structures. Repeat surgery does not significantly improve the outcome, making further therapies, including irradiation, medical therapy, and even bilateral adrenalectomy, necessary *(91,103)*.

The complication rate of transsphenoidal surgery for the treatment of pituitary adenomas is low, with a perioperative mortality of less than 2% (major causes being: pulmonary embolism and myocardial infarction). Most frequently (<20% of patients), postoperative transient hyponatremia develops as part of the sydrome of inappropriate secretion of antidiuretic hormone (SIADH). Transient postoperative diabetes insipidus (<15% of patients) and CSF rhinorrhea (<5%) are also seen. Permanent diabetes insipidus develops in <3% of patients, usually in those who require more extensive surgery such as hemihypophysectomy or hypophysectomy. Meningitis is rarely seen and related to a CSF leak that usually is easily treated. Hypopituitarism occurs in less than 2% *(4,80,101,104)*.

A second transsphenoidal operation may be indicated if CD persists and/or the first surgery was performed by an inexperienced surgeon *(91)*. Providing that ectopic ACTH syndrome has been excluded, this surgery often involves a hemihypophysectomy or total hypophysectomy and only rarely a selective adenomectomy. If dura invasion was present at the first surgical exploration, no further transsphenoidal surgeries should be undertaken (except for debulking in rare cases), and radiation, medical therapy, and, in refractory cases, bilateral adrenalectomy should be employed.

Radiotherapy (see also Chapter 13)

The second line of therapy is pituitary irradiation with 4500 to 5000 cGy (rad), administered in daily fractions of 180 cGy, delivered during a period of 6 wk. This type of pituitary radiation involves an external beam irradiation from a high-energy linear accelerator.

Radiation delivery can also be achieved by high-voltage cobalt-60 particle irradiation, heavy particle beam radiotherapy, and stereotactic radiosurgery. Primary radiotherapy results in CD remission in up to 85% of patients *(105,106)*. Hypercortisolism in these patients may persist up to 3 yr after radiation before a decline to normal cortisol levels can be seen. Radiation in association with mitotane therapy (*o-p*'DDD), can produce a remission rate of approx 80% in the first year *(107)*. This can increase further in the second year, but the sustained remission rate after discontinuing mitotane therapy drops significantly to less than 60% of the patients. Mitotane can be discontinued after 1 yr, if UFC has normalized. It can be reinitiated if hypercortisolemia recurs. By 3 yr, 80% to 90% of patients will have achieved biochemical remission of CS and will no longer need mitotane, because the effects of irradiation become established. If mitotane therapy is not tolerated by or fails to cure the patient, the final line of treatment is bilateral open or laparascopic adrenalectomy *(108)*. This procedure is uniformly effective at the expense, however, of a commitment to hormone replacement for life, and a significant risk (10%–15%) for subsequent development of Nelson's syndrome *(109–111)*.

Proton beam pituitary radiotherapy (12,000–14,000 rad) exposes the hypothalamus only to approx 500 rad, and thus rarely leads to anterior pituitary hormone deficiencies *(105)*. Gamma Knife radiosurgery (gamma irradiation from cobalt-60 administered stereotactically in a single dose) may achieve long-term remission rates of 82% after multiple treatments *(103,112)*. Approx 20% of patients develop pituitary insufficiency requiring hormone replacement therapy. If there is no chiasmal involvement and the adenoma is intrasellar, Gamma Knife radiosurgery may be an alternative treatment to conventional radiotherapy *(113–115)*.

Radiotherapy usually is used in patients with persistent or recurrent CD after pituitary surgery. For patients with microadenomas treated with second-line radiotherapy, the remission rate at 3-yr follow-up can be up to 80% *(103,106,115,116)*. For patients with macroadenomas, the response to radiotherapy is less favorable. In children, radiotherapy usually is rarely necessary and is more problematic than in adults, given the special need of pituitary hormones during the prepubertal and pubertal periods.

Long-term complications of (conventional) pituitary radiotherapy include hypopituitarism, memory deficits, brain necrosis, optic nerve or optic chiasm injury, and carcinogenesis *(117,118)* (and Chapter 13). When surgery and radiotherapy are combined, hypopituitarism may occur in as many as 50% of patients during a 10-yr period *(119, 120)*. At 8 year follow-up, the incidence of deficiencies in TSH, ACTH, gonadotropins, and growth hormone was 49%, 84%, 96%, and 100%, respectively *(117)*. Therefore, patients who undergo pituitary radiotherapy need lifelong follow-up with routine testing for hypopituitarism and CD recurrence. Such testing should include periodic MRI brain/pituitary scanning and visual field testing.

Medical Therapy

If surgical cure is impossible, blockade of steroidogenesis is indicated and combination chemotherapy and/or radiation therapy may be administered. Ketoconazole is the most useful agent. It blocks adrenal steroidogenesis at several levels, the most important being the 20–22 desmolase step, which catalyzes the conversion of cholesterol to pregnenolone, thus avoiding accumulation of steroid biosynthesis intermediates that can cause or worsen hypertension and/or hirsutism *(121)*. To control CD, doses of 400–1200 mg/d po are usually required. One might start ketoconazole at 200 mg once a day, gradually increasing the dose over 2 to 3 wk, with frequent assessment of serum cortisol levels before and after administering the drug. Reversible side effects, including elevations of hepatic transaminases and gastrointestinal irritation, may occur and may be dose limiting. In this case, metyrapone can be added to achieve normocortisolemia *(13,122)*. Other blocking agents that may be used alone or in combination with ketoconazole and/or metyrapone include aminoglutethimide and trilostane *(122)*.

Metyrapone is a selective inhibitor of 11-β-hydroxylase. Monotherapy is limited by salt retention with development of hypertension and virilization *(123)*. Aminoglutethimide inhibits the conversion from cholesterol to pregnenolone and thus leads to decline of all adrenal and gonadal steroids. Monotherapy is less efficacious for treating CD than combination therapy with other inhibitors of steroidogenesis. Side effects include nausea, sedation, and rash *(122)*.

Mitotane, an adrenolytic agent, can produce short-term remission in approx 83% of patients with CD *(107)*. Trilostane, an inhibitor of the 3-β-hydroxysteroid dehydrogenase, is less effective in treating CD than other agents.

If iv administration of inhibitors of steroidogenesis becomes necessary, etomidate can be given. This anesthetic agent is an imidazole derivative and inhibits 11-β-hydroxylase, thereby reducing cortisol levels *(124)*.

Octreotide, cyproheptadine, bromocriptine, and valproic acid have all been used to inhibit ACTH secretion but are not effective *(122)*.

Bilateral Adrenalectomy

Although commonly used in the past for treating patients with CD/CS to control hypercortisolemia, bilateral adrenalectomy is now reserved for patients who did not respond to pituitary surgery and/or radiotherapy as well as medical treatment. Currently, perioperative morbidity is less than 32% and mortality less than 2% *(109,125,126)*. Laparoscopic adrenalectomy led to a further decline in perioperative morbidity *(127)*. Recurrence rates on long-term follow-up are less than 4%. Postoperatively, patients require lifelong glucocorticoid and mineralocorticoid replacement therapy and evaluation for residual (ectopic) adrenal tissue, as well as the development of Nelson's syndrome.

Corticosteroid Replacement

Glucocorticoid replacement should be started after a successful pituitary adenomectomy (approx on d 5 after low or undetectable serum and urinary cortisol levels have been obtained). The action is undertaken because in those patients the HPA axis is suppressed by the chronic exposure to excess glucocorticoids and fails to function for several months after the removal of normal corticotroph inhibition, such as an ACTH-secreting pituitary adenoma *(128)*. Hydrocortisone should be replaced at a rate of 12 to 15 mg/m^2/d by mouth, with appropriate increases in minor stress (two-fold) and major stress (up to 10-fold) for appropriate lengths of time. The recovery of the suppressed HPA axis can be monitored with a short ACTH test every 3 mo. When the 30-min plasma cortisol exceeds 18 μg/dl, hydrocortisone can be discontinued. After a bilateral adrenalectomy, corticosteroid replacement will be necessary for life and includes both glucocorticoids and mineralocorticoids.

NELSON'S SYNDROME

In 1958, Nelson and colleagues *(110)* reported the rapid enlargement of ACTH-secreting pituitary adenomas after bilateral adrenalectomy. Historically, these patients develop hyperpigmentation by excessive ACTH elevation (the ACTH molecule contains α-MSH) and radiologic demonstration of pituitary enlargement *(129)*. Although the incidence of Nelson's syndrome has been reported to be as high as 38% in patients with CD who underwent bilateral adrenalectomy *(109,130–133)*, it is encountered only rarely these days, because bilateral adrenalectomy is now reserved for patients who did not respond to pituitary surgery and/or radiotherapy. Because many ACTH-secreting pituitary adenomas respond to CRH stimulation, it is conceivable that, in analogy to some patients with severe hypothyroidism (TSH >100 U/mL, TRH elevation unknown) and subsequent pituitary enlargement, in patients after bilateral adrenalectomy the CRH stimulus causes enlargement of some but not all ACTH-secreting adenomas, with a subset having a more aggressive potential (those that might have recurred anyway, if pituitary surgery had been performed as first-line therapy).

Children with CD who underwent bilateral adrenalectomy as first-line treatment have a higher incidence of Nelson's syndrome than do adults, because they have more years of life to live and thus a longer follow-up period *(134,135)*.

Whether pituitary irradiation before adrenalectomy can prevent the development of Nelson's syndrome is unknown *(109,136)*. ACTH levels in patients with Nelson's syndrome frequently exceed 1000 pg/mL. Headaches and visual field defects may be present *(131)*. The majority of Nelson's syndrome tumors are macroadenomas and invasive.

Recurrent hypercortisolism after adrenalectomy may be seen by cortisol production from adrenal rest tumors, usually residing in the testes *(137)*.

If possible, patients with Nelson's syndrome in whom vision is threatened should undergo pituitary surgery to remove or debulk the tumor. Pituitary irradiation is the only currently available second-line therapy, because medical treatment does not have a significant role in treating Nelson's syndrome *(106,133,138,139)*.

SUMMARY

Excess and prolonged endogenous glucocorticoid production, whether ACTH-dependent or ACTH-independent, results in the classic clinical and biochemical picture of CS. The diagnosis requires demonstration of an increased cortisol secretion rate, best achieved by determination of 24-h UFC excretion levels. In mild or confusing cases, distinction from the hypercortisolism of pseudo-Cushing states may prove difficult. A dexamethasone/ oCRH test or close monitoring of the patient for a few months may be helpful. Most cases of primary adrenal CS can be ruled out by undetectable basal and/or CRH-stimulated plasma ACTH and negative adrenal imaging procedures. ACTH-dependent CS can then be differentiated by an oCRH test and imaging procedures. A discrete pituitary lesion on gadolinium-enhanced MRI and a standard oCRH with stimulated ACTH levels consistent with such a lesion are usually sufficient to proceed to transsphenoidal surgery. If no visible pituitary lesion is present, or if the oCRH test is equivocal, bilateral simultaneous inferior petrosal or cavernous sinus sampling with oCRH administration are necessary to distinguish between a pituitary and an ectopic ACTH source. Surgical ablation is the treatment of choice for all types of CS. In the approx 5%–10% of cases with CD in whom transsphenoidal surgery fails and in the 5% of cases in whom the disease recurs, repeat transsphenoidal surgery or radiation therapy in association with mitotane treatment are reasonable alternatives. Bilateral adrenalectomy effectively cures hypercortisolism if resection of the ACTH-secreting tumor is unsuccessful and radiation/medical therapy fail.

REFERENCES

1. Cushing H. The basophil adenomas of the pituitary body and their clinical manifestations (pituitary basophilism). Bull Johns Hopkins Hosp 1932;50:137–195.
2. Mindermann T, Wilson CB. Age-related and gender-related occurrence of pituitary adenomas. Clin Endocrinol (Oxf) 1994;41(3):359–364.

3. Aron DC, Findling JW, Tyrrell JB. Cushing's disease. Endocrinol Metab Clin North Am 1987;16(3):705–730.
4. Mampalam TJ, Tyrrell JB, Wilson, CB. Transsphenoidal microsurgery for Cushing disease. A report of 216 cases. Ann Intern Med 1988;109(6):487–493.
5. Carey RM, et al. Ectopic secretion of corticotropin-releasing factor as a cause of Cushing's syndrome. A clinical, morphologic, and biochemical study. N Engl J Med 1984;311(1):13–20.
6. Auchus RJ, et al. Corticotropin-releasing hormone production by a small cell carcinoma in a patient with ACTH-dependent Cushing's syndrome. J Endocrinol Invest 1994;17(6):447–452.
7. Newell-Price J, et al. The diagnosis and differential diagnosis of Cushing's syndrome and pseudo-Cushing's states. Endocr Rev 1998;19(5):647–672.
8. Yanovski JA, Cutler GB, Jr. Glucocorticoid action and the clinical features of Cushing's syndrome. Endocrinol Metab Clin North Am 1994;23(3):487–509.
9. Magiakou MA, et al. Cushing's syndrome in children and adolescents. Presentation, diagnosis, and therapy. N Engl J Med 1994;331(10):629–636.
10. Magiakou MA, Mastorakos G, Chrousos GP. Final stature in patients with endogenous Cushing's syndrome. J Clin Endocrinol Metab 1994;79(4):1082–1085.
11. Robyn JA, et al. Cushing's syndrome in childhood and adolescence. J Pediatr Child Health 1997;33(6):522–527.
12. Savage MO, et al. Cushing's disease in childhood: presentation, investigation, treatment and long-term outcome. Horm Res 2001;55(Suppl 1):24–30.
13. Koch CA, et al. Spinal epidural lipomatosis in a patient with the ectopic corticotropin syndrome. N Engl J Med 1999;341(18):1399–400.
14. Orth DN, Cushing's syndrome. N Engl J Med 1995;332(12):791–803.
15. Koch CA, et al. Cushing's disease presenting with avascular necrosis of the hip: an orthopedic emergency. J Clin Endocrinol Metab 1999;84(9):3010–3012.
16. Bouzas EA, et al. Posterior subcapsular cataract in endogenous Cushing syndrome: an uncommon manifestation. Invest Ophthalmol Vis Sci 1993;34(13):3497–3500.
17. Dorn LD, et al. The longitudinal course of psychopathology in Cushing's syndrome after correction of hypercortisolism. J Clin Endocrinol Metab 1997;82(3):912–919.
18. Sapolsky RM. Glucocorticoids and hippocampal atrophy in neuropsychiatric disorders. Arch Gen Psychiatry 2000;57(10):925–935.
19. Starkman MN. et al. Hippocampal formation volume, memory dysfunction, and cortisol levels in patients with Cushing's syndrome. Biol Psychiatry 1992;32(9):756–765.
20. Bailey RE. Periodic hormonogenesis—a new phenomenon. Periodicity in function of a hormone-producing tumor in man. J Clin Endocrinol Metab 1971;32(3):317–327.
21. Atkinson AB, et al. Five cases of cyclical Cushing's syndrome. Br Med J (Clin Res Ed) 1985;291(6507):1453–1457.
22. Brown RD, et al. Cushing's disease with periodic hormonogenesis: one explanation for paradoxical response to dexamethasone. J Clin Endocrinol Metab 1973;36(3):445–451.
23. Hocher B, et al. Hypercortisolism with non-pigmented micronodular adrenal hyperplasia: transition from pituitary-dependent to adrenal-dependent Cushing's syndrome. Acta Endocrinol (Copenh) 1993;128(2):120–125.
24. Liebowitz G, et al. Fluctuating hyper-hypocortisolaemia: a variant of Cushing's syndrome. Clin Endocrinol (Oxf) 1997;46(6):759–763.
25. Oates TW, et al. Cushing's disease with cyclic hormonogenesis and diabetes insipidus. Neurosurgery 1979;5(5):598–603.
26. Atkinson AB, et al. Cyclical Cushing's disease: two distinct rhythms in a patient with a basophil adenoma. J Clin Endocrinol Metab 1985;60(2):328–332.
27. Liberman B, et al. Periodic remission in Cushing's disease with paradoxical dexamethasone response: an expression of periodic hormonogenesis. J Clin Endocrinol Metab 1976;43(4): 913–918.

28. Mosnier-Pudar H, et al. Long-distance and long-term follow-up of a patient with intermittent Cushing's disease by salivary cortisol measurements. Eur J Endocrinol 1995;133(3): 313–316.
29. Vagnucci AH, Evans E. Cushing's disease with intermittent hypercortisolism. Am J Med 1986;80(1):83–88.
30. Sakiyama R., Ashcraft MW, Van Herle AJ. Cyclic Cushing's syndrome. Am J Med 1984; 77(5):944–946.
31. Carson DJ, et al. Cyclical Cushing's syndrome presenting as short stature in a boy with recurrent atrial myxomas and freckled skin pigmentation. Clin Endocrinol (Oxf), 1988;28(2):173–180.
32. Koch CA, et al. (Primary pigmented nodular adrenocortical dysplasia (PPNAD) within the scope of Carney complex as the etiology of Cushing syndrome). Med Klin 2000;95(4):224–230.
33. Reincke M. Subclinical Cushing's syndrome. Endocrinol Metab Clin North Am 2000; 29(1):43–56.
34. Krieger DT. Physiopathology of Cushing's disease. Endocr Rev 1983;4(1):22–43.
35. Biller BM. Pathogenesis of pituitary Cushing's syndrome. Pituitary versus hypothalamic. Endocrinol Metab Clin North Am 1994;23(3):547–554.
36. Gertz BJ, et al. Chronic administration of corticotropin-releasing factor increases pituitary corticotroph number. Endocrinology 1987;120(1):381–388.
37. Schnall AM, et al. Pituitary Cushing's disease without adenoma. Acta Endocrinol (Copenh) 1980;94(3):297–303.
38. Horvath E, Kovacs K, Scheithauer BW. Pituitary hyperplasia. Pituitary 1999;1(3–4):169–179.
39. Saeger W, Ludecke DK. Pituitary hyperplasia. Definition, light and electron microscopical structures and significance in surgical specimens. Virchows Arch 1983;399(3):277–287.
40. Scheithauer BW, et al. Pituitary carcinoma: an ultrastructural study of eleven cases. Ultrastruct Pathol 2001;25(3):227–242.
41. Ratliff JK, Oldfield EH. Multiple pituitary adenomas in Cushing's disease. J Neurosurg 2000;93(5):753–761.
42. Stenzel-Poore MP, et al. Development of Cushing's syndrome in corticotropin-releasing factor transgenic mice. Endocrinology 1992;130(6):3378–3386.
43. Dahia PL, Grossman AB. The molecular pathogenesis of corticotroph tumors. Endocr Rev 1999;20(2):136–155.
44. Schulte HM, et al. Clonal composition of pituitary adenomas in patients with Cushing's disease: determination by X-chromosome inactivation analysis. J Clin Endocrinol Metab 1991;73(6):1302–1308.
45. Biller BM, et al. Clonal origins of adrenocorticotropin-secreting pituitary tissue in Cushing's disease. J Clin Endocrinol Metab 1992;75(5):1303–1309.
46. Shimon I, Melmed S. Genetic basis of endocrine disease: pituitary tumor pathogenesis. J Clin Endocrinol Metab 1997;82(6):1675–1681.
47. Gicquel C, et al. Monoclonality of corticotroph macroadenomas in Cushing's disease. J Clin Endocrinol Metab 1992;75(2):472–475.
48. Herman V, et al. Clonal origin of pituitary adenomas. J Clin Endocrinol Metab 1990;71(6):1427–1433.
49. Buckley N, et al. p53 Protein accumulates in Cushings adenomas and invasive non- functional adenomas. J Clin Endocrinol Metab 1994;79(5):1513–1516.
50. Karl M, et al. Cushing's disease preceded by generalized glucocorticoid resistance: clinical consequences of a novel, dominant-negative glucocorticoid receptor mutation. Proc Assoc Am Physicians 1996;108(4):296–307.
51. Karl M, et al. Nelson's syndrome associated with a somatic frame shift mutation in the glucocorticoid receptor gene. J Clin Endocrinol Metab 1996;81(1):124–129.

52. Contreras LN, Hane S, Tyrrell JB. Urinary cortisol in the assessment of pituitary-adrenal function: utility of 24-hour and spot determinations. J Clin Endocrinol Metab 1986;62(5):965–969.
53. Gomez MT, et al. Urinary free cortisol values in normal children and adolescents. J Pediatr 1991;118(2):256–258.
54. Pavlatos FC, Smilo RP, Forsham PH. A rapid screening test for Cushing's syndrome. JAMA 1965;193:96–99.
55. Tsigos C, Papanicolaou DA, Chrousos GP. Advances in the diagnosis and treatment of Cushing's syndrome. Baillieres Clin Endocrinol Metab 1995;9(2):315–336.
56. Newell-Price J, et al. A single sleeping midnight cortisol has 100% sensitivity for the diagnosis of Cushing's syndrome. Clin Endocrinol (Oxf) 1995;43(5):545–550.
57. Liddle GW. Tests of pituitary-adrenal suppressibility in the diagnosis of Cushing's syndrome. J Clin Endocrinol Metab 1960;20:1539–1561.
58. Raff H, Raff JL, Findling JW. Late-night salivary cortisol as a screening test for Cushing's syndrome. J Clin Endocrinol Metab 1998;83(8):2681–2686.
59. Papanicolaou DA, et al. A single midnight serum cortisol measurement distinguishes Cushing's syndrome from pseudo-Cushing states. J Clin Endocrinol Metab 1998;83(4):1163–1167.
60. Tsigos C, Chrousos GP. Physiology of the hypothalamic-pituitary-adrenal axis in health and dysregulation in psychiatric and autoimmune disorders. Endocrinol Metab Clin North Am 1994;23(3):451–466.
61. Gold PW, et al. Responses to corticotropin-releasing hormone in the hypercortisolism of depression and Cushing's disease. Pathophysiologic and diagnostic implications. N Engl J Med 1986;314(21):1329–1335.
62. Yanovski JA, et al. Corticotropin-releasing hormone stimulation following low-dose dexamethasone administration. A new test to distinguish Cushing's syndrome from pseudo-Cushing's states. Jama 1993;269(17):2232–2238.
63. White A, Clark AJ. The cellular and molecular basis of the ectopic ACTH syndrome. Clin Endocrinol (Oxf) 1993;39(2):131–141.
64. Chrousos GP, et al. The corticotropin-releasing factor stimulation test. An aid in the evaluation of patients with Cushing's syndrome. N Engl J Med 1984;310(10):622–626.
65. Nieman LK, et al. A simplified morning ovine corticotropin-releasing hormone stimulation test for the differential diagnosis of adrenocorticotropin-dependent Cushing's syndrome. J Clin Endocrinol Metab 1993;77(5):308–312.
66. Flack MR, et al. Urine free cortisol in the high-dose dexamethasone suppression test for the differential diagnosis of the Cushing syndrome. Ann Intern Med 1992;116(3):211–217.
67. Tyrrell JB, et al. An overnight high-dose dexamethasone suppression test for rapid differential diagnosis of Cushing's syndrome. Ann Intern Med 1986;104(2):180–186.
68. Dichek HL, et al. A comparison of the standard high dose dexamethasone suppression test and the overnight 8-mg dexamethasone suppression test for the differential diagnosis of adrenocorticotropin-dependent Cushing's syndrome. J Clin Endocrinol Metab 1994;78(2):418–422.
69. Biemond P, de Jong FH, Lamberts SW. Continuous dexamethasone infusion for seven hours in patients with the Cushing syndrome. A superior differential diagnostic test. Ann Intern Med 1990;112(10):738–742.
70. Avgerinos PC, et al. The metyrapone and dexamethasone suppression tests for the differential diagnosis of the adrenocorticotropin-dependent Cushing syndrome: a comparison. Ann Intern Med 1994;121(5):318–327.
71. Doppman JL, et al. Macronodular adrenal hyperplasia in Cushing disease. Radiology 1988;166(2):347–352.

72. Doppman JL, et al. Adrenocorticotropin-independent macronodular adrenal hyperplasia: an uncommon cause of primary adrenal hypercortisolism. Radiology 2000;216(3):797–802.
73. Buchfelder M, et al. The accuracy of CT and MR evaluation of the sella turcica for detection of adrenocorticotropic hormone-secreting adenomas in Cushing disease. AJNR Am J Neuroradiol 1993;14(5):1183–1190.
74. Hall WA, et al. Pituitary magnetic resonance imaging in normal human volunteers: occult adenomas in the general population. Ann Intern Med 1994;120(10):817–820.
75. Doppman JL, et al. Gadolinium DTPA enhanced MR imaging of ACTH-secreting microadenomas of the pituitary gland. J Comput Assist Tomogr 1988;12(5):728–735.
76. Oldfield EH, et al. Petrosal sinus sampling with and without corticotropin-releasing hormone for the differential diagnosis of Cushing's syndrome. N Engl J Med 1991;325(13):897–905.
77. Doppman JL, Oldfield EH, Nieman LK. Bilateral sampling of the internal jugular vein to distinguish between mechanisms of adrenocorticotropic hormone-dependent Cushing syndrome. Ann Intern Med 1998;128(1):33–36.
78. Doppman JL, et al. The hypoplastic inferior petrosal sinus: a potential source of false-negative results in petrosal sampling for Cushing's disease. J Clin Endocrinol Metab 1999;84(2):533–540.
79. Miller DL. Neurologic complications of petrosal sinus sampling. Radiology 1992; 183(3):878.
80. Semple PL, Laws ER, Jr. Complications in a contemporary series of patients who underwent transsphenoidal surgery for Cushing's disease. J Neurosurg 1999;91(2):175–179.
81. Mamelak AN, et al. Venous angiography is needed to interpret inferior petrosal sinus and cavernous sinus sampling data for lateralizing adrenocorticotropin- secreting adenomas. J Clin Endocrinol Metab 1996;81(2):475–481.
82. Graham KE, et al. Cavernous sinus sampling is highly accurate in distinguishing Cushing's disease from the ectopic adrenocorticotropin syndrome and in predicting intrapituitary tumor location. J Clin Endocrinol Metab 1999;84(5):1602–1610.
83. Sasaki A, et al. Immunoreactive corticotropin-releasing hormone in human plasma during pregnancy, labor, and delivery. J Clin Endocrinol Metab 1987;64(2):224–229.
84. Buescher MA, McClamrock HD, Adashi EY. Cushing syndrome in pregnancy. Obstet Gynecol 1992;79(1):130–137.
85. Chrousos GP, Detera-Wadleigh SD, Karl M. Syndromes of glucocorticoid resistance. Ann Intern Med 1993;119(11):1113–1124.
86. Friedman TC, Chrousos GP. Transsphenoidal resection in Cushing's disease: definition of success. Clin Endocrinol (Oxf) 1993;39(6):701.
87. Wilson CB. A decade of pituitary microsurgery. The Herbert Olivecrona lecture. J Neurosurg 1984;61(5):814–833.
88. Pluta RM, et al. Extrapituitary parasellar microadenoma in Cushing's disease. J Clin Endocrinol Metab 1999;84(8):2912–2923.
89. Watson JC, et al. Localization of pituitary adenomas by using intraoperative ultrasound in patients with Cushing's disease and no demonstrable pituitary tumor on magnetic resonance imaging. J Neurosurg 1998;89(6):927–932.
90. Oldfield EH, et al. Preoperative lateralization of ACTH-secreting pituitary microadenomas by bilateral and simultaneous inferior petrosal venous sinus sampling. N Engl J Med 1985; 312(2):100–103.
91. Ram Z, et al. Early repeat surgery for persistent Cushing's disease. J Neurosurg 1994;80(1):37–45.
92. Simmons NE, et al. Serum cortisol response to transsphenoidal surgery for Cushing disease. J Neurosurg 2001;95(1):1–8.
93. Chee GH, et al. Transsphenoidal pituitary surgery in Cushing's disease: can we predict outcome? Clin Endocrinol (Oxf) 2001;54(5):617–626.

94. Nishizawa S, et al. What can predict postoperative "endocrinological cure" in Cushing's disease? Neurosurgery 1999;45(2):39–44.
95. Avgerinos PC, et al. The corticotropin-releasing hormone test in the postoperative evaluation of patients with cushing's syndrome. J Clin Endocrinol Metab 1987;65(5):906–913.
96. Losa M, et al. Desmopressin stimulation test before and after pituitary surgery in patients with Cushing's disease. Clin Endocrinol (Oxf) 2001;55(1):61–68.
97. Sheehan JM, et al. Results of transsphenoidal surgery for Cushing's disease in patients with no histologically confirmed tumor. Neurosurgery 2000;47(1):33–36; discussion 37–39.
98. Nieman LK, et al. Prediction of long-term remission of Cushing's disease after successful transsphenoidal resection of ACTH-secreting tumor. In: *Program & Abstracts of the Annual Meeting of the Endocrine Society*. San Diego, CA:1999.
99. McCance DR, Besser M, Atkinson AB. Assessment of cure after transsphenoidal surgery for Cushing's disease. Clin Endocrinol (Oxf) 1996;44(1):1–6.
100. McCance DR, et al. Assessment of endocrine function after transsphenoidal surgery for Cushing's disease. Clin Endocrinol (Oxf) 1993;38(1):79–86.
101. Bochicchio D, Losa M, Buchfelder M. Factors influencing the immediate and late outcome of Cushing's disease treated by transsphenoidal surgery: a retrospective study by the European Cushing's Disease Survey Group. J Clin Endocrinol Metab 1995;80(11):3114–3120.
102. Wilson CB. The long-term results following pituitary surgery for Cushing's disease and Nelson's syndrome. In: *Secretory Tumors of the Pituitary Gland*. Black PM, et al., eds. New York: Raven Press; 1984;287–294.
103. Sheehan JM, et al. Radiosurgery for Cushing's disease after failed transsphenoidal surgery. J Neurosurg 2000;93(5):738–742.
104. Olson BR, et al. Isolated hyponatremia after transsphenoidal pituitary surgery. J Clin Endocrinol Metab 1995;80(1):85–91.
105. Kjellberg RN, et al. Proton beam therapy of Cushing's disease and Nelson's syndrome. In: *Secretory Tumors of the Pituitary Gland*. Black BM, et al., eds. New York: Raven Press; 1984;294–307.
106. Howlett TA, et al. Megavoltage pituitary irradiation in the management of Cushing's disease and Nelson's syndrome: long-term follow-up. Clin Endocrinol (Oxf) 1989;31(3):309–323.
107. Luton JP, et al. Treatment of Cushing's disease by O,p'DDD. Survey of 62 cases. N Engl J Med 1979;300(9):459–464.
108. Zeiger MA, et al. Effective reversibility of the signs and symptoms of hypercortisolism by bilateral adrenalectomy. Surgery 1993;114(6):1138–1143.
109. Nagesser SK, et al. Long-term results of total adrenalectomy for Cushing's disease. World J Surg 2000;24(1):108–113.
110. Nelson DH, et al. ACTH-producing tumor of the pituitary gland. N Engl J Med 1958;259:161–164.
111. Nelson DH, Meakin JW, Thorn GW. ACTH-producing pituitary tumors following adrenalectomy for Cushing's syndrome. Ann Intern Med 1960;52:560–569.
112. Rahn T, Thoren M, Werner S. Stereotactic radiosurgery in pituitary adenomas. In: *Pituitary Adenomas: New Trends in Basic and Clinical Research*. Faglia G, et al., eds. New York: Elsevier Science; 1991;303–312.
113. Ganz JC. Gamma knife treatment of pituitary adenomas. In: *Pituitary Adenomas*. Landolt AM, Vance ML, Reilly PL, eds. New York, NY: Churchill-Livingstone; 1996;461–474.
114. Izawa M, et al. Gamma knife radiosurgery for pituitary adenomas. J Neurosurg 2000;93 (suppl 3):19–22.
115. Hoybye C, et al. Adrenocorticotropic hormone-producing pituitary tumors: 12- to 22-year follow-up after treatment with stereotactic radiosurgery. Neurosurgery 2001;49(2):284–291;discussion 291–292.
116. Estrada J, et al. The long-term outcome of pituitary irradiation after unsuccessful transsphenoidal surgery in Cushing's disease. N Engl J Med 1997;336(3):172–177.

117. Littley MD, et al. Hypopituitarism following external radiotherapy for pituitary tumours in adults. Q J Med 1989;70(262):145–160.
118. Hughes MN, et al. Pituitary adenomas: long-term results for radiotherapy alone and post-operative radiotherapy. Int J Radiat Oncol Biol Phys 1993;27(5):1035–1043.
119. Snyder PJ, et al. Hypopituitarism following radiation therapy of pituitary adenomas. Am J Med 1986;81(3):457–462.
120. Halberg FE, Sheline GE. Radiotherapy of pituitary tumors. Endocrinol Metab Clin North Am 1987;16(3):667–684.
121. Engelhardt D, Weber MM. Therapy of Cushing's syndrome with steroid biosynthesis inhibitors. J Steroid Biochem Mol Biol 1994;49(4–6):261–267.
122. Miller JW, Crapo L. The medical treatment of Cushing's syndrome. Endocr Rev 1993;14(4):443–458.
123. Verhelst JA, et al. Short and long-term responses to metyrapone in the medical management of 91 patients with Cushing's syndrome. Clin Endocrinol (Oxf) 1991;35(2):169–178.
124. Krakoff J, et al. Use of a parenteral propylene glycol-containing etomidate preparation for the long-term management of ectopic Cushing's syndrome. J Clin Endocrinol Metab 2001;86(9):4104–4108.
125. Jenkins PJ, et al. The long-term outcome after adrenalectomy and prophylactic pituitary radiotherapy in adrenocorticotropin-dependent Cushing's syndrome. J Clin Endocrinol Metab 1995;80(1):165–171.
126. McCance DR, et al. Bilateral adrenalectomy: low mortality and morbidity in Cushing's disease. Clin Endocrinol (Oxf) 1993;39(3):315–321.
127. Bax TW, et al. Laparoscopic bilateral adrenalectomy following failed hypophysectomy. Surg Endosc 1996;10(12):1150–1153.
128. Doherty GM, et al. Time to recovery of the hypothalamic-pituitary-adrenal axis after curative resection of adrenal tumors in patients with Cushing's syndrome. Surgery 1990;108(6): 1085–1090.
129. Weinstein M, Tyrrell B, Newton TH. The sella turcica in Nelson's syndrome. Radiology 1976;118(2):363–365.
130. Kelly WF, et al. Cushing's disease treated by total adrenalectomy: long-term observations of 43 patients. Q J Med 1983;52(206):224–231.
131. Kasperlik-Zaluska AA, et al. Nelson's syndrome: incidence and prognosis. Clin Endocrinol (Oxf) 1983;19(6):693–698.
132. Cohen KL, Noth RH, Pechinski T. Incidence of pituitary tumors following adrenalectomy. A long-term follow-up study of patients treated for Cushing's disease. Arch Intern Med 1978;138(4):575–579.
133. Kemink SA, et al. Management of Nelson's syndrome: observations in fifteen patients. Clin Endocrinol (Oxf) 2001:54(1):45–52.
134. Kemink L, et al. Patient's age is a simple predictive factor for the development of Nelson's syndrome after total adrenalectomy for Cushing's disease. J Clin Endocrinol Metab 1994;79(3):887–889.
135. Thomas CG, Jr, et al. Nelson's syndrome after Cushing's disease in childhood: a continuing problem. Surgery 1984;96(6):1067–1077.
136. Moore TJ, et al. Nelson's syndrome: frequency, prognosis, and effect of prior pituitary irradiation. Ann Intern Med 1976;85(6):731–734.
137. Hamwi GJ, et al. Activation of testicular adrenal rest tissue by prolonged excessive ACTH production. J Clin Endocrinol Metab 1963;23:861–869.
138. Wislawski J, et al. Results of neurosurgical treatment by a transsphenoidal approach in 10 patients with Nelson's syndrome. J Neurosurg 1985;62(1):68–71.
139. Pivonello R., et al. Complete remission of Nelson's syndrome after 1-year treatment with cabergoline. J Endocrinol Invest 1999;22(11):860–865.

5 Nonfunctioning Pituitary Tumors

Mary H. Samuels, MD

Contents

DEFINITION

Pituitary adenomas are commonly divided into "functioning" tumors (those that secrete pituitary hormones and cause clinical syndromes) and "nonfunctioning" tumors (those that do not secrete a pituitary hormone that leads to a clinical syndrome) *(1)*. Tumors that do not secrete growth hormone (GH), adrenocorticotropic hormone (ACTH), prolactin, or thyroid-stimulating hormone (TSH) constitute the nonfunctioning pituitary tumors. Approximately 30% of pituitary adenomas are considered nonfunctioning by these criteria.

PATHOPHYSIOLOGY

Microscopic examination of clinically nonfunctioning tumors reveals a spectrum of structural differentiation, from those with well-developed endoplasmic reticulum and Golgi complexes to those with poorly developed cytoplasmic organelles. The latter are often classified as null cell tumors or oncocytomas. In most cases, electron microscopic studies of clinically silent tumors reveal the presence of small secretory granules, suggesting that at least a small amount of each of the several hormones is produced by these tumors *(2)*.

From: *Management of Pituitary Tumors: The Clinician's Practical Guide, Second Edition*
Edited by: M. P. Powell, S. L. Lightman, and E. R. Laws, Jr.

Further in-vivo and in-vitro studies of nonfunctioning pituitary adenomas reveal that most do produce pituitary hormones, in most cases one or more of the pituitary gonadotropins (follicle stimulating hormone [FSH] and luteinizing hormone [LH]) *(2-4)*. The most common hormone produced is FSH, with production of LH or the α-subunits of FSH and LH being less common. Production of these hormones from nonfunctioning pituitary tumors can sometimes be inferred by careful interpretation of basal serum hormone levels. For example, suppressed LH and elevated FSH levels in a patient with a known pituitary tumor indicates an FSH-secreting tumor, because almost all other causes of elevated FSH levels are accompanied by elevated LH levels. In other cases, measurement of the hormones during various stimulation tests reveals abnormal responses that indicate tumoral secretion of these hormones *(5)*. Pathologic analysis of nonfunctioning tumors often shows immunostaining for FSH β-subunit, LH β-subunit, and/or α-subunit, and *in situ* hybridization shows the presence of gonadotropin subunit mRNA species *(6,7)*. Finally, most nonfunctioning tumors produce intact gonadotropins and/or gonadotropin subunits when placed in cell culture *(6,8,9)*. Serum hormone levels, immunocytochemical staining intensity, mRNA levels, and hormone production in cell culture are not always well correlated in these tumors, illustrating the difficulty in preoperative diagnosis *(10)*.

There are several reasons why these tumors appear nonfunctioning, even though they usually make at least one of the pituitary hormones. The first reason is that FSH and LH excess, unlike the pituitary hormones listed in the first paragraph, do not usually cause any specific symptoms, although rare exceptions exist. For example, a small subgroup of men with FSH-secreting tumors may present with testicular enlargement caused by FSH-induced hypertrophy of the seminiferous tubules. As another example, men rarely have elevated testosterone levels attributable to LH secreting tumors. The second reason is that often only the α- or β-subunits of the hormone are produced, and the uncombined subunits are not active. The third reason is that the hormones are often only secreted into the blood in small amounts, and, therefore, blood levels are often normal.

CLINICAL PRESENTATION

By definition, nonfunctioning tumors do not have a clinical syndrome caused by hormone overproduction. Instead, nonfunctioning pituitary tumors present in patients with symptoms resulting from the size and location of the tumor, or symptoms of pituitary hormone deficiency, or a combination of these two effects *(1)*.

When diagnosed, most of these tumors are macroadenomas (>1 cm in diameter), because there is no syndrome of hormone excess to bring them to medical attention when they are smaller.

Symptoms Resulting from the Size and Location of the Tumor

Headache

Any pituitary adenoma (or any other tumor or disease affecting the pituitary region, for that matter) can cause headaches. The headaches may vary from mild to severe, and the severity is not always proportional to tumor size. The headaches are commonly retro-orbital but may be more generalized and can be mistaken for other types of headaches, such as tension or migraine headaches. Because these tumors usually grow slowly and can become quite large before they are discovered, the headaches are often present for many years. On the other hand, some patients with very large tumors are surprisingly free of headaches. Rarely, patients will have sudden onset of a severe headache or give a history of a severe headache that spontaneously resolved. Such a history raises the possibility of acute hemorrhage or infarction of the tumor.

Vision

Another common symptom caused by the size and location of the tumor is decreased vision. This usually presents as temporal visual field defects, although other visual field loss may also occur. It is caused by the tumor growing upward out of the sella and pressing on the optic chiasm. The decrease in peripheral vision may be quite extensive without the patient realizing it, because people tend to rely on central, rather than peripheral, vision for most daily activities. Other less common vision complaints include diplopia. This results from the tumor extending laterally into the cavernous sinus and compressing the cranial nerves controlling extraocular muscle function.

Symptoms of Normal Pituitary Hormone Loss

As nonfunctioning pituitary tumors grow, they compress the pituitary gland, pituitary stalk, and hypothalamus and interfere with normal pituitary hormone production. This can lead to partial or complete anterior pituitary hormone deficiency *(11)*.

The first hormone to become deficient is usually GH. Therefore, children with growing masses in the pituitary region usually have growth failure. Adults with GH deficiency do not have specific symptoms, although GH deficiency does have some nonspecific effects on energy and sense of well-being in adults (*see* Chapter 12).

The next hormones to become deficient are usually the gonadotropins. Prepubertal children have no effects from gonadotropin deficiency, but adults develop oligoamenorrhea, impotence, and/or infertility. Deficiencies of TSH, which leads to hypothyroidism, and ACTH, which leads to hypoadrenalism, are less common, even with large tumors. Deficiency of prolactin (PRL) is also uncommon and only presents in the postpartum period as a failure to lactate. Diabetes insipidus as a result of deficiency of the posterior pituitary hormone vasopressin (antidiuretic hormone [ADH]) is much less common, even with very large pituitary adenomas. The presence of diabetes insipidus should raise the suspicion that the lesion is not a pituitary adenoma.

The clinical presentation of a patient with hypopituitarism is nonspecific and thus may lead to confusion. Many of the symptoms of hypopituitarism are vague, and patients can be misdiagnosed with chronic fatigue or psychiatric illness before the true diagnosis is known. In addition, symptoms of one hormone deficiency may mask those of another hormone deficiency. For example, weight gain is expected with hypothyroidism and weight loss with hypoadrenalism. If a patient has both TSH and ACTH deficiencies, weight may be increased, decreased, or unchanged from baseline.

Finally, routine screening for individual hormones may not uncover pituitary hormone deficiency. For example, the recommended screening test for hypothyroidism is a TSH level, which is highly sensitive for primary hypothyroidism but useless in hypopituitarism. Patients with central hypothyroidism caused by a pituitary tumor may have low, normal, or even mildly elevated TSH levels. To diagnose central, rather than primary, hypothyroidism, a free T4 level must be interpreted in conjunction with suggestive symptoms.

One pituitary hormone that can be nonspecifically elevated by nonfunctioning tumors is PRL. It is not unusual to see mild to moderate hyperprolactinemia (up to 200 μg/dL or 4,000 mU/L) in patients with large nonfunctioning pituitary tumors or other pituitary-hypothalamic diseases. The source of the PRL is not the tumor, but normal lactotrophs that produce excess PRL when there is an interruption of hypothalamic input of dopamine, the PRL inhibitory factor. This can cause confusion or misdiagnosis if the tumor is mistakenly believed to be a prolactinoma. Prolactinomas are almost always treated medically with dopamine agonists, which are highly effective in lowering PRL levels, resolving symptoms, and reducing tumor size in prolac-tinoma patients (*see* Chapter 2).

Dopamine agonists will also lower PRL levels in patients with nonfunctioning tumors but do not treat the tumor mass itself. In that case, the tumor may continue to grow while the patient and care provider are falsely reassured by the lower PRL levels and sometimes even a return of a normal menstrual cycle. For this reason, PRL levels must be interpreted cautiously in patients with large tumors, and mild elevations in patients with large tumors are most consistent with a nonspecific PRL elevation, rather than a prolactinoma.

It should be noted that the symptoms listed for nonfunctioning pituitary adenomas are nonspecific. Any large mass or infiltrative process in the pituitary/hypothalamic region can produce identical symptoms of mass effect and/or hypopituitarism. Therefore, the differential diagnosis of these lesions includes craniopharyngiomas, meningiomas, gliomas, metastatic tumors, and other tumorous or infiltrative processes. In some cases, magnetic resonance imaging (MRI) characteristics or elevated serum gonadotropin levels can help with the differential diagnosis, but pathologic examination of tumor tissue may be needed for the final diagnosis.

CLINICAL EVALUATION

Imaging

Patients who are suspected of having a nonfunctioning pituitary adenoma should ideally have a high-resolution MRI study directed toward the pituitary gland. An MRI provides the best assessment of tumor size, location, extent, and relationship to important surrounding structures and is essential for the neurosurgeon to adequately plan surgery and to monitor treatment. A general brain MRI is often inadequate to image the pituitary region, and a specific pituitary MRI done with a magnet of adequate strength is optimal.

If an MRI is not available, a computed tomography (CT) study directed at the pituitary region may be done. Fine-cut reconstruction or coronal CT can give good enough image quality to make many clinical decisions.

Visual Assessment

If the tumor is seen on MRI to be abutting or distorting the optic chiasm, a formal assessment of vision should be done, to include visual field measurements (to assess damage to the optic chiasm) and careful inspection of the optic discs (*see* Chapter 6). Automated visual field measurements can also be helpful in the follow-up of these tumors, because they can be more sensitive to minor changes in tumor size than the MRI.

Endocrine Assessment

In addition to the tests performed to assess tumor anatomy, it is important that patients with pituitary tumors be evaluated for pituitary hormone status by an experienced endocrinologist, to overcome the difficulties in diagnosis discussed. The biochemical evaluation should to some extent depend on the patient's complaints, but the patient may have minimal symptoms even with significant hormone loss. For that reason, all patients with large tumors should have at least a basic evaluation for each of the pituitary hormones *(11,12)*. Preoperative evaluation should include the following (*see* Table 1):

1. PRL level. All patients with pituitary tumors in whom an operation is considered must have a preoperative PRL level. PRL deficiency is not an issue, because it is not treated, but elevated PRL levels are important to document. Markedly elevated PRL levels indicate the presence of a prolactinoma, which is important because in most cases it obviates the need for surgery.

Table 1
Suggested Preoperative Endocrine Evaluation of Pituitary Tumors

Hormone	*Preoperative Testing*	*Postoperative Testing*	*Comment*
Prolactin	PRL level	None	Rule out prolactinoma; PRL deficiency not routinely evaluated
Thyroid hormone	Free-T4 level	Free T4	TSH levels are not useful
Cortisol	Not routinely tested if no suggestive clinical findings and surgery planned	Low-dose ACTH stimulation test	Can cover with empiric low-dose glucocorticoids until surgery if clinically indicated; further evaluation occurs postoperatively
Gonadal hormones	FSH, LH, α-subunit, testosterone (men) or estradiol (women)	Testosterone (men); FSH, LH, α-subunit levels if preoperative levels elevated	Rule out gonadotropin secreting tumor; gonadal deficiency not routinely evaluated preoperatively
Growth hormone	IGF-1 level	GH stimulation testing if indicated	Rule out silent GH-secreting tumor; GH deficiency not routinely evaluated preoperatively
Antidiuretic hormone	Not routinely tested if no symptoms	Not routinely tested if no symptoms	Glucocorticoid deficiency can mask symptoms of diabetes insipidus

Prolactinomas are usually easily diagnosed with a basal PRL measurement. As discussed, mild hyperprolactinemia in the context of a large tumor does not indicate a prolactinoma. There is a rough direct correlation between tumor size and PRL level in prolactinomas, so the PRL level must be interpreted in relation to the tumor size.

2. Thyroid hormone levels. Each patient with a clinically nonfunctioning pituitary tumor should have a free-T4 level measured. A low free-T4 level indicates the need for L-thyroxine replacement therapy. The goal of therapy is a midnormal free-T4 level. As mentioned, it is not helpful to follow TSH levels. Free T4 should be measured before surgery to provide necessary L-thyroxine replacement before the induction of general anesthesia, because hypothyroid patients may have problems with clearance of anesthetic agents and other postoperative complications. If possible, surgery should be delayed for at least 1 wk. In dire

emergency, rapid thyroid replacement can be achieved with triiodothyronine, but this can involve cardiac dangers.

3. Adrenal axis evaluation. In general, if the patient does not have symptoms of hypoadrenalism, and surgery is planned in the near future, there is no need to routinely evaluate the adrenal axis preoperatively, because evaluation of the adrenal axis is more complicated than the other pituitary axes.

   In addition, it is our practice that all patients receive perioperative coverage with glucocorticoids, and the adrenal axis is evaluated after surgery in any case. This, however, is not the case in all centers (*see* Chapter 11). If patients have suggestive symptoms or a low cortisol level, it is appropriate to place them on a replacement dose of hydrocortisone until surgery. This low dose protects them from adrenal insufficiency without causing side effects related to overtreatment.

   We do not routinely evaluate patients with large clinically nonfunctioning tumors for ACTH excess. Although there are reports of "silent" ACTH-secreting tumors, macroadenomas making ACTH are quite rare. This is a histologic diagnosis, and such patients need surgery and postoperative reevaluation regardless of the presence of ACTH secretion.

4. Gonadal hormones. We measure FSH, LH, α-subunit, and testosterone (in men) or estradiol (in women) routinely, although this is not the rule in all centers. Our goal is not to evaluate the patient for hypogonadism, because this will need to be addressed postoperatively. However, based on the discussion under "Pathophysiology" earlier, many nonfunctioning tumors make one or more of the gonadotropins, and preoperative elevated levels can provide a tumor marker for postoperative monitoring.

5. Growth hormone. Adults do not need an evaluation for GH deficiency before surgery. However, it is sensible to routinely measure the insulin-like growth factor 1 (IGF-1) level in all patients with large nonfunctioning pituitary tumors. IGF-1 is a good screening test for GH excess, and there are a few reports of silent GH-secreting tumors *(13)*. Such tumors make GH but do not present clinically as acromegaly. They still require surgery for the tumor mass, but it is helpful to know that the tumor is making GH, because medical therapies are available postoperatively for GH-secreting tumors. Children with large pituitary tumors are often evaluated for growth failure as their presenting symptom of the pituitary tumor.

6. ADH. Patients are not routinely evaluated preoperatively for ADH deficiency, because it is rare in patients with nonfunctioning tumors and should present with polyuria, polydipsia, and nocturia. Therefore, if a patient does not have those symptoms, one can wait until after the surgery to evaluate the patient's ADH status. If a patient does have symptoms, treatment is not needed unless the polyuria and nocturia are severe or unless the patient has trouble with access to water. Note that ADH deficiency symptoms may be masked by adrenal insufficiency, and treatment of such patients with glucocorticoids may lead to the first appearance of symptomatic diabetes insipidus.

TREATMENT

There are four treatment options for nonfunctioning pituitary tumors: observation, neurosurgery, radiation therapy, and medical therapy. These options are described in detail in Chapters 8 and 13 and will be briefly summarized here.

Observation

Observation without specific treatment is sometimes appropriate for patients with nonfunctioning pituitary tumors, but this decision must be made carefully, and the patient must be closely followed. Observation is most appropriate for smaller tumors that do not threaten vision or cause headaches or other symptoms. Such tumors are often found incidentally when MRIs or CTs are performed for unrelated reasons *(12)*. Most of these tumors grow slowly and can safely be monitored with serial MRIs. In fact, a recent cost-effectiveness analysis suggests that a single PRL level, without repeated MRIs, may be appropriate for incidentally discovered microadenomas *(14)*. Observation may also be appropriate in older patients with large tumors who have other serious medical problems and do not have a long life expectancy, because the slow-growing tumor may not cause any problems in the patient's lifetime. In most cases, however, large tumors should be treated.

Surgery

In almost all cases, neurosurgery is the initial treatment of choice for nonfunctioning pituitary tumors. The surgery is usually performed via the transsphenoidal route, which avoids a craniotomy. The goal in most cases of large tumors is to debulk the tumor, rather than to completely remove it. In the case of smaller tumors, complete cure is a reasonable goal.

The single most important factor in achieving optimal surgical results with large pituitary tumors (good debulking, few or no side effects, no damage to the normal pituitary gland and other structures) is an experienced surgeon with a good track record. Transsphenoidal surgery is best done by surgeons who perform many such operations every year and have documented good results with low complication rates.

Surgical success rates and complication rates are critically dependent on tumor size *(1,15;* and *see* Chapter 8*)*. In the most experienced centers, initial gross total tumor resection for nonfunctioning tumors is as high as 90%, although these numbers probably underestimate the presence of residual tumor. Improvement in vision and/or visual field defects are seen in 60% to >80% of patients in published surgical series. However, worsening of vision can also be seen in 3% to 11% of these patients.

Recurrence rates after surgery without irradiation for nonfunctioning pituitary tumors is reported to be between 10% and 75%, usually after many months or years of follow-up. However, these data include many studies that used cranial, rather than transsphenoidal, surgery and included tumors of heterogeneous size, invasiveness, and completeness of resection. In one study of patients who had apparently complete transsphenoidal resection without evidence of tumor invasion or rapid growth, the recurrence rate without irradiation was 10% *(16)*. These data suggest that many patients with nonaggressive tumors can be followed after complete resection without adjuvant therapy. New surgical techniques, such as endoscopic surgery, hold promise for improved cure rates with fewer complications and are currently under study (*see* Chapter 10).

Radiation Therapy

Pituitary tumors are rarely treated primarily with external beam radiotherapy, because radiation takes many years to work, is not extremely effective in controlling size, and usually leads to pituitary hormone deficiencies. However, in some cases, primary radiation therapy may be considered for these tumors. More commonly, radiation therapy is used as an adjuvant treatment after surgery to prevent tumor regrowth *(16)*. Conventional radiation therapy is administered to the tumor area via a linear accelerator through multiple ports to deliver 45 Gy throughout 5-6 wk (*see* Chapter 13). With this technique, there is a slow and variable tumor response in terms of stabilization or decrease in tumor size. Published reports indicate a 3% to 26% tumor recurrence rate with postoperative radiotherapy *(16)*. However, these studies include heterogenous patient groups, radiation doses, and tumor characteristics, and it is difficult to extrapolate these results to individual patients. There is also a high incidence of the eventual development of hypopituitarism, anecdotal evidence of adverse neuropsychologic effects, and case reports of second brain tumors or other central nervous system complications after conventional radiotherapy *(16,17)*.

More recently, stereotactic radiosurgery has been used in pituitary tumors to circumvent some of these problems *(18-20)*. This uses a high dose of ionizing radiation delivered in a precisely defined, tightly concentrated field with a steep fall-off and little radiation to surrounding tissue. Details of this technique are described in Chapter 14. To date, there are limited data regarding efficacy and side effects of stereotactic radiosurgery applied to nonfunctioning pituitary adenomas. The procedure is effective in stabilizing tumor size in most patients, with frequent reports of actual tumor shrinkage. Rates of development of hypopituitarism were initially stated to be low, but further follow-up of treated patients has revealed increasing rates of hypopituitarism with time. It should be noted that hypopituitarism occurs more quickly with stereotactic radiosurgery compared with conventional radiotherapy, and these patients must be followed closely for this side effect.

Because many nonfunctioning pituitary tumors are large and cannot be completely removed by surgery, the question of postoperative radiation therapy often arises. In many cases, the tumor has been sufficiently debulked and can be monitored without further treatment, even with known residual tumor present. In these cases, MRI scans can be recommended to be performed 6 mo after surgery and then repeated on an annual basis or according to similar protocols. If the tumor shows signs of regrowth, repeat surgery or radiation therapy can be considered. This decision is based on patient characteristics, as well as the size, location, and expected aggressiveness of the residual tumor.

Medical Therapy

Medical therapy has become important for the treatment of some functioning pituitary tumors, primarily PRL and GH-secreting tumors. Unfortunately, despite several clinical studies, no clearly effective medical therapy for nonfunctioning pituitary tumors has emerged. The following therapies have been evaluated *(2,15)*.

Dopamine Agonist Therapy

The presence of dopamine receptors has been established in clinically nonfunctioning and gonadotropin tumors, and administration of dopamine agonists can lead to decreases in serum levels of gonadotropins. Based on these findings, several patients with such tumors have been given bromocriptine or other dopamine agonists *(21-23)*. Results of long-term therapy of these tumors with dopamine agonists have been variable. There are case reports of improvements in visual fields and/or tumor shrinkage with dopaminergic agents administered for 6 wk to 7 yr, although reduction of tumor size was quite variable (0% to 50%). In addition, these patients often required high doses of dopamine agonists, which are difficult to tolerate. Based on these data, dopamine agonists can be tried in unusual cases when other treatment options have failed or are refused.

Somatostatin Analog Therapy

Somatostatin regulates gonadotropin and subunit secretion in healthy subjects and in many disease states. Many endocrine tumors, including nonfunctioning and gonadotropin adenomas, contain somatostatin receptors. In-vitro incubation of gonadotropin adenomas with somatostatin or its analogs suppresses gonadotropin or subunit secretion in up to two thirds of tumors, although this is variable. Somatostatin analogs also appear to inhibit cell growth of nonfunctioning tumors in vitro.

To date, several reports have been published regarding octreotide therapy of patients with clinically nonfunctioning, gonadotropin, or α-subunit tumors *(24,25)*. These studies have shown heterogeneous clinical and biochemical responses, with individual reports of decreased serum gonadotropin levels, improved visual fields, and/or decreased tumor size. Visual improvements have been reported to be more common than reduction in tumor size, suggesting an independent effect on the visual pathway. Based on these findings, octreotide, like dopamine agonists, may be tried in select patients with refractory tumors. Whether to use octreotide or dopamine agonists as adjuvant therapy is unclear; acute responses to dopamine or somatostatin infusions do not necessarily predict chronic effects of these agents. One study suggests that combination therapy with octreotide and a dopamine agonist may be effective, but this study included only 10 patients who were followed for 6 mo *(26)*.

GnRH Analog Therapy

Recently, long-acting gonadotropin-releasing hormone (GnRH) analogs have been developed to treat many sex-steroid-dependent conditions. In normal subjects, these drugs initially act as GnRH agonists by binding to GnRH receptors, but eventually cause GnRH-receptor downregulation, with decreases in gonadotropin secretion and bioactivity. Subsets of nonfunctioning pituitary tumors contain GnRH receptors at levels comparable to those in normal human pituitaries. These findings form the basis of attempts to treat gonadotroph adenomas with GnRH agonists.

A small number of patients with gonadotropin tumors have been given GnRH agonists to reduce tumorous hormone secretion and tumor size after surgical resection *(27-31)*. GnRH agonists were given at various doses for periods of time ranging between 3 wk and 3 mo. A few patients had decreases in serum FSH and LH levels during treatment, but most had increased gonadotropin subunit levels. Cell culture studies confirm these clinical findings, showing persistent stimulation of gonadotropin secretion in adenomatous cells during continuous GnRH exposure. The mechanism for this chronic agonist effect is unknown, but may indicate that GnRH agonists are not effective in downregulating GnRH receptors on adenomatous tissue. In any case, these drugs are usually not effective in treating gonadotropin tumors and may be deleterious.

More promising are the GnRH antagonists, which do not have an initial agonist effect in normal subjects. To date, one study has reported results of 3-12 mo of GnRH antagonist treatment of five men with FSH secreting tumors *(32)*. All five had normalization of serum FSH levels, but α-subunit levels were not reported. None of the patients had any change in pituitary volume, and one had worsening visual fields. These preliminary data suggest that GnRH antagonists may be useful as adjuvant therapy for persistent or recurrent gonadotropin tumors but do not support their use to control tumor size. However, more extensive long-term studies are clearly necessary to adequately assess the role of these new agents in gonadotropin adenomas.

Post-Therapy Evaluation and Treatment of Hormone Deficiencies

Imaging

After surgery for nonfunctioning pituitary adenomas, patients should be followed for recurrence or incomplete resection with MRI scanning. We recom-

Table 2
Suggested Postoperative Treatment and Monitoring of Patients with Nonfunctioning Pituitary Tumors

Hormone	*Replacement Therapy*	*Monitoring*
Prolactin	None	None
Thyroid hormone	L-thyroxine	Check free T4 every 6-8 wk until mid-normal free-T4 level achieved; then check free T4 yearly (TSH not useful)
Cortisol	Hydrocortisone or equivalent	Biochemical testing not helpful for dose adjustment; avoid long-acting glucocorticoids
Gonadal hormones	Estrogen/progestin (premenopausal women); testosterone (men)	Safety monitoring on a yearly basis
Growth hormone	GH	IGF-1 levels; ? Measures of body composition
Antidiuretic hormone	dDAVP	Clinical; Na levels

mend postponing the first postoperative MRI until 4-6 mo after surgery, since earlier MRI does not adequately assess the extent of tumor resection *(33)*. After a postoperative baseline has been established, MRI can be repeated every year for 3-5 years, and then less frequently if the tumor size is stable.

Endocrinology

Patients should also have a thorough endocrine evaluation, with treatment of any hormone deficiencies. This includes patients who were diagnosed with preoperative hormone deficiencies, because they can sometimes be reversed by the surgery *(34,35)*. Our recommended evaluation is similar to that discussed earlier under "Endocrine Assessment" for preoperative patients, with a few exceptions (*see* Table 1). In patients who have postoperative pituitary hormone deficiencies, recommended endocrine treatment and monitoring strategies are listed in Table 2.

Prolactin

No postoperative testing for PRL is needed in patients who do not have prolactinomas.

Thyroid Hormones

A free-T4 level should be measured at least 6 wk after surgery, and L-thyroxine therapy started if the free-T4 level is low. The goal of L-thyroxine therapy is a mid-normal free-T4 level, and TSH levels are not helpful. Measuring free-T4 levels before 6 wk postoperatively is not helpful, because insufficient time has elapsed to assess the thyroid axis. Thyrotropin-releasing hormone (TRH) stimulation tests are not indicated. If L-thyroxine is started, repeated free-T4 levels should be measured every 6-8 wk until a mid-normal level is achieved. After this, the free-T4 level should be repeated yearly for a stable patient.

Adrenal Axis

Patients are usually sent home after pituitary surgery on replacement doses of hydrocortisone (15-30 mg/d according to protocol) or its equivalent to prevent symptomatic hypoadrenalism in case of pituitary damage. Higher doses or longer acting glucocorticoids are inappropriate, because they will lead to adrenal suppression.

Six weeks after surgery, patients should be instructed to withold their hydrocortisone dose on the day of testing, and a short ACTH stimulation test should be performed. Waiting 6 wk means that the adrenal glands will atrophy if there is ACTH deficiency, and an ACTH stimulation test will show a blunted cortisol response. In the past, high-dose ACTH (250 μg) was used in this test, but recent publications suggest that low-dose (1 μg) tests are more accurate in diagnosing ACTH deficiency *(36)*. A cortisol response of <18 μg/dL (500 nmol/L) 30 or 60 min after injection of 1 μg of ACTH is consistent with ACTH deficiency, and the patient needs hydrocortisone replacement therapy. We tailor the amount of hydrocortisone to the patient's size and degree of ACTH deficiency. Smaller patients and those with mildly blunted ACTH stimulation tests do not always need traditional full dose (15-30 mg/d) hydrocortisone replacement.

Once a patient has been started on hydrocortisone, blood or urine tests are not particularly helpful in assessing dose adequacy, and clinical judgment is key to adjusting hydrocortisone doses to avoid symptoms of hypoadrenalism or exogenous Cushing's syndrome.

Gonadal Hormones

Postoperatively, loss of menses in a premenopausal woman is diagnostic of hypogonadism, and no further biochemical evaluation is needed. Young hypogonadal women require estrogen replacement therapy (oral contraceptives or equivalent therapy) to maintain well-being and bone mass.

Postmenopausal women with pituitary adenomas do not need an evaluation for gonadal deficiency, and decisions regarding estrogen replacement therapy are independent of the presence of tumor.

Men should have a testosterone level measured 6 wk after surgery. If the testosterone level is low, testosterone therapy should be initiated to maintain sexual function, body composition, and bone mass. There are four ways to administer testosterone therapy to hypogonadal men: (1) intramuscular injections every 2–3 wk, (2) daily transdermal patch, (3) daily testosterone gel, and

(4) in Europe some patients are given 2 or 3 200-mg pellets inserted subcutaneously every 3–6 mo. Each delivery system has advantages and disadvantages, and the type of testosterone therapy should be individualized for each patient.

Once a patient is taking testosterone, yearly monitoring should be done for blood pressure, hemoglobin levels, lipid levels, and prostate disease, but testosterone levels do not need to be measured unless there is a clinical problem with efficacy. In the past, GnRH tests were used to evaluate patients with pituitary tumors and suspected gonadotropin deficiency, but this test does not add any useful information to the clinical evaluation and basal serum hormone levels.

In younger patients with pituitary tumors who desire fertility, hypogonadism is a more serious problem, because fertility is more difficult to achieve than sex steroid replacement. When fertility is required, such patients will need injections of exogenous gonadotropins, which have varied success in inducing fertility. A careful discussion should occur preoperatively with patients who desire future fertility to determine the extent of surgery and to review the options for preoperative sperm retrieval and storage.

Growth Hormone

Until recently, adults with pituitary tumors were not evaluated for GH deficiency. However, numerous reports now provide convincing evidence that adults with GH deficiency have health consequences owing to lack of GH, including decreased well-being, changes in body composition and strength, adverse effects on lipids, and bone loss *(37,38;* and *see* Chapter 12*)*. For that reason, many patients are now evaluated and treated for GH deficiency. However, the long-term consequences of treating patients with GH, sometimes for decades, are not known. For that reason, we individualize the decision to evaluate for GH deficiency after careful discussion with the patient.

Once the decision is made to evaluate the patient's GH axis, a stimulation test must be done, because basal GH or IGF-1 levels are not usually diagnostic. The most sensitive stimulation test for GH deficiency is an insulin tolerance test, in which subjects are rendered hypoglycemic with an insulin injection and the GH response is measured. However, this is a cumbersome test and is not recommended in older patients or those with cardiac disease or seizures. There is no consensus as to an acceptable alternative test, although a recent direct comparison of five commonly used tests (including the insulin tolerance test) suggests that a combination of arginine and growth hormone-releasing hormone (GHRH) provides the greatest reliability *(38,39)*.

If a patient elects to begin GH therapy, the initial dose should be low to avoid side effects that are common when starting GH. The dose is then gradually increased based on IGF-1 levels, so as to reach a mid- to high-normal level for the patient's age. The optimal monitoring tests for a patient on GH are not standardized but can include measures of body composition, lipids, and bone density in addition to the IGF-1 levels.

Antidiuretic Hormone

Some patients will develop diabetes insipidus within a few days of surgery resulting from surgical damage and will require either temporary or permanent therapy with 1-deamino-D-arginine vasopression (dDAVP, a V2-receptor-selective vasopression agonist).

In most cases, these patients have significant polyuria, polydipsia, and hypernatremia if they are denied access to free water. Aside from these patients, who are, fortunately, uncommon in expert surgical centers, we do not routinely evaluate or treat patients for diabetes insipidus (*see* Chaper 12).

If a patient complains of polyuria or significant nocturia after surgery, we usually begin with a simple 24-h urine collection for volume. If the 24-h volume is normal or high-normal, we do not pursue the evaluation. If the volume is high, the patient may need a water deprivation test to prove the presence of diabetes insipidus. Patients who do require dDAVP can be monitored clinically and with occasional serum sodium measurements.

CONCLUSION

In summary, we see a patient 6 wk after pituitary surgery and perform a clinical evaluation. At that time, we measure free-T4 and testosterone level (in men) and perform a low-dose ACTH stimulation test for cortisol levels. We replace any of these deficient hormones and recheck levels as appropriate for the individual hormone. If a patient decides that GH therapy is an option, a GH stimulation test is performed on a separate visit once the other hormones are adequately replaced.

If a patient has had pituitary surgery but no other treatment directed at the tumor, the postoperative evaluation listed in the previous paragraph only needs to be done once, unless the tumor regrows and new symptoms develop. However, patients who undergo radiation therapy require repeated monitoring for pituitary hormone deficiencies that can develop years after radiation (*see* Chapter 12). In published studies, partial or complete hypopituitarism occurred in up to 85% of patients within 10 yr of conventional radiation therapy *(40,41)*. In patients who have received radiation therapy, the evaluation summarized in the preceding paragraph is repeated yearly.

Most patients with clinically nonfunctioning pituitary tumors have large tumors and symptoms related to mass and/or pituitary hormone deficiencies. In most cases, initial treatment is surgical, with adjuvant radiotherapy or medical therapy prescribed on an individual basis. Careful hormonal follow-up of patients is needed to accurately diagnose and treat hormone deficiencies attributable to the tumor or its treatment.

REFERENCES

1. Aron DC, Tyrrell JB, Wilson CB. Pituitary tumors - current concepts in diagnosis and management. West J Med 1995;162:340-352.
2. Katznelson L, Alexander JM, Klibanski A. Clinical Review 45: Clinically nonfunctioning pituitary adenomas. J Clin Endocrinol Metab 1993;76:1089–1094.
3. Young WF, Scheithauer BW, Kovacs KT, Horvath E, David DH, Randall RV. Gonadotroph adenoma of the pituitary gland: a clinicopathologic analysis of 100 cases. Mayo Clin Proc 1996;71:649–656.
4. Ho DM, Hsu CY, Ting LT, Chiang H. The cliniopathological characteristics of gonadotroph cell adenoma: a study of 118 cases. Hum Pathol 1997;28:905–911.
5. Snyder PJ. Gonadotroph cell adenomas of the pituitary. Endocr Rev 1985;6:552–563.
6. Katznelson L, Alexander JM, Bikkal HA, Jameson JL, Hsu DW, Klibanski A. Imbalanced follicle-stimulating hormone β-subunit hormone biosynthesis in human pituitary adenomas. J Clin Endocrinol Metab 1992;74:1343–1351.
7. Jameson JL, Klibanski A, Black PM, et al. Glycoprotein hormone genes are expressed in clinically nonfunctioning pituitary adenomas. J Clin Invest 1987;80:1472–1478.
8. Snyder PJ, Bashey HM, Phillips JL, Gennarelli TA. Comparison of hormonal secretory behavior of gonadotroph cell adenomas in vivo and in culture. J Clin Endocrinol Metab 1985;61:1061–1065.
9. Asa SL, Cheng Z, Ramyar L, et al. Human pituitary null cell adenomas and oncocytomas in vitro: effects of adenohypophysiotropic hormones and gonadal steroids on hormone secretion and tumor cell morphology. J Clin Endocrinol Metab 1992;74:1128–1134.
10. Samuels MH, Henry P, Kleinschmidt-DeMasters BK, Lillehei K, Ridgway EC. Pulsatile glycoprotein hormone secretion in glycoprotein-producing pituitary tumors. J Clin Endocrinol Metab 1991;73:1281–1288.
11. Vance ML. Hypopituitarism. N Engl J Med 1994;330:1651–1662.
12. Molitch ME, Russell EJ. The pituitary "incidentaloma." Ann Int Med 1990;112:925–931.
13. Yamada S, Sano T, Stefaneanu L, et al. Endocrine and morphological study of a clinically silent somatotroph adenoma of the human pituitary. J Clin Endocrinol Metab 1993;76: 352–356.
14. King JT, Justice AC, Aron DC. Management of incidental pituitary microadenomas: a cost-effectiveness analysis. J Clin Endocrinol Metab 1997;82:3625–3632.
15. Lamberts SWJ, deHerder WW, van der Lely AJ, Hofland LJ. Imaging and medical management of clinically nonfunctioning pituitary tumors. Endocrinologist 1995;5:448–450.
16. Hansen LK, Molitch ME. Postoperative radiotherapy for clinically nonfunctioning pituitary adenomas. The Endocrinologist 1998;8:71–78.
17. Guinan EM, Lowy C, Stanhope N, Lewis PD, Kepelman MD. Cognitive effects of pituitary tumours and their treatments: two case studies and an investigation of 90 patients. J Neurol Neurosurg Psychiatry 1998;65:870–876.
18. Mitsumori M, Shrieve DC, Alexander E, et al. Initial clinical results of LINAC-based stereotactic radiosurgery and stereotactic radiotherapy for pituitary adenomas. Int J Radiat Oncol Biol Phys 1998;42:573–580.
19. Laws ER, Vance ML. Radiosurgery for pituitary tumors and craniopharyngiomas. Neurosurg Clin North Am 1999;10:327–336.
20. Izawa M, Hayashi M, Nakaya K, et al. Gamma knife radiosurgery for pituitary adenomas. J Neurosurg 2000;93 (Suppl 3):19–22.
21. Colao A, Ferone D, Lastoria S, et al. Hormone levels and tumour size response to quinagolide and cabergoline in patients with prolactin-secreting and clinically nonfunctioning pituitary adenomas: predictive value of pituitary scintigraphy with ^{123}I-methoxybenzamide. Clin Endocrinol 2000;52:437–445.

22. Giusti M, Bocca L, Glorio T, et al. Cabergoline modulation of α-subunit and FSH secretion in a gonadotroph adenoma. J Endocrinol Invest 2000;23:463–466.
23. Nobels FR, de Herder WW, van den Brink WM, et al. Long-term treatment with the dopamine agonist quinagolide of patients with clinically nonfunctioning pituitary adenoma. Eur J Endocrinol 2000;143:615–621.
24. Plockinger U, Reichel M, Fett U, Seager W, Quabbe HJ. Preoperative octreotide treatment of growth hormone-secreting and clinically nonfunctioning pituitary macroadenomas: effect on tumor volume and lack of correlation with immunohistochemistry and somatostatin receptor scintigraphy. J Clin Endocrinol Metab 1994;79:1416–1423.
25. Warnet A, Harris AG, Renard E, Martin D, James-Deidier A, Chaumet-Riffaud P. A prospective multicenter trial of octreotide in 24 patients with visual defects caused by nonfunctioning and gonadotropin-secreting pituitary adenomas. Neurosurgery 1997;41:786–795.
26. Andersen M, Bjerre P, Schroder HD, et al. In vivo secretory potential and the effect of combination therapy with octreotide and cabergoline in patients with clinically nonfunctioning pituitary adenomas. Clin Endocrinol 2001;54:23–30.
27. Roman SH, Goldstein M, Kourides IA, et al. The luteinizing hormone-releasing hormone (LHRH) agonist (D-trp^6-pro^9-NEt) LHRH increased rather than lowered LH and α-subunit levels in a patient with an LH-secreting pituitary tumor. J Clin Endocrinol Metab 1984;58: 313–319.
28. Sassolas G, LeJeune H, Trouillas J, et al. Gonadotropin-releasing hormone agonists are unsuccessful in reducing tumoral gonadotropin secretion in two patients with gonadotropin-secreting pituitary adenomas. J Clin Endocrinol Metab 1988;67:180–185.
29. Zarate A, Fonseca ME, Mason M, et al. Gonadotropin-secreting pituitary adenoma with concomitant hypersecretion of testosterone and elevated sperm count. Treatment with LRH agonist. Acta Endocrinol 1986;113:29–34.
30. Chapman AJ, MacFarlane IA, Shalet SM, et al. Discordant serum α-subunit and FSH concentrations in a woman with a pituitary tumor. Clin Endocrinol 1984;21:123–129.
31. Klibanski A, Jameson JL, Biller BMK, et al. Gonadotropin and α-subunit responses to chronic LHRH analogue administration in patients with pituitary tumors. J Clin Endocrinol Metab 1989;68:81–86.
32. McGrath GA, Goncalves RJ, Udupa JK, et al. New technique for quantitation of pituitary adenoma size: use in evaluating treatment of gonadotroph adenomas with a gonadotropin-releasing hormone antagonist. J Clin Endocrinol Metab 1993;76:1363–1368.
33. Rodriguez O, Mateos B, de la Pedraja R, et al. Postoperative follow-up of pituitary adenomas after transsphenoidal resection: MRI and clinical correlation. Neuroradiology 1996;38: 747–754.
34. Arafah BM. Reversible hypopituitarism in patients with large nonfunctioning pituitary adenomas. J Clin Endocrinol Metab 1986;62:1173–1179.
35. Webb SM, Rigla M, Wagner A, Oliver B, Bartumeus F. Recovery of hypopituitarism after neurosurgical treatment of pituitary adenomas. J Clin Endocrinol Metab 1999;84: 3696–3700.
36. Abdu TA, Elhadd TA, Neary R, Clayton RN. Comparison of the low dose short synacthen test (1 microg), the conventional dose short synacthen test (250 microg) and the insulin tolerance test for assessment of the hypothalamo-pituitary-adrenal axis in patients with pituitary disease. J Clin Endocrinol Metab 1999;84:838–843.
37. Vance ML, Mauras N. Growth hormone therapy in adults and children. N Engl J Med 1999;341:1206–1216.
38. Ho KK. Diagnosis and management of adult growth hormone deficiency. Endocrine 2000;12:189–196.
39. Biller BMK, Samuels MH, Zagar A, et al. Sensitivity and specificity of six tests for the diagnosis of adult GH deficiency. J Clin Endocrinol Metab 2002;87:2067–2079.

40. Snyder PJ, Fowble BF, Schatz NJ, Savino PJ, Gennarelli TA. Hypopituitarism following radiation therapy of pituitary adenomas. Am J Med 1986;81:457–462.
41. Tominaga A, Uozumi T, Arita K, Kurisu K, Yano T, Hirohata T. Anterior pituitary function in patients with nonfunctioning pituitary adenoma: results of longitudinal follow-up. Endocr J 1995;42:421–427.

6 Visual Manifestations of Pituitary Tumors

Ian MacDonald, BMedSc, MB, ChB, PhD, FRCAP, FRCP, FRCOphth,
and Michael P. Powell, MB, BS, FRCS

CONTENTS

INTRODUCTION

Visual loss is the mode of presentation in approx one third of patients, and thus one of the most common ways in which pituitary tumors are discovered, and some understanding of the signs of chiasmatic compression are known to most reasonably alert medical students from their early neuroanatomy studies! A clearer understanding of the ways in which the visual system is affected by tumors arising from the sella is important for two reasons. First, all pituitary tumors—functional, nonfunctional and nonadenomatous—can affect the eyesight once they extend outside the fossa, either upward, as is more common, or sideways. Secondly, detection of asymptomatic involvement of the visual pathways can provide important evidence about the extent of pituitary tumors presenting in other ways and improve outcome by timely intervention.

From: *Management of Pituitary Tumors: The Clinician's Practical Guide, Second Edition*
Edited by: M. P. Powell, S. L. Lightman, and E. R. Laws, Jr. © Humana Press Inc., Totowa, NJ

Because many patients are first seen with the symptoms attributable to damage of the afferent visual system, an approach to the patient with visual failure is considered first. Individual manifestations will be considered in detail after this.

APPROACH TO THE PATIENT WITH VISUAL FAILURE

Two questions must be answered when a patient with visual failure is seen: Where is the lesion? and What is its pathologic nature? Clinical answers to the second question come mainly from the patient's history, and the physical examination should answer the first question.

The first step, then, is the detailed history of the mode of onset and evolution of the symptoms. The second step is then to search for evidence to localize the lesion, involving one or both eyes, and to establish a baseline for monitoring progression of the disease and the treatment effects. The second step involves the rigorous examination of the first six cranial nerves, followed by the remainder of the standard neurologic examination to detect spread of the tumor beyond the sella region.

The final stage of the neurologic assessment involves selecting appropriate investigations to confirm clinical localization and diagnosis, to provide more evidence about the pathologic nature of the compressing lesion, and to plan treatment. Magnetic resonance imaging (MRI) and, to a lesser extent, computed X-ray tomography (CT) provide invaluable and sometimes complementary evidence. MRI usually with and without gadolinium-DPTA (diethylenetriaminepenta acetic acid) enhancement, is the method of choice for delineating the extent of the lesion and its relationship to neural structures. CT gives information about bone involvement and calcification, which may be difficult to interpret on MRI. The presence of calcification is important to differential diagnosis, because it is common in craniopharyngiomas, occasionally seen in meningiomata, and only rarely seen in pituitary adenomas. MRI should be the first imaging investigation whenever possible, and other imaging is seldom required. Plain-skull X-rays and cerebral angiography are now virtually never required. Postoperatively, MRI is the clear imaging choice for following progress.

Other physiologic examinations, such as visual evoked potentials with half-field stimulation, had a brief place in the investigative armamentarium, but imaging techniques have advanced to such an extent that their place in now questionable.

VISUAL SYMPTOMATOLOGY

Symptoms Attributable to Optic Nerve Fiber Damage

Visual loss is a common mode of presentation. Although it can be assumed that the majority of tumors that present this way are nonfunctioning adenomas, all adenomas, particularly prolactinomas in men, frequently giant somatotrophs and rarely, Cushing's tumors and thyrotrophs can present with visual loss. A common symptom of chiasmal compression is the patent's tendency to bump into objects on the side of the temporal field loss, either unilaterally or bilaterally. When central vision is affected early, usually through direct compression of the optic nerve particularly where there is a þost- fixed' chiasm, patients complain of blurred vision often with scotomatous central field loss. On occasion, severe visual loss is discovered in one eye when the "good" eye is covered, leading to a false report of sudden visual loss. That the loss has been more gradual is usually suggested by the presence of optic atrophy, which takes a month or more to develop.

It is noteworthy that patients do not complain that the abnormal visual field is black but rather that it is blank: they are unaware of visual stimuli. A positive complaint of blackness is more likely to accompany retinal disease and not lesions of the optic nerve fibers at any level.

Several unusual symptoms may be encountered as a consequence of bitemporal hemianopias. Postfixational blindness occurs when there is a bitemporal field defect that precisely splits the middle of the field *(1,2)*. In these circumstances, when a patient converges on a relatively close object, more distant objects fall into the blind hemifields behind the object of attention and therefore are not seen. Symptomatically this is manifested, for instance, by difficulty in cutting finger nails—focusing on the scissors results in disappearance of the nails—or occasionally in driving when focusing on near objects, such as the driving instruments, causes important distant objects, such as traffic lights or pedestrians, to disappear.

The presence of postfixational blindness is readily demonstrated by confrontation. The patient is asked to focus on one of two objects held 30 cm from the face. The other object is then moved toward the examiner. When it enters the blind fields, the patient no longer sees it.

A second group of symptoms derives from the phenomenon of retinal slip. The relationship between the fields contributed by each eye is normally preserved by a neurophysiologic mechanism that depends on the stimulation of corresponding points in the homonymous hemifields. With a bitemporal field loss this is impossible. The patient's visual perception depends on the function of two nasal fields that are not locked together. Slippage can thus occur. In the vertical plane, the slippage results in a tendency when reading to drop to the next lower line. In the horizontal plane, slippage can result in words either running into each other or expanding: door may become *dor* or *dooor*. Slippage can have most unfortunate consequences, as when a patient who was a bank clerk was reprimanded for making errors on several orders of magnitude because he lost or added several zeros to clients' balance sheets without being aware of what was happening.

Unusually, an abnormal increase in separation of the nasal fields can be reported as diplopia. Clearly its cause must be distinguished from defects in eye movements.

Positive Visual Symptoms

The symptoms thus far described are attributed to loss of function of the axons derived from the retinal ganglion cells. Occasionally patients experience spontaneous flashes of blue, yellow or white light. Such symptoms are infrequently mentioned, and their occurrence may be more often ascertained from direct questioning. The flashes are probably attributable to abnormal excitability, which has been shown in central nerve fibers passing through a demyelinating lesion *(3)*. As described in the following section, incomplete compressive lesions result in focal demyelination at the site of the compression.

Neighborhood Symptoms

Diplopias are caused by paresis of one or more of the extraocular muscles. Cranial nerves III, IV, and VI when passing through the cavernous sinus, lateral to the fossa, may be engulfed in lateral extension of pituitary adenomas, yet their function is almost never not lost except in pituitary apoplexy. When this occurs this usually presents predominately as a oculomotor nerve palsy; however, sporadic reports of isolated abducens nerve palsies have been made. In the absence of apoplexy, oculomotor nerve palsies are more commonly caused by other parasella pathologies, particularly, meningiomas of the cavernous sinus and trigeminal neuromas.

Headache is probably the most common neighborhood symptom. It is present in three quarters of patients at some stage in their histories on careful questioning. It is believed that headache results from stretching of the dural lining of the pituitary fossa and diaphragma sellae. As in many headaches caused by mass intracranial lesions, the pattern is more common in the early morning but is usually not severe, except in apoplexy. It may, however, dominate some patients' lives, particularly in acromegaly and, to a lesser extent, in prolactinoma. In the latter it may complicate dopamine agonist therapy (q.v.); in the former, somatostatin analogs have a surprising effect not related to lowering of growth hormone and insulin-like growth hormone factor (IGF)-1 levels. In all patients with headache, it is essential to take a careful drug use history, because regular use of non prescription medication containing paracetamol may lead to so-called analgesia headache. Changing to nonsteroidal anti-inflammatory medication is the first line of management for analgesia headache.

Rarely a patient may present with temporal lobe epilepsy when a giant tumor spreads laterally to involve the brain (Fig. 1). Major and minor seizures may occur, the latter involving olfactory hallucinations, an intense déjà vu experi-

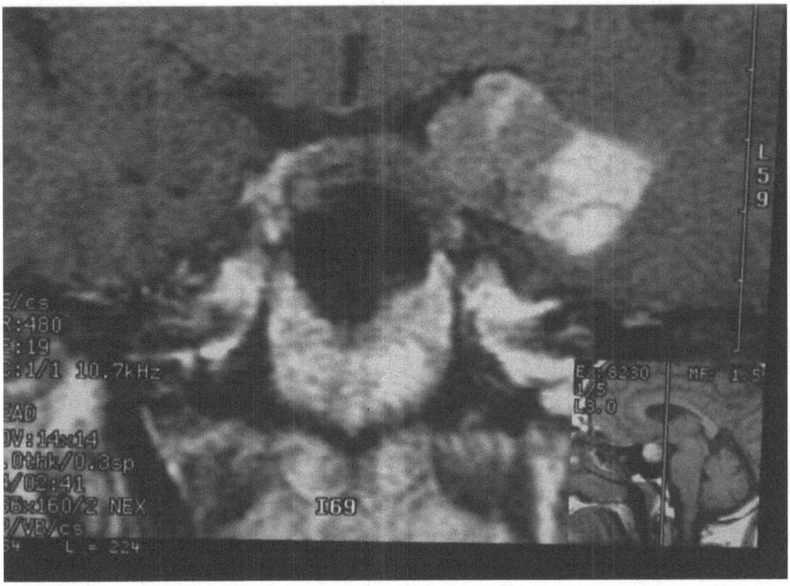

Fig. 1. Coronal enhanced T1 magnetic resonance imaging (MRI) showing a massive prolactinoma that has extended laterally through the cavernous sinus on the left. The patient presented with temporal lobe epilepsy and a history of impotence.

ence, and a rising epigastric sensation. These features may appear as an aura preceding a major attack.

FINDINGS ON EXAMINATION

The most important part of the examination is that of the optic nerves and the eye.

Visual Acuity

The visual acuity of each eye corrected with a pinhole (or by current corrective refraction, remembering that not all people keep their vision testing current) must be recorded for reading and for distance. The latter is particularly important, because many reading charts in use are not standardized. The severity of impairment varies widely, and acuity is often normal in the early stages of chiasmal compression when only the peripheral field is affected. When field loss splits macular vision, the acuity is usually preserved, but the patient may only read letters on the nasal side of the chart. A reduction of acuity in the absence of refractive error or incidental abnormalities in the media indicates that the field defect has crossed the midline.

Color Vision

Testing color vision with each eye separately may provide invaluable evidence of subtle pathologic changes in the fibers of the anterior visual pathways. Impairment of color vision is exceptional in retinal disease, and a unilateral defect is almost always acquired; a bilateral defect is useful diagnostically if it is known (as it often is) that color vision was previously normal.

Visual Fields

The most useful piece of evidence for localization of the site of compression is that provided by examination of the visual fields. *(4)*. Although the fields must always be recorded for future comparison, confrontation with a small red object can provide invaluable immediate evidence of hemianopsias (bitemporal or homonymous) and scotomata.

In examining the fields by confrontation, it is important to test both the peripheral and the central areas. The latter is done best by holding a small red object halfway between the patient's and the examiner's eyes and asking the patient to compare the quality of the color when the object is moved quickly from a few degrees within the nasal field to a few degrees into the nasal field. Desaturation of the color within the temporal field is an early sign of chiasmal compression.

Fields are now most commonly plotted using the Humphrey automated perimeter system. Regardless of where it is performed, the automation ensures a reliable uniformity of response that is easily compared regardless of where the original was performed, with the follow-up from one's own unit. Goldman fields may remain the gold standard in difficult cases, and in experienced hands the tangent screen is invaluable for revealing the details of field loss. Comparison of fields over time is facilitated by using the same symbols and colors on successive occasions—an obvious point surprisingly often forgotten. Who checks that the Humphrey visual field test is the same stimulus (our unit uses the Goldman I4e)? Failure to compare like with like is a known cause of urgent referral to our pituitary clinic.

Bitemporal hemianopia is one of the most common findings with pituitary tumors and indicates chiasmal compression (Fig. 2). The completeness of the hemianopia varies and depends on the size of the tumor and position of the chiasm. When the latter is markedly postfixed, quite a large suprasellar extension of a tumor may produce minimal, if any, loss.

The field loss often begins unilaterally, when the intracranial optic nerve is compressed close to its junction with the chiasm. Early involvement of the

---

Fig. 2. (opposite page) (A) Goldmann field assessment. Typical bitemporal hemianopia resulting from chiasmal compression. (B) Humphrey field assessment. Only the full threshold picture is shown, illustrating a dense left temporal field loss and a lesser degree of upper right quadrantic field loss.

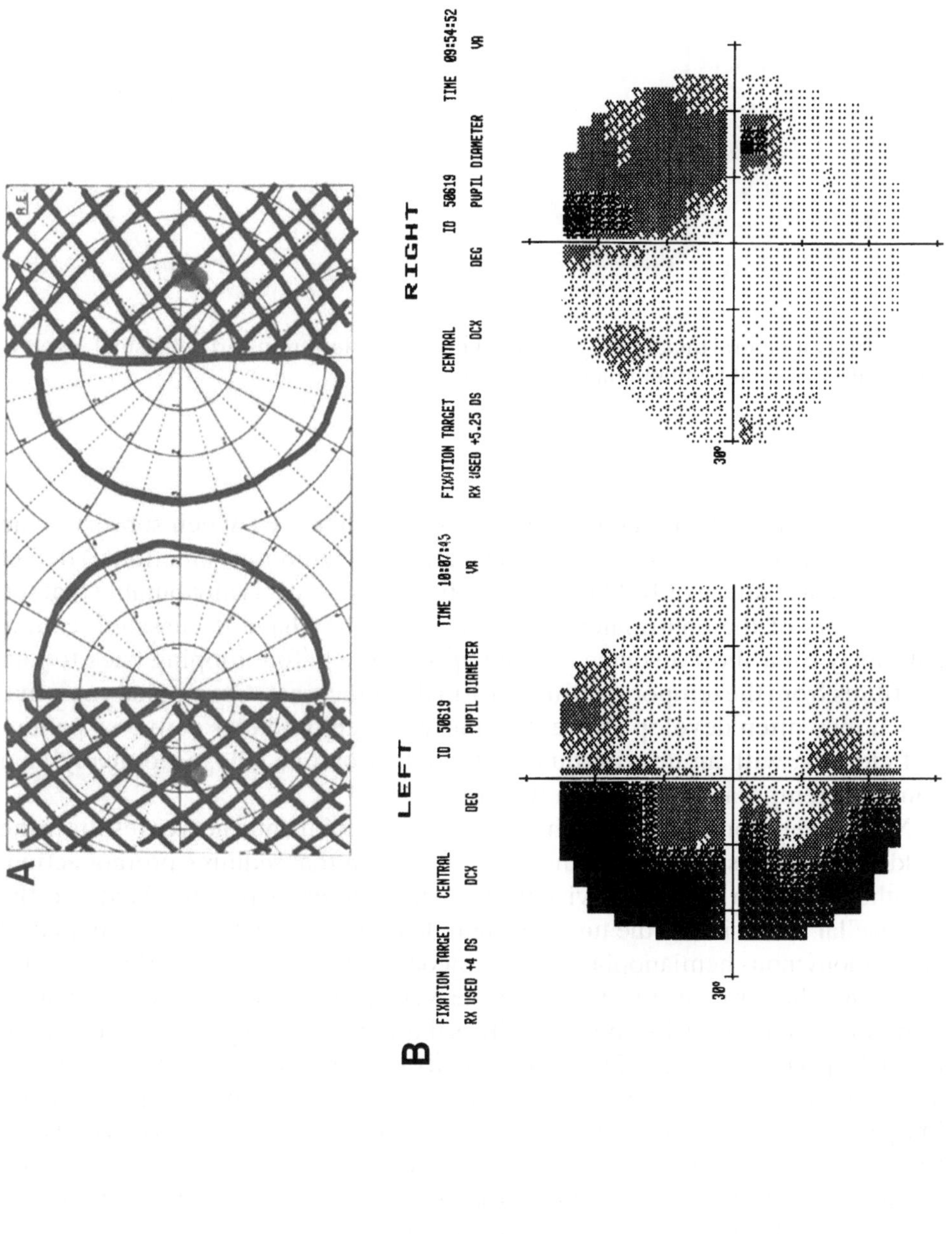
A
R.E.
B
LEFT
FIXATION TARGET CENTRAL
RX USED +4 DS
DCX
DEG
ID 50619
PUPIL DIAMETER
TIME 10:07:45
VA
30°
RIGHT
FIXATION TARGET CENTRAL
RX USED +5.25 DS
DCX
DEG
ID 50619
PUPIL DIAMETER
TIME 09:54:52
VA
30°

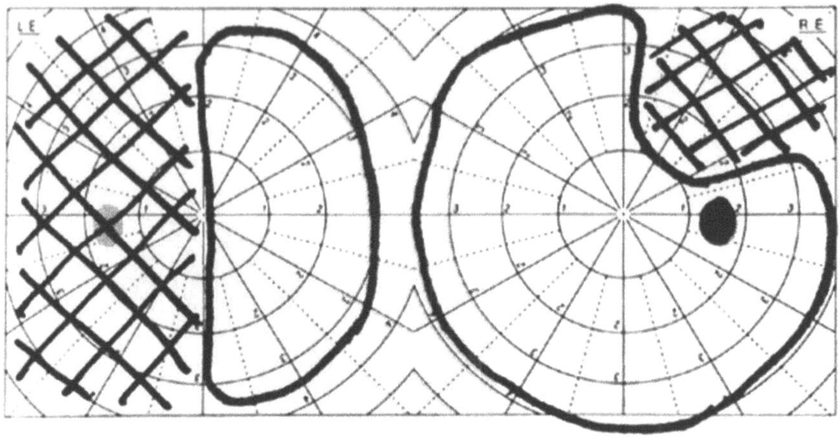

Fig. 3. Early temporal quadrantic junctional loss on the left from early chiasmal involvement with temporal hemianopia on the right.

decussating fibers from the nasal retina of the other eye (which subserves the temporal field) is often signaled by a small upper temporal (junctional) defect (Fig. 3). This pattern of field loss, it is believed by some, is attributable that the nasal fibers of the contralateral eye that, after they have decussated, course anteriorly for a short distance into the optic nerve before looping back to join the fibres from the temporal retina to form the optic tract. Craniopharyngioma, which may often develop above the chiasm, often produces converse pattern of field loss, with an inferior quadrantic defect on one side, accompanying a complete temporal field loss on the other (Fig. 4).

More severe compression of chiasm and intracranial optic nerves results in the field defects crossing the midline—a serious sign that requires prompt action. Another common pattern of visual loss when the chiasm is prefixed and the suprasellar extension of the tumor is more laterally rather than centrally placed is a homonymous hemianopia, which is incongruous, indicating optic tract compression. The surgeon must beware the very prefixed chiasm which makes transcranial surgery risky and difficult, as the approach is blocked by the lack of 'normal' space below the chiasm and vitrually no space between the optic nerves and cartoids laterally. This situation can be anticipated on even poor quality imaging when, in the sagittal images, the mass of the lesion is directed backwards toward or even into the posterior fossa. Attempting tumor removal transcranially in this situation may lead to rapid surgical confusion and abandonment of the procedure with the tumor hiding behind the chiasm and carotids in the same way as a difficult craniopharyngioma.

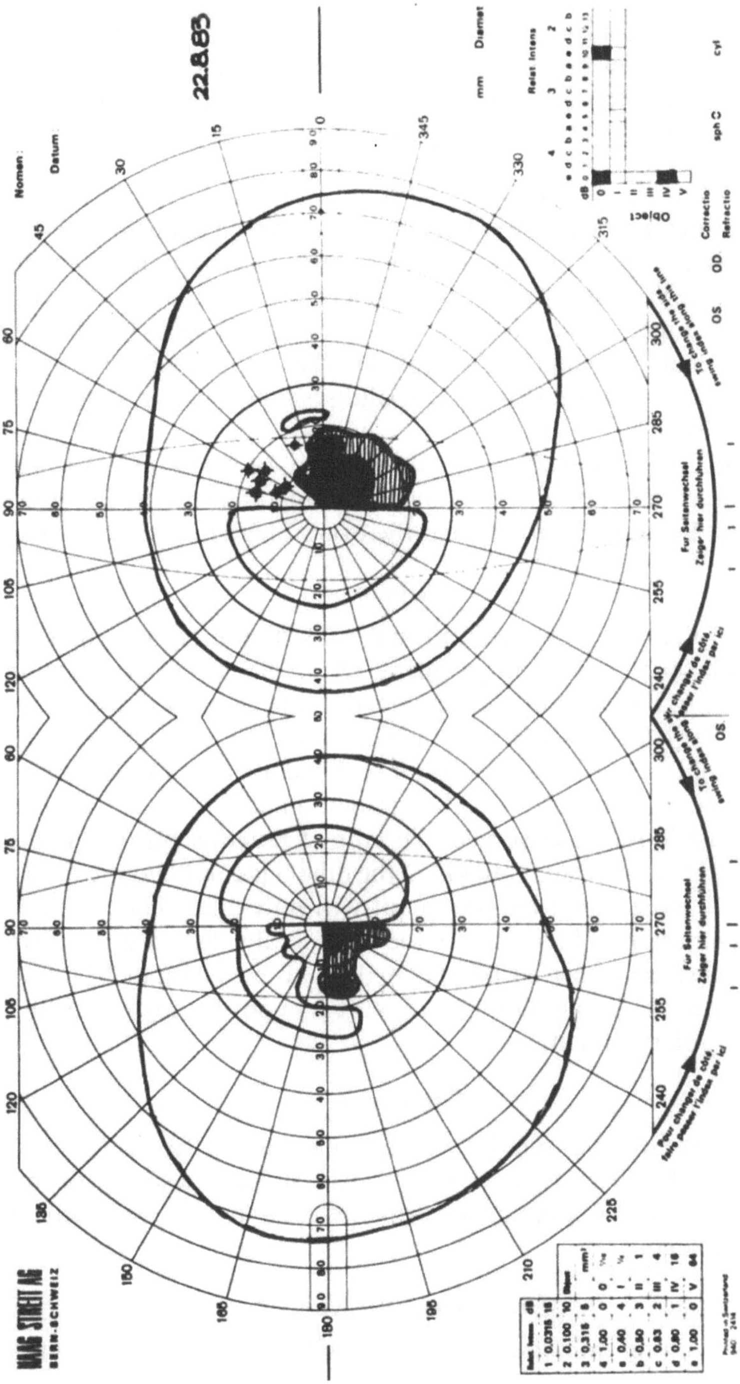

Fig. 4. Temporal field defect on the right with a lower junctional defect on the left from a craniopharyngioma.

Occasionally patients present with homonymous or bitemporal defects affecting only the central few degrees of vision, the latter pattern being attributable to involvement of the decussating fibers from the maculae at the posterior inferior part of the chiasm.

Fundi

Fundal examination may reveal optic atrophy, which indicates that compression is long-standing, or may show normal discs, which indicate a potentially good prognosis for vision. Optic atrophy does not necessarily indicate a poor outcome from surgery as is shown in one of the surgical series *(9)*. The observation of an opticociliary shunt vessel provides strong evidence against a pituitary tumor as a cause of the visual loss and, in adults, suggests the presence of an optic nerve meningioma.

Papilledema is excessively rare, although may be rarely seen when a tumor extends to block the foramina of Monro. The importance of tilted discs is discussed under "Results of Surgery and Recovery of Vision" following.

Pupils

A poor response to light with normal constriction on accommodation is expected with severe visual impairment. Of greater value in detecting more subtle damage of the optic nerves or chiasm is the demonstration of a relative afferent papillary defect which is found with unilateral or asymmetric involvement. The simplest way to demonstrate such a defect is as follows: the direct and consensual light reactions are examined on each side in the usual way. Pupillary constriction is observed. The direct reaction on one side is then retested, and the light swung quickly to the other side. If the optic nerve on the second side is more abnormal, the pupil will now dilate because the neural input to the superior colliculus from the ipsilateral side is less powerful (as a result of damage to the nerve fibers) than the consensual input. The test is best performed with low ambient illumination. It is important to exclude hippus as a cause of papillary dilatation.

The Orbit

The position of the eyes relative to one another and to the orbital rims should always be recorded. The presence of proptosis suggests a cause for the visual symptoms other than a pituitary tumor, most commonly a meningioma in the wing of the sphenoid.

Other Cranial Nerves

Anosmia resulting from the involvement of the olfactory tract is rarely seen with pituitary tumors, at least before transcranial surgery. Its presence suggests another cause for visual loss, most often a subfrontal meningioma extending backward, causing downward pressure on the chiasm and even involvement of the optic nerves. Ocular palsies and involvement of the trigeminal nerve (of which a sensitive indicator of involvement is depression of the corneal reflex) provide presumptive evidence of lateral extension of the tumor into the cavernous sinus, where the nerves may be compressed. As mentioned, this is extremely rare in adenomas, except in apoplexy, but is much more common in meningiomas of the sinus.

A striking finding with long-standing compression of the oculomotor nerve is elevation of the eyelid on attempted adduction because of aberrant re-innervation of the levator palpebrae superioris by regenerating fibers properly destined for the medial rectus. Because spontaneous occurrence of this sign is commonly seen with meningiomas involving the cavernous isinus and infraclinoid aneurysms of the carotid artery, its presence counts against a diagnosis of a pituitary adenoma.

RESULTS OF SURGERY AND RECOVERY OF VISION

Decompression of the anterior visual pathways can result in a remarkably rapid and complete recovery of vision, provided not too many of the optic nerve fibers have degenerated. The risk of irreversible change is increased by both abrupt compression (as in apoplexy) and by prolonged compression, when severe optic atrophy reflects the severity of the nerve fiber loss. Although this seems remarkably obvious, it is difficult to prove from the various surgical series on postsurgical visual recovery in the literature. Furthermore, it is far from clear how quickly surgical intervention must be performed once chiasmatic compression from a tumor mass has been or should have been demonstrated. When most physicians discover a mass, they clamor to have the mass removed at the next available opportunity by the best possible surgeon, a luxury that in these days of healthcare rationing is not immediately available to every patient. In the protocol established at our hospital, the maximum period of delay should be 6 wk, but even this is far too long in some cases and not ideal. Nevertheless, despite horrific-looking scans, minimal visual loss in some patients often stablizes over many months.

When recoverable, visual fields may start to open in the recovery area immediately after surgery and further open in the following days, which questions the mechanisms of vision recovery after decompression, which have been investigated experimentally *(5,6)*. It is probable that the immediate recovery depends on the reversal of ischemic conduction block in demyelinated, remyelinated and morphologically intact fibers. The slower phase probably depends on progressive remyelination and adaptive synaptic mechanisms to compensate for axonal loss *(7)*. Complete recovery may continue for months, and, in our clinic, improvement after 2 or 3 yr is not unknown. Recovery of vision in the five major surgical series is given in Table 1 *(8–12)*.

Table 1
Recovery of Vision: *Surgical Series Results*

Reference	*Pt No.*	*Recovery and type*	*Comments*
Symon, 1979 *(10)*	101	57% Full/37% partial	Craniotomy series with "giant" tumors excepted
Cohen, 1985 *(11)*	100	79% Acuity/74% fields	Best overall data
Findlay, 1983 *(12)*	34	85% Improved	Complex field assesment
Laws, 1977 *(8)*	62	16.7% Full fields, 69% improved	
Powell, 1995 *(9)*	67	34% Full/43% partial fields	

Unusual incomplete bitemporal bitemporal or binasal defects are occasionally found in asymptomatic individuals being examined for some other purpose, most often in the course of assessment for corrective lenses. Such defects are often associated with anomalously shaped (tilted) or hypoplastic optic discs (Fig. 5), and are of no pathologic significance. If, however, there is any doubt about the cause of such defects, compression of the chiasm must be excluded by appropriate imaging.

FOLLOW-UP

A patient who has had the neurologic manifestations of a pituitary tumor must be followed up indefinitely (*see* Chapter 12), because recurrence can occur even 25 yr or more after surgery. Once the postoperative period and radiotherapy (if given) are complete and hormonal replacement stabilized, patients are best followed up in a multidisciplinary clinic with endocrinological, neurosurgical, and radiotherapy input and with ophthalmological assessment available.

REFERENCES

1. Nachtigäller H, Hoyt WF. Stöungen des Seheindruckes bei bitemporaler Hemianopsie und Verscheibung der Sehachsen. Klin Monatsbl Augenheilk 1970;156:821–836.
2. Kirkham TH. The ocular symptamatology of pituitary tumors. Proc R Soc Med 1972;65:517–518.
3. Smith KJ, MacDonald WI. Spontaneous and evoked discharges from a central demyelinating lesion. J Neurol Sci 1982;55:39–47.
4. Glaser JS. *Neuro-opthalmology*, 2nd ed. Philadelphia: Lipincott; 1990.
5. Kayan A, Earl CJ. Compressive lesions of the optic nerves and chiasm: pattern of recovery of vision following surgical treatment. Brain 1975;98:13–28.
6. Clifford-Jones RE, MaDonald WI, Landon DN. Chronic optic compression: an experimental study. Brain 1985;108:241–262.

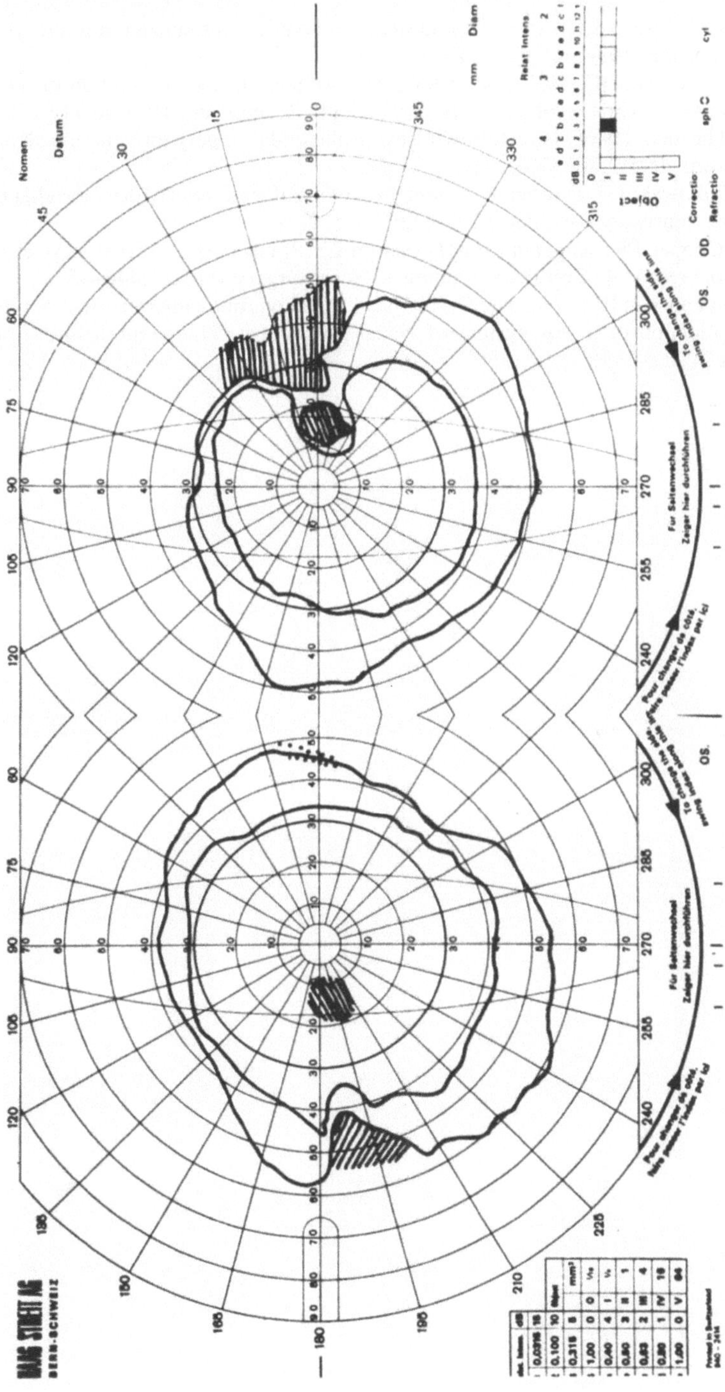

Fig. 5. Field defects associated with anomalous discs.

7. Darian-Smith C, Gilbert CD. Axonal sprouting accompanies reorganization in the adult cat striate cortex. Nature 1994;368:737–740.
8. Laws ER Jr, Trautman JC, Mollenhorst RW. Transsphenoidal decompression of the optic nerve and chiasm—visual results in sixty-two patients. J Neurosurg 1977;46:717–722.
9. Powell MP. The recovery of vision following transsphenoidal surgery for pituitary adenomas. Brit J Neurosurg 1995;9:367–373.
10. Symon L, Jakubowski J. Transcranial management of pituitary tumors with suprasellar extension. J Neurol Neurosurg Psychiatry 1979;42:123–133.
11. Cohen AR, Cooper PR, Kupersmith MJ, Flamm ES, Ransohoff J. Visual recovery after transsphenoidal removal of pituitary adenomas. Neurosurgery 1985;17:446–452.
12. Findlay G, McFadzean RM, Teasdale G. Recovery of vision following treatment of pituitary tumours: application of a new system of visual assessment. Trans Ophthalmol Soc UK 1983;103 (Pt 2):212–216.

7 Surgical Assessment and Anesthetic Management of the Pituitary Patient

Michael P. Powell, MB, BS, FRCS
and Nicholas P. Hirsch, MB, BS, FRCA

Contents

INTRODUCTION

The aim of this chapter is to assist the surgeon and the anesthetist in the preoperative assessment of the pituitary patient and in planning the operation. We also clarify the aims of surgery and discuss how to manage the patient with pituitary apoplexy.

SURGICAL ASSESSMENT

Clinical Presentation

The patient with a pituitary lesion usually presents in a combination of one or more of four ways.

- Endocrine dysfunction. Overproduction is most commonly seen in prolactinoma, for which surgery is not usually first-line therapy. It is also seen in acromegaly, Cushing's disease (CD), and, rarely, secondary hyperthyroid-

From: *Management of Pituitary Tumors: The Clinician's Practical Guide, Second Edition*
Edited by: M. P. Powell, S. L. Lightman, and E. R. Laws, Jr. © Humana Press Inc., Totowa, NJ

ism. Underproduction may result from the presence of a large nonfunctioning tumor.

- Local pressure symptoms, especially with impairment of visual fields or visual acuity, and more rarely with dysfunction of cranial nerves III to VI, including trigeminal neuralgia.
- Headache, sometimes related to dural distortion around the pituitary fossa. Infrequently it is associated with other raised intracranial pressure symptoms, such as drowsiness. Headache is also prevalent in patients with small adenomas without mass effect, and there is emerging evidence of a neurovascular pattern to this headache that may suggest a neuroendocrine cause (Levy M, Goadsby P, personal communication). In pituitary apoplexy, subarachnoid hemorrhage may contribute to acute headache.
- Incidental discovery during scanning for some other purpose.

The Aim of Surgery

The surgeon must decide what it is he or she wishes to achieve by operating and make this aim clear to the patient. Surgery usually has one of four aims that sometimes overlap:

- Total tumor removal to produce an endocrine cure.
- Debulking of a large multilobular tumor before radiotherapy.
- Decompression of the chiasm and optic nerves to either treat existing visual failure or prevent further encroachment of tumor that lies adjacent to the optic apparatus.
- Biopsy alone, which may sometimes be required without debulking when the radiologic diagnosis is unclear and further therapy undecided. An example of this is an operation to differentiate between sellar neurosarcoid and tuberculosis.

For microadenomas with hormone overproduction, the goal is early and permanent control of elevated hormone levels. This can only be achieved with total surgical removal. Subtotal removal of tumor in such cases may achieve temporary improvement in symptoms, but recurrence is inevitable unless some other adjuvant therapy is used, such as radiotherapy or medical therapy. Such a compromise delays control of elevated hormone levels and increases the inconvenience to the patient and also the cost of treatment. Therefore, there is often a good case for re-exploration if a microadenoma is not cured at the first operation, provided the endocrine diagnosis is certain. This is especially worthwhile where pathologic evidence of an adenoma is confirmed at the first operation.

For macroadenomas, complete resection is also the aim, but in practice, the ability to achieve complete removal of large tumors may be limited by lateral extensions or true pathologic invasion of the cavernous sinus or the dura.

Debulking of a large macroadenoma with visual symptoms may achieve considerable improvement in vision even without a complete resection. Headache may also improve with debulking, although curiously, headache related to small growth hormone (GH) secreting tumors may persist if the acromegaly is not cured, even when there is no residual tumor seen on scanning.

Tumors discovered as incidental radiologic findings require hormonal and visual assessment to assess the potential benefits of surgical treatment. Radiologic signs that are atypical for an adenoma suggest that surgery should be carried out to obtain a diagnosis. A subclinical field defect may be discovered, which warrants surgery to prevent progression. Evidence of subclinical hypopituitarism may be an added indication for surgery, as tumor removal can result in restoration of normal pituitary function. This contrasts with the commonly held and voiced view of endocrinologists in the 1980s and 1990s that surgery results in loss of function. Where these investigations are normal, surgery should be considered if the tumor is closely juxtaposed to the chiasm, to remove the risk of visual deterioration, or if serial magnetic resonance imaging (MRI) demonstrates progression.

Preoperative Workup

Once the need for surgery has been determined the minimum surgical workup for every patient includes the following.

Endocrine Assessment

Endocrine assessment has two goals:

1. First, the surgeon and the endocrinologist must be sure of an accurate endocrine diagnosis before proceeding with surgery. In cases of hormone excess, it is essential to have adequate evidence of a pituitary source. It should not be assumed that all referring physicians will have completed the appropriate tests before referral. Aside from the risks to the patient of unnecessary pituitary exploration, the surgeon aquires an apparent surgical failure which is really a failure to investigate.
   Measurement of serum prolactin (PRL) is mandatory. This is required to identify hyperprolacinemia attributable to a prolactinoma that usually responds to medical treatment with a dopamine agonist and spares the patient an operation.
   Thyroid function must also be assessed. It is dangerous to operate on a hypothyroid patient (*see* next paragraph). Also, rarely, a large pituitary lesion, apparently a tumor, may result from thyrotroph hyperplasia secondary to primary hypothyroidism. The MRI appearances in Fig. 1 were seen in such a case and resolved after thyroid replacement.
2. Second, the identification and treatment of hormone deficiency is required to optimize the safety of the anesthetic. Thyroxine and cortisol levels are the most important variables. The patient with myxoedema is at risk for a perioperative thyroid crisis if not placed on adequate replacement. If preoperative hypocortisolemia is present, then hydrocortisone replacement is essential.

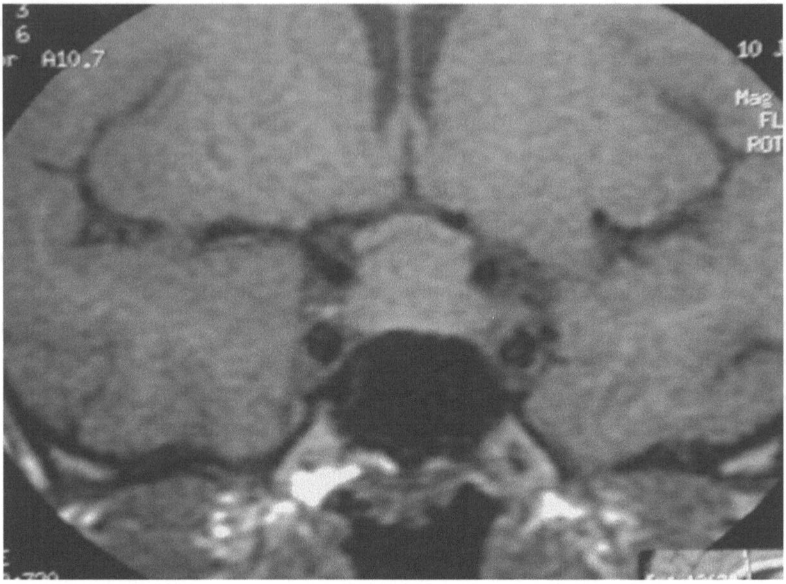

Fig. 1. Coronal T1 MRI shows a mass extending into the suprasellar space and displacing the chiasm. A 16-yr-old girl with a pituitary lesion confirmed as thyrotroph hyperplasia on histology. TSH was 27.1 mU/L.

Charting Visual Fields

Unless the tumor is entirely intrasellar, charting visual fields should always be done to both detect subclinical field defects and to act as a baseline investigation for the future. The automated Humphrey chart is internationally standardized and is satisfactory for identifying the bitemporal hemianopia characteristic of field loss from a chiasmal cause or more subtle quadrantic defects.

Imaging

Apart from its diagnostic role, preoperative imaging provides anatomical information to ensure a safe approach to the fossa from either below or above. The shape and consistency of the surgical target must be known and any atypical anatomy, especially a deviated midline sphenoid septum, recognized.

A high-quality MRI should always be obtained. The normal gland seen on MRI can change throughout life. Through most of life the normal gland is contained within the fossa without any upward bowing of the upper surface of the gland (Fig. 2).

In pregnancy and during the teenage growth spurt, the gland enlarges and it is quite possible to extend into the suprasellar space and even touch the chiasm. Hypertrophy from other causes also occurs rarely, for instance in primary hypothyroidism (Fig. 1). The gland may also be squeezed up into the suprasel-

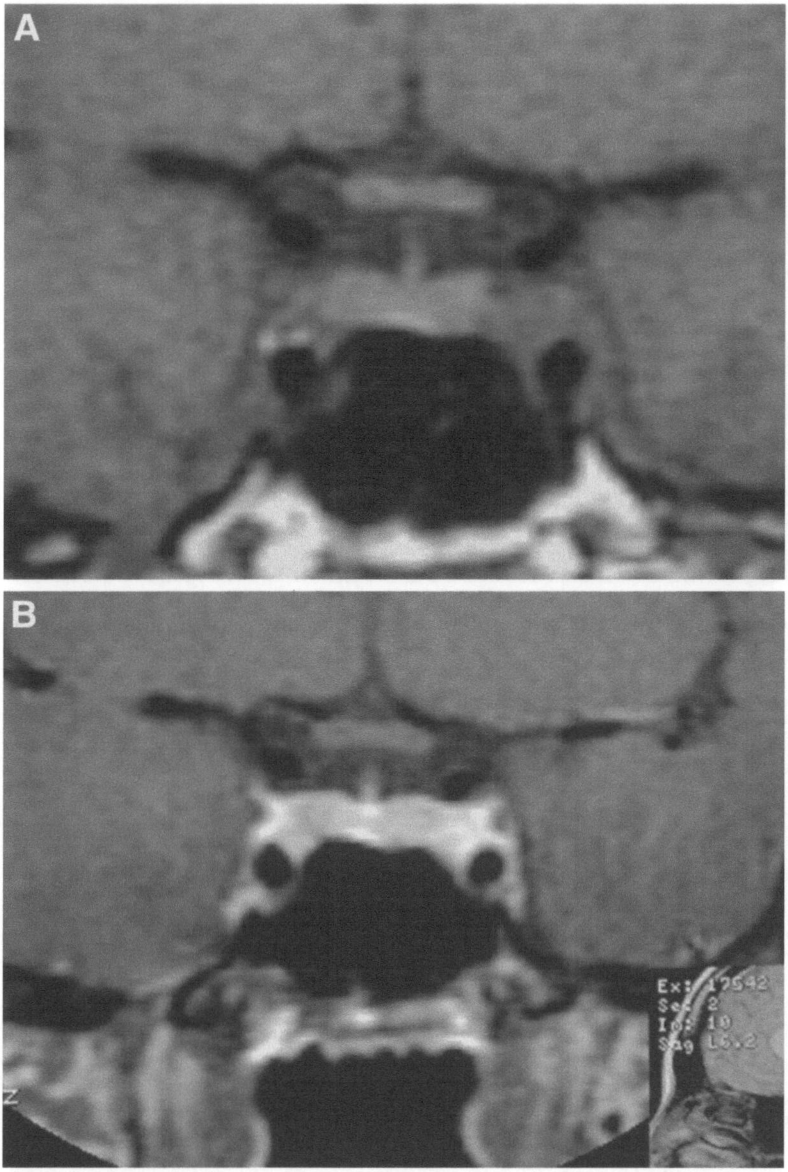

Fig. 2. (A) Normal gland in 32-yr-old woman. MRI T1 coronal image. Note small cavernous sinus meningioma on left. (B) T1 coronal with gadolinium, 1 mm posterior, to image (A). Note the pituitary stalk.

lar space by inturning of the carotid syphon in the cavernous sinus, the so-called kissing carotids (Fig. 3).

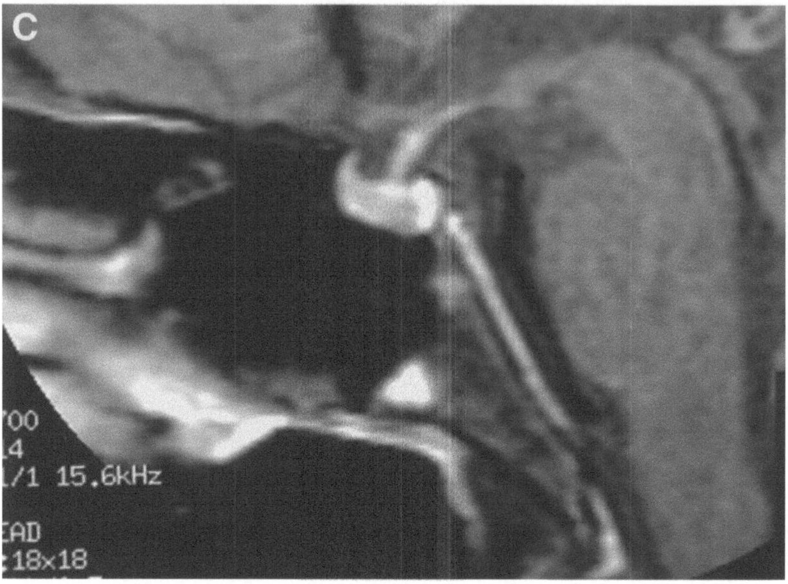

Fig. 2. (C) Sagittal T1 MRI with enhancement of same patient, note posterior lobe is hyperintense.

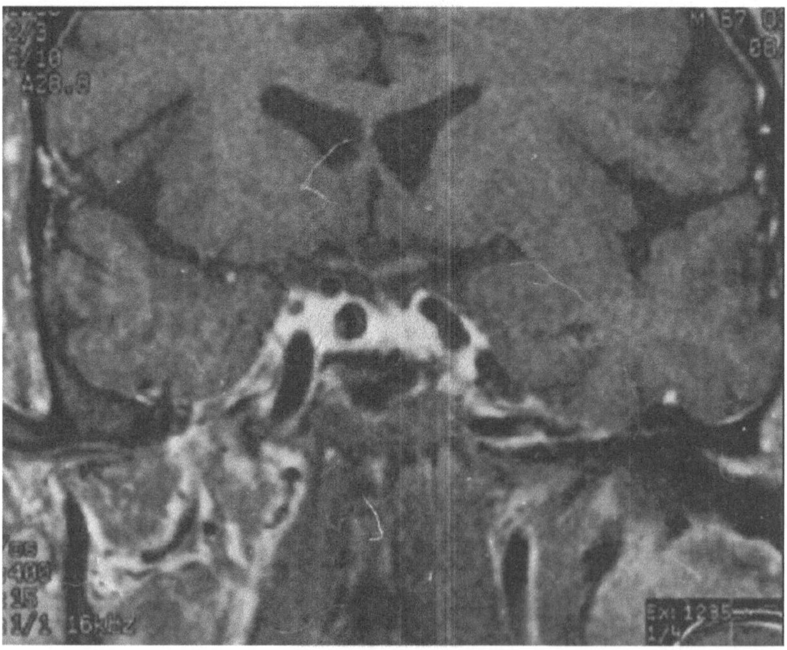

Fig. 3. T-enhanced coronal MRI. Right internal carotid extending to midline in the pituitary fossa.

It is also possible to have completely normal pituitary function with an enlarged "ballooned" fossa, such as may be found in macroadenomas. Whether this reflects a tumor that has at some stage infarcted, leaving the normal gland intact or ballooning through chronic raised pressure of mild asymptomatic pseudo-tumor cerebri, is unknown. The posterior lobe has high signal intensity on T1-weighted images. Although it is customary to give contrast medium, it often adds little to the value of the images.

Computed tomography (CT) is useful in difficult cases, particularly where there has been bone removal at a previous operation. The lateral skull radiograph is obsolete as part of the workup, being of low sensitivity, but the skill of interpreting the skull radiograph is essential to the surgeon when using intraoperative fluoroscopy. For all our revision cases, we employ an interactive image guidance system.

A Note on Pituitary Apoplexy

Because they present with acute symptoms, patients with pituitary apoplexy are commonly referred directly to the neurosurgical unit with minimum prior investigation. The key point regarding these patients is that they require the same high standard of preparation as elective cases, including identification and correction of any hormone deficit and satisfactory imaging. Steroids are administered to both treat deficiency of the hypothalamic-pituitary-adrenal (HPA) axis and diminish peritumoral swelling. Patients are sometimes gravely ill with a combination of panhypopituitarism, subarachnoid hemorrhage, and oculomotor palsies; it is misguided to embark on an urgent decompression without a full workup to minimize the risks of surgery. An operation within 24 to 48 h is satisfactory once endocrine and electrolyte abnormalities are corrected; emergency surgery out of hours is almost never indicated.

Once the patient is prepared, an operation promotes resolution of headache and recovery of cranial nerve deficits. The outlook for visual acuity after surgery is good. In a study of 35 patients by Randeva et al., complete restoration of visual acuity occurred in all patients operated on within 8 d *(1)*.

When headache alone is the predominant symptom it is sometimes advisable to await a natural recovery. This may be the correct course, even when there is a coexisting third nerve palsy. The third nerve is surprisingly robust and can sometimes recover over days without any operative intervention. There may then be a role for a delayed operation to remove the tumor remnant and confirm the diagnosis.

Perioperative Medications

Corticosteroids

Symptoms of secondary adrenal insufficiency in pituitary patients may be subtle, and the best way to guard against perioperative adrenal insufficiency is to give prophylactic hydrocortisone cover to all patients. This is a safe policy, but in selective adenomectomy hydrocortisone is unnecessary so long as the HPA axis is normal. Hout et al. studied 82 patients with microadenomectomy with a normal HPA axis *(2)*. Only two patients showed evidence of HPA insufficiency in the postoperative period, in whom it was clinically evident and replacement was given safely. Our policy is to administer 100 mg of hydrocortisone on induction only to patients with evidence of cortisol insufficiency.

Antibiotic Prophylaxis

During transsphenoidal surgery, the operative field is exposed to commensals present in the sphenoid sinus and the operation is therefore contaminated. Despite this, and probably because of the extra-arachnoid nature of most transsphenoidal surgery, the infection rate after surgery is low. We use antibiotic prophylaxis in the form of a single dose of 1.5 g cefuroxime iv on induction, although some surgeons consider this unnecessary.

The Choice of Operative Approach

Tumor size is the main factor in selecting the surgical route. The Hardy Classification (*3*; Table 1) is based on radiologic appearances and remains a satisfactory system, although alternatives have been suggested.

Microadenomas (Grades 0 and 1) should only be approached via the transsphenoidal route. It is impossible to perform the microdissection required to separate the tumor from the normal gland transcranially. Any attempt to do so runs a significant risk of damage, not only to the normal gland but also to the posterior lobe (Fig. 4).

Tumors occupying the whole sella (Grades II and III) are also best approached from below (Fig. 5).

Occasionally, in a significantly expanded fossa a reasonable decompression can be carried out from above. It is difficult to justify such an approach because significant tumor clearance and preservation of endocrine function is far less easy to achieve. Tumors that extend laterally into the cavernous sinus (Grade E) or further into the subtemporal area are always a difficult surgical problem, because it is difficult to reach this area by either route (Fig. 6).

Cavernous sinus surgery is now an established division of skull-base surgery, but it is questionable whether a formal extradural approach to the sella via the cavernous sinus is warranted in pituitary adenoma because of the benign nature of the tumor. The response to radiotherapy is usually favorable, although slow. In our view, however, this approach is never a first-line option. It is of historical interest that both Sir Victor Horsley and Harvey Cushing, the pioneers of pituitary surgery, began their attempts to approach the pituitary by using the subtemporal route and abandoned it because of unacceptable complications.

Table 1
The Hardy Classification of Pituitary Adenomas

Grade	
Sella turcica	
Enclosed adenoma	
0	Intact with normal contour
I	Intact with bulging floor
II	Intact, enlarged fossa
Invasive adenoma	
III	Localized sellar destruction
IV	Diffuse destruction
Suprasellar	
A	Suprasellar cistern only
B	Recesses of third ventricle
C	Whole anterior third ventricle
D	Intracranial extradural
E	Extracranial extradural (lateral cavernous)

Endoscopic pituitary surgery employing an angled endoscope may provide the most promising way to approach an adenoma extending into the cavernous sinus.

With suprasellar tumors (Grades A, B, C, and D) good results can also be achieved with transsphenoidal surgery for both chiasmal decompression and endocrine preservation. This is particularly true for those tumors of Grades A, B, and C. Increasing experience with the extended transsphenoidal approach (Couldwell and Weiss, 1998; Kaptain et al., 2001) means that most experienced pituitary surgeons have extended the range of suprasellar tumors for which they will consider an inferior approach as a first option. Even for multilobulated suprasellar tumors of higher grade, transsphenoidal surgery can still be effective if used as part of a staged procedure. The large tumor cavity often fails to collapse initially, appearing as a mass of saline with clot on early postoperative scans. These appearances can be misleading; it is important to rescan the patient before the second transcranial procedure, at which time the residual tumor has usually reduced markedly in size.

ANESTHETIC MANAGEMENT

Successful pituitary surgery depends not only on surgical expertise but also on careful anesthetic management. The latter requires accurate preoperative assessment and meticulous perioperative and postoperative care common to all intracranial procedures.

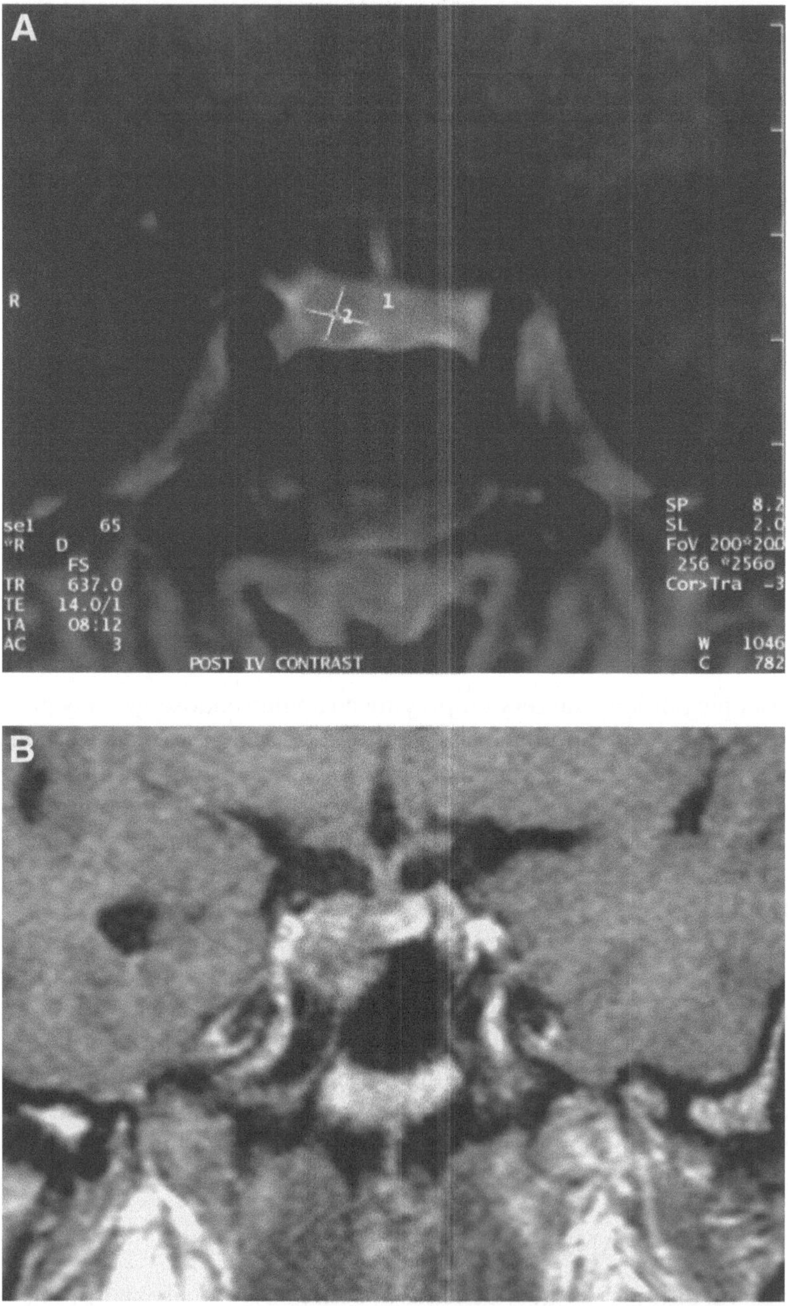

Fig. 4. (A) T1 gadolinium-enhanced coronal MRI. Note the radiologist's measurement of widest diameter of the lesion. (B) Coronal MRI of a GH-secreting microadenoma obscured by a small Rathke's cleft cyst.

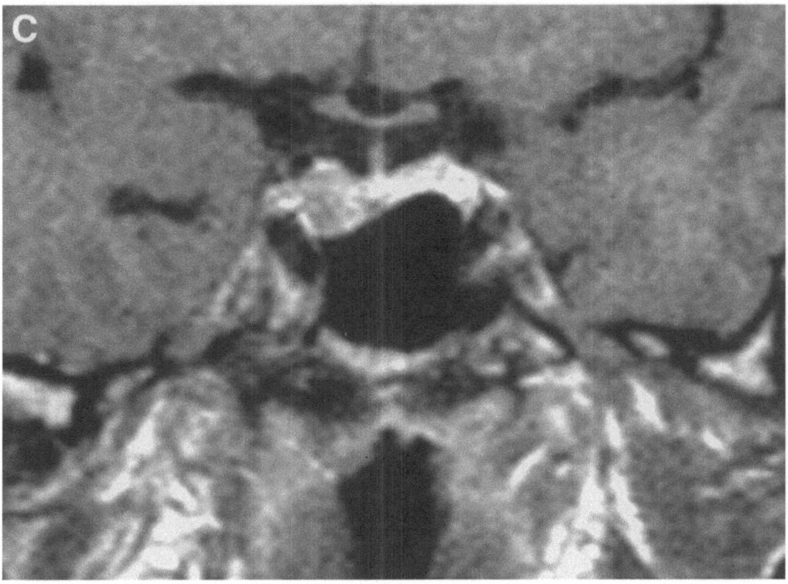

Fig. 4. (C) Same patient as in (B). Small microadenoma revealed behind Rathke's cleft cyst.

Preoperative Management

In general, nonfunctioning pituitary tumors present when they are of sufficient size to produce chiasmal compression with or without compression syndromes of the cavernous sinus or suprachiasmal structures. It is essential for the anesthetist to be aware that raised intracranial pressure (ICP) may be present because of either the large size of the tumor or hydrocephalus resulting from obstruction of cerebrospinal fluid (CSF) at the third ventricle. In contrast, functioning pituitary tumors are usually microadenomas and the anesthetist's attention should be directed toward assessment of the clinical effects of hormonal hypersecretion.

It therefore follows that, in addition to the routine preoperative assessment performed on patients undergoing a neurosurgical procedure, the anesthetist must specifically assess the patient's visual function and endocrine status, the clinical effects of hormonal hypersecretion (or hyposecretion), as well as looking for signs of raised ICP.

Patients with acromegaly and CD are likely to be suffering from co-existing systemic complications of their disease and must be assessed accordingly (*see* Chapters 3 and 4).

Acromegaly

GH hypersecretion affects not only the extremities but also the tissues of the mouth, tongue, pharnyx, and larynx. In addition to the almost invariable prog-

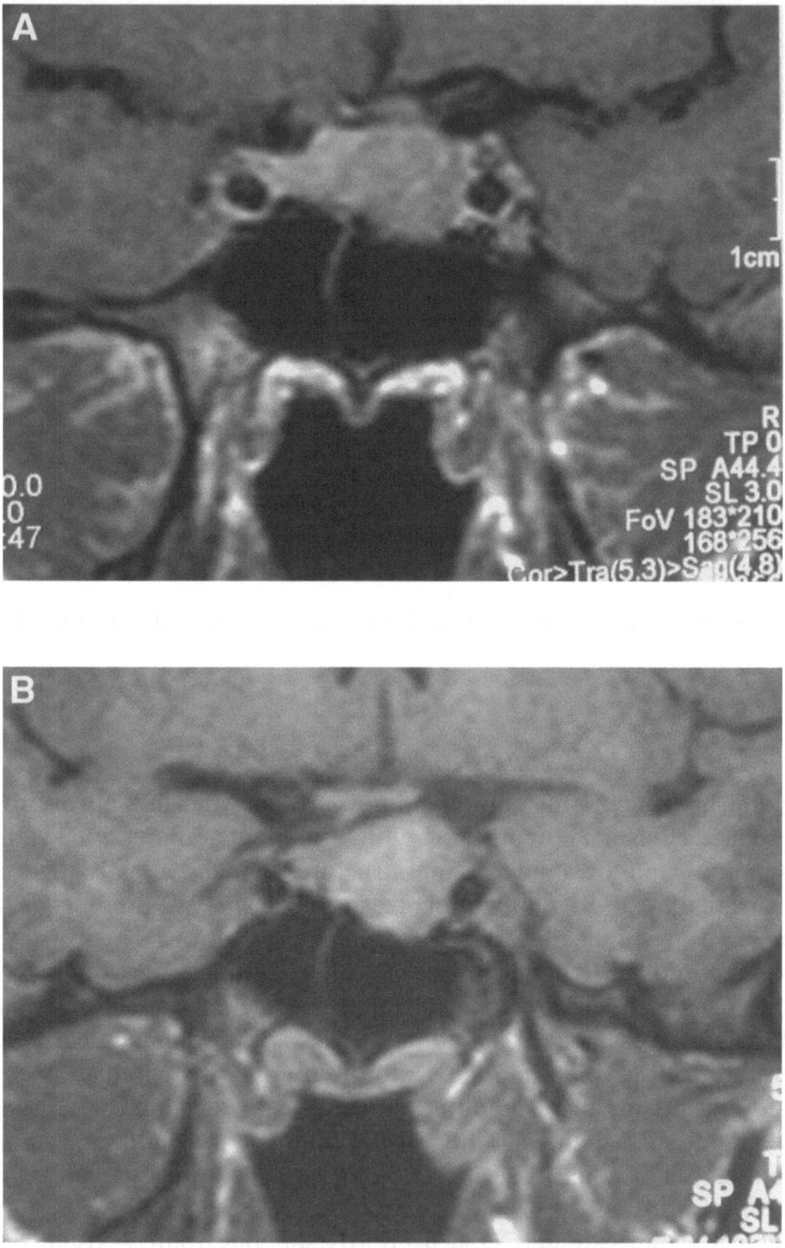

Fig. 5. (A) Unenhanced coronal T1 MRI of >10 mm GH-secreting adenoma. (B) Enhanced coronal T1 MRI of the lesion in (A).

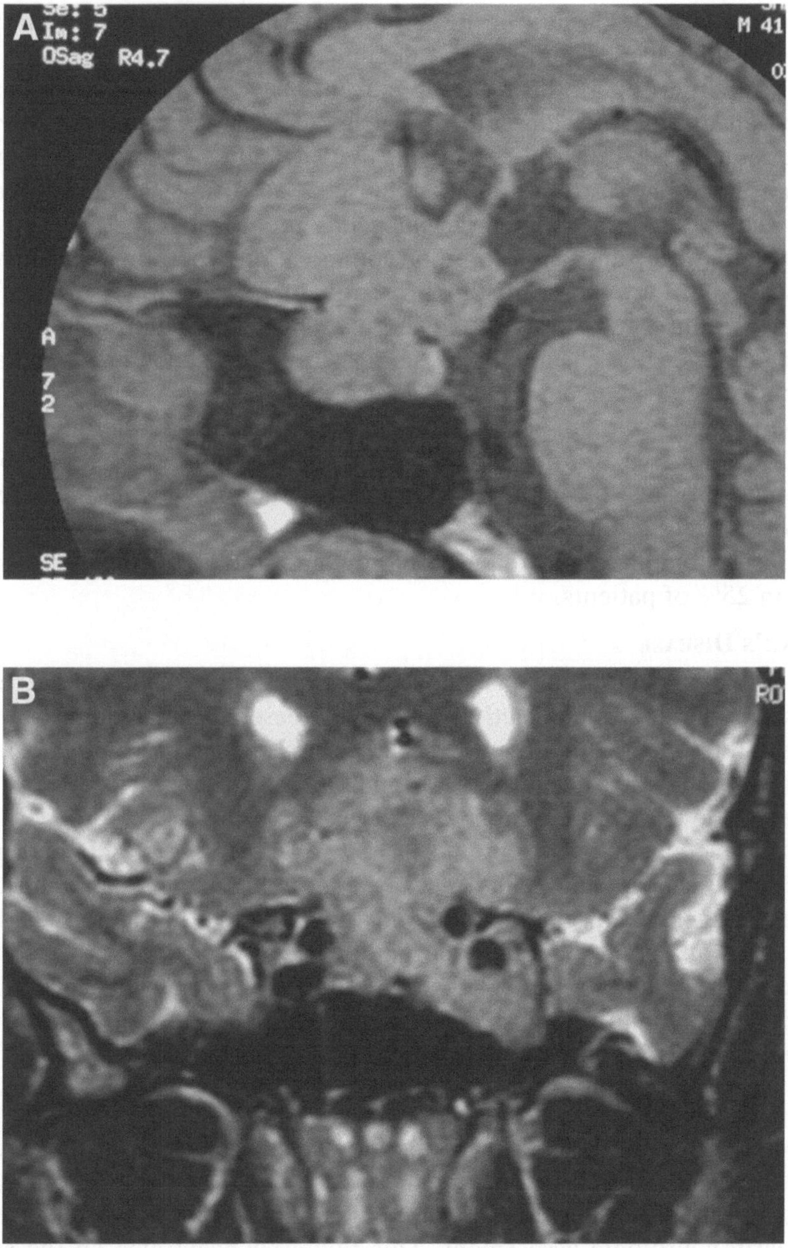

Fig. 6. Sagittal unenhanced T1 MRI (A) and coronal unenhanced T2 MRI (B) of a massive multilobed growth hormone (GH)-secreting tumor presenting with loss of vision. Chiasmal compression is best seen in (B). Note, too, the invasion of the cavernous sinus with engulfing of the left carotid. A tumor like this is a challenge by any route and is best tackled by both transcranial and transsphenoidal approaches, followed by radiotherapy.

nathism and macroglossia seen in acromegaly, the pharyngeal and laryngeal tissues are thickened, resulting in a decreased laryngeal aperture and hypertrophy of the peri-epiglottic folds. Recurrent laryngeal nerve palsy has been reported, and the thyroid enlargement seen in 25% of patients may cause tracheal compression. It is therefore not surprising that difficulties of airway management and tracheal intubation are commonly reported. Careful assessment of the airway is vital and may require indirect laryngoscopy preoperatively.

Obstructive sleep apnea is a common complication of acromegaly and reflects the airway pathology and results in a three-fold increase in the risk of death from respiratory failure. A history of loud snoring, apnea, and daytime hypersomnolence should alert the anesthetist of the possibility of sleep apnea, and a sleep study performed if indicated.

Hypertension occurs in 30% of patients with acromegaly, but, unlike CD, it is usually responsive to antihypertensive treatment. Ventricular hypertrophy and interstitial fibrosis are common in long-standing acromegaly and may result in reduced ventricular function.

Glucose intolerance is a frequent finding, and frank diabetes mellitus (DM) occurs in 25% of patients.

Cushing's Disease

Hypertension occurs in approx 85% of patients with CD and is the result of increased mineralocorticoid activity and an increased plasma volume. It is often relatively refractive to treatment. The left ventricular hypertrophy seen in the condition is believed to be partially attributable to the effects of hypertension and to excessive levels of circulating cortisol.

Obstructive sleep apnea is found in 30% of patients with CD and may be related to the centripetal obesity that occurs; the latter may also contribute to gastroesophageal reflux that is commonly encountered. Preoperative administration of H_2 antagonists is often warranted.

Glucose intolerance or frank diabetes mellitus (DM) occurs in 60% of patients and, with the immunosuppressive action of the high levels of circulating glucocorticoids, coexisting infection is common.

Perioperative Anesthetic Management

Anesthesia for pituitary surgery follows the same principles as those for general neuroanesthesia and includes maintenance of cerebral perfusion and oxygenation while providing suitable surgical conditions and rapid emergence to allow early neurologic assessment. This review concentrates on the specific issues regarding pituitary surgery.

Premedication

Sedative premedication is often withheld in patients undergoing neurosurgical procedures. However, if anxiolysis is deemed necessary, a small dose of benzodiazepine is appropriate. It must be remembered that all sedative drugs exacerbate obstructive sleep apnea and should be avoided in those patients suspected of having the condition. It is common practice to administer hydrocortisone (100 mg) on induction of anesthesia, although the need for this is being increasingly questioned.

Airway Management

Maintenance of the airway and ventilation with a bag and mask is generally straightforward in patients with acromegaly although large face pieces and oral airways are necessary. Similarly, tracheal intubation, in our experience, is usually uneventful if long-bladed laryngoscopes are used. However, severe involvement of laryngeal mucosa and vocal cords may make tracheal intubation impossible with conventional laryngoscopes. In such cases, fiber-optic tracheal intubation is a safe alternative. Some authorities suggest tracheostomy for such patients, and equipment for this procedure should be available should the need arise. After intubation, the tracheal tube must be securely fixed in a suitable position and the mouth and pharynx packed to prevent passage of blood into the glottis and stomach.

Preparation of Nasal Mucosa

Adequate vasoconstriction of the nasal mucosa is essential for providing reasonable conditions for transsphenoidal surgery. This need becomes even more important if an endoscopic technique is being used. Traditionally, mixtures of cocaine and epinephrine have been used, but the high incidence of subsequent arrhythmias has resulted in the search for safer alternatives; a mixture of the sympathomimetic xylometazoline and lidocaine produces effects equivalent to those of cocaine.

Subarachnoid Drain

A subarachnoid lumbar drain may be inserted in patients with macroadenomas with significant suprasellar extension. This has two purposes. Introduction of 10 mL aliquots of 0.9% saline during surgery increases pressure within the lateral ventricles and produces prolapse of the suprasellar portion of the tumor into the operative field. In addition, should the dura be breached during the procedure, CSF can be drained postoperatively through the catheter.

Maintenance of Anesthesia

The choice of anesthetic technique used falls outside the remit of this chapter but follows that used for other neurosurgical procedures. There are periods of intense surgical stimulation while the surgeon gains access to the pituitary fossa, and these are accompanied by episodes of hypertension. The short-acting opioid drug remifentanil is ideally suited to offset the blood pressure changes and its short context-sensitive half-life ensures rapid recovery. However, if this agent is used, it is vital to administer a long-acting analgesic (such as morphine) before the end of surgery to provide adequate analgesia on emergence. Patients should be monitored as for all neurosurgical procedures.

After surgery, extubation of the trachea is carried out after return of spontaneous ventilation, removal of the throat pack, and careful suctioning of the pharynx.

Patients undergoing uncomplicated transsphenoidal surgery generally return to the general ward after a period in the recovery room; those who have undergone cranial surgery are nursed in the intensive care unit for 24 h.

Postoperative Management

Postoperative management consists of careful airway management, provision of adequate postoperative analgesia, appropriate fluid and hormone replacement, and careful monitoring for postoperative complications. The latter include the development of diabetes insipidus, (DI) and hyponatremia and are discussed in Chapter 11 and 12.

Airway Management

Maintenance of a clear airway in those patients undergoing transsphenoidal surgery may be difficult in the immediate postoperative period. The presence of blood within the pharynx, the distorted upper airway anatomy of the patient with acromegaly patient and the use of nasal packs all contribute to compromise airway patency. Acute pulmonary edema after extubation has been reported in this group of patients. It is therefore vital that patients with compromised airways are nursed in a high-dependency area where close monitoring of ventilation can be carried out.

Postoperative Analgesia

Although traditionally codeine phosphate has been the drug of choice to produce postoperative analgesia after neurosurgery, recent work has shown that morphine produces more effective and longer lasting analgesia; in addition,morphine is not associated with an increased rate of side effects. It is rapidly replacing codeine as the first-line drug postoperatively.

Hormone Replacement

Most centers continue to prescribe regular hydrocortisone during the postoperative period, although this may be unnecessary for some patients. Most units performing several hypophysectomies have their own protocols (drawn up with their endocrinology colleagues) for hormone replacement.

REFERENCES

1. Randeva HS, Schoebel J, Byrne J, Esiri M, Adams CB, Wass JA. Classical pituitary apoplexy: clinical features, management and outcome. Clin Endocrinol (Oxf) 1999;51(2):181–188.
2. Hout WM, Arafah BM, Salazar R, Selman W. Evaluation of the hypothalamic-pituitary-adrenal axis immediately after pituitary adenomectomy: is perioperative steroid therapy necessary? J Clin Endocrinol Metab 1988;66(6):1208–1212.

3. Hardy J, Vezina JL. Transphenoidal neurosurgery of intracranial neoplasm. In: Thompson RA, Green JR, eds, *Advances in Neurology*. New York:Raven Press;1976.

ADDITIONAL READING

Bradley KM, Adams CB, Potter CP, Wheeler DW, Anslow PJ, Burke CW. An audit of selected patients with non-functioning pituitary adenoma treated by transsphenoidal surgery without irradiation. Clin Endocrinol (Oxf) 1994;41(5):655–659.

Couldwell WT, Weiss MH. The transnasal transphenoidal approach. In: Apuzzo MLJ, ed. *Surgery of the Third Ventricle.* 2nd ed. Baltimore: Williams and Wilkins;1998, pp. 553–574.

Kaptain GJ, Vincent DA, Sheehan JP, Laws ER, Jr. Transsphenoidal approaches for the extracapsular resection of midline suprasellar and anterior cranial base lesions. Neurosurgery 2001;49(1):94–100; discussion 100–101.

Pituitary Tumors. Recommendations for service provision and guidelines for management of patients. Consensus statement of a working party. London: Royal College of Physicians of London;1997.

Smith M, Hirsch NP. Pituitary disease and anaesthesia. Brit J Anaesth 2000;85(1):3–14.

8 Transsphenoidal Surgery

Kamal Thapar, MD, PhD, FRCS (C)
and Edward R. Laws, Jr., MD, FACS

CONTENTS

INTRODUCTION

In this chapter, surgery of pituitary tumors and associated sellar lesions is reviewed. Because much of contemporary pituitary surgery is the development of techniques of transsphenoidal surgery, this approach is reviewed in detail. Surgical indications, evaluation of surgical strategy and technique, surgical complications, and new technical developments are discussed.

INDICATIONS FOR SURGERY

Although there are significant developments in the medical treatment of pituitary tumors, the only unquestionably successful therapy is that applied to prolactinomas. The majority of other symptomatic pituitary lesions are managed surgically. The classic surgical indications for sellar lesions include the following:

From: *Management of Pituitary Tumors: The Clinician's Practical Guide, Second Edition*
Edited by: M. P. Powell, S. L. Lightman, and E. R. Laws, Jr. © Humana Press Inc., Totowa, NJ

1. The most urgent indication for surgical intervention relates to instances of pituitary apoplexy *(1)*. Patients may present with either hemorrhage into an existing pituitary tumor or with acute necrosis of the tumor with subsequent swelling (Fig. 1). In the most florid of examples, the presentation includes sudden headache, visual loss, ophthalmoplegia, altered level of consciousness, and collapse from adrenal insufficiency. This is discussed in Chapter 7.
2. A second clear indication for surgery is progressive mass effect (usually visual loss) from a large macroadenoma or other sellar mass (Fig. 1). These patients should always have a serum prolactin (PRL) determination because prompt and dramatic shrinkage of prolactinomas can occur with appropriate pharmacologic management. More often, the PRL level is only modestly elevated and the patient has a clinically nonfunctioning pituitary tumor or other sellar mass. Such patients are in need of surgical decompression.
3. Among the hyperfunctioning pituitary adenomas, surgery is the treatment of choice for Cushing's disease (CD), acromegaly, and secondary hyperthyroidism. In CD, medical management is invariably suboptimal and surgery provides the best means of obtaining prompt and lasting remission. In somatotroph and thyrotroph adenomas, some latitude exists for the use of somatostatin analogs as the initial intervention; however, surgery remains the preferred, primary, and definitive treatment for these conditions. For prolactinomas, however, medical therapy is the preferred initial option in most instances.
4. Failure of previous therapy is an increasingly common indication for surgical intervention and usually occurs in one of several situations. The most straightforward are those patients with symptomatic recurrence in whom previous therapy resulted in a satisfactory remission. Other patients will have been treated with radiotherapy and, after a favorable initial response, now present with recurrence of symptoms, in the form of either mass effect or recurrent hormonal hypersecretion. Others will have been treated with medical therapy, with suboptimal response.
5. A final occasional surgical indication is the need for a tissue diagnosis. Although seldom required in the case of functioning pituitary adenomas, this indication may be important when the surgeon is confronted with a nonfunctioning sellar mass whose pathologic identity cannot be confirmed without histologic examination *(2)*.

CONTRAINDICATIONS TO SURGERY

Contraindications for surgery are very few, and most are relative rather than absolute. The most important contraindications relate to the general medical condition of the patient, which, in the face of florid CD, acromegaly, or secondary hyperthyroidism, can pose a significant anesthetic risk. In most cases, however, the medical condition of the patient can be stabilized without undue delay. Similarly, profound hypopituitarism can also be a temporary contraindication to surgery, although it should be fully responsive to steroid and thyroid replacement. Active

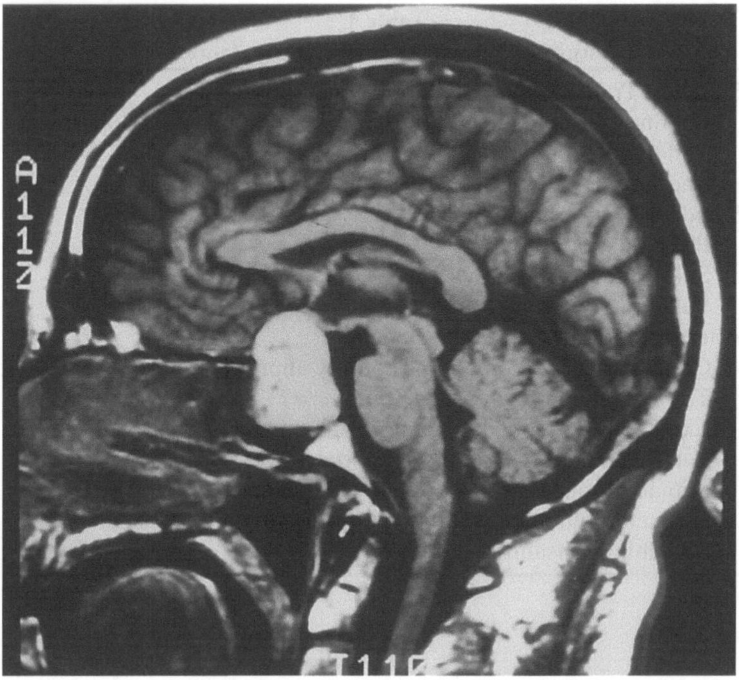

Fig. 1. Sagittal MRI (T1) of pituitary apoplexy with sudden enlargement of a preexisting pituitary macroadenoma.

sinus infection may also contraindicate the transsphenoidal approach, although this is generally responsive to appropriate antibiotic therapy. Very rarely MRI may reveal ectatic and tortuous carotid arteries that protrude from the region of the cavernous sinus and obstruct transsphenoidal access.

CHOICE OF SURGICAL APPROACH

Surgical approaches to the sellar region can be broadly categorized into three basic groups: (1) transsphenoidal approaches, (2) conventional craniotomy, and (3) alternative skull-base approaches (Table 1). Within each of the three groups, there is one or more standard procedures, as well as a variety of technical variations and options that allow the operation to be tailored to the situation at hand. Currently, 96% of all pituitary adenomas can be approached through one or another variation of the transsphenoidal approach. The remainder require transcranial approaches, consisting of either standard pterional or subfrontal craniotomy or various skull-base approaches, which may be transcranial, extracranial, or a combination of the two.

Table 1
Surgical Approaches for Pituitary Tumors

Standard Transsphenoidal Approaches
Endonasal, submucosal, transseptal transsphenoidal approach
Endonasal, submucosal, septal pushover approach
Endoscopic transsphenoidal approach
Standard Transcranial Approaches
Pterional craniotomy
Subfrontal craniotomy
Subtemporal craniotomy
Alternative Skull base Approaches
Cranio-orbito-zygomatic osteotomy approach
Transbasal approach of Dcerome
Extended transsphenoidal approach
Lateral rhinotomy/paranasal approaches
Sublabial transseptal approach with nasomaxillary osteotomy
Transethmoidal and extended transethmoidal approaches
Sublabial transantral approach

The surgical approach depends on a several factors. The most important of these include: (1) the size of the sella, (2) its degree of mineralization, (3) the size and pneumatization of the sphenoid sinus, (4) the position and tortuosity of the carotid arteries, (5) the presence and direction of any intracranial tumor extensions, (6) whether any uncertainty exists about the pathology of the lesion, (7) whether any previous therapy has been administered (surgery, pharmacologic, or radiotherapeutic), and (8) the surgeon's experience .

As general guidelines, a transsphenoidal approach is preferred in all but the following circumstances: (1) a tumor with significant anterior extension into the anterior cranial fossa or lateral and/or posterior extension into the middle or posterior cranial fossae, (2) a tumor with suprasellar extension and an hour-glass configuration that is constrained by a small diaphragmatic aperture, (3) when there is reason to believe that the consistency of a tumor having suprasellar extension is sufficiently fibrous to prevent its collapse and descent into the sella when resected from below, and (4) if there is doubt about the actual nature of the pathology (for example, meningioma). If any of these features is present, a transcranial procedure is preferred. It is important to recognize that these classic guidelines are less absolute today than they were in the past. The development of the extended transsphenoidal approach has now provided transsphenoidal access to several lesions that, in light of our guidelines, would have previously been considered accessible by transcranial approaches only. The spectrum of lesions accessible to transsphenoidal surgery is widening.

Occasionally the configuration of the tumor is such that a single approach, either transsphenoidal or transcranial, is insufficient to remove the tumor. This is uncommon and is typically associated with dumb-bell shaped tumors with a significant intrasellar component that has grown up through and has been narrowed by the diaphragmatic aperture. The suprasellar component in such cases may be inaccessible from below, whereas the infrasellar component may not be safely and readily accessible from above. Similarly, such bicompartimentalization occurs when an intrasellar component is associated with anterior, lateral, and retrosellar intracranial extensions into the anterior, middle, and posterior cranial fossae.

ESTABLISHING SURGICAL GOALS AND AN OVERALL PROGRAM OF MANAGEMENT

After presurgical assessment and before surgery, the surgical objective and its role in the overall management plan should always be considered. This is usually simple. For example, in the otherwise healthy patient in whom a clinically nonfunctioning macroadenoma is compromising vision, the surgical objectives would be decompression of the optic apparatus and an attempt at gross total tumor resection. The management plan would include long-term postoperative surveillance for and treatment of hypopituitarism and possible tumor recurrence. However, treatment decisions can be more complicated. For example, in the patient with acromegaly with a macroadenoma whose size and invasiveness are too great for a surgical cure, the aim would be decompression of neural structures and maximal reduction of tumor burden. The management plan would include normalization of growth hormone (GH)/insulin-like growth hormone factor (IGF)-1 levels with various forms of pharmacotherapy, consideration of radiation therapy (radiosurgery or conventional irradiation), and long-term surveillance/treatment of acromegaly-related complications (secondary neoplasms, cardiovascular disease, and so forth). The surgical objectives, the surgical management alternatives, and the potential need of additional therapy should be understood by both surgeon and patient at the outset.

TRANSSPHENOIDAL SURGERY

For the majority of pituitary tumors, some form of transsphenoidal surgery is the most appropriate route *(3–4)*. Usually this is a standard microsurgical submucosal transseptal transsphenoidal procedure. There are many virtues of the transsphenoidal approach. Most importantly, it is the least traumatic route of surgical access to the sella, providing excellent visualization of the pituitary gland and adjacent pathology. The lack of visible scars, lower morbidity and mortality as compared with transcranial procedures, the necessity of only a brief hospital stay, the relatively brief recuperative period, and the overall safety of the procedure add to the procedure's appeal.

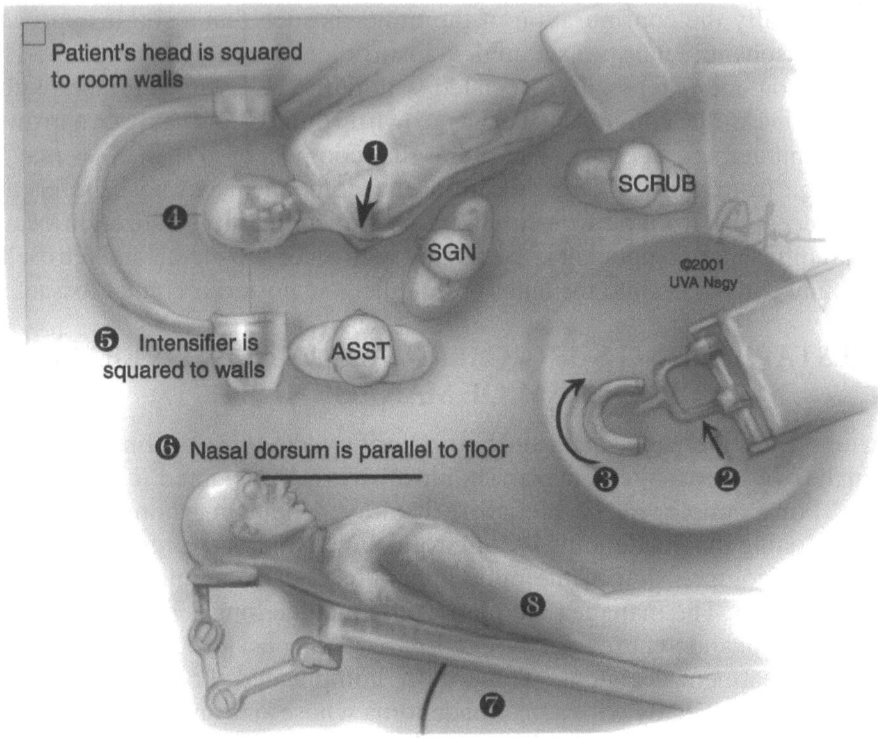

Fig. 2. (A) Positioning of patient for transsphenoidal surgery. *1*, Right shoulder at the top of right edge of table. *2*, Mayfield headrest. *3*, Horseshoe support for head angled to the left. *4*, Head parallel to the walls of the room. *5*, C-arm image intensifier perpendicular to the walls of the room. *6*, Bridge of nose parallel to floor. *7*, Thorax elevated 20–30°. *8*, Right lower quadrant of abdomen exposed and "prepped" for fat graft.

Procedure

The procedure is performed under general anesthesia, with the patient placed in a semirecumbent position (Fig. 2A). Some surgeons prefer to operate from the head of the table, with the patient's head in extension, facing toward the patient's feet (Fig. 2B). Because pituitary reserve for the pituitary-adrenal axis may be impaired, it is customary to administer a regimen of "stress dose" exogenous corticosteroids both during surgery and in the immediate postoperative period. The indications for this are reviewed in Chapters 7 and 9. Antibiotic prophylaxis is usually employed, although many leading surgeons dispense with this.

The procedure requires some form of navigational guidance to ensure a safe trajectory to the sella. The standard apparatus for this has been, and continues to be, videofluoroscopy. More recently, there has been increasing reliance on com-

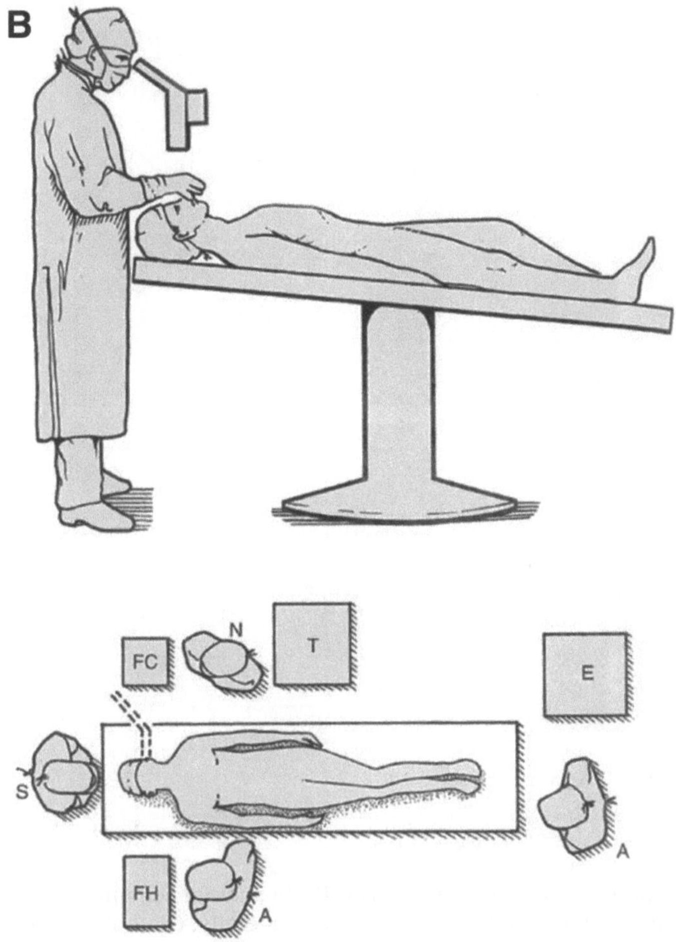

Fig. 2. (B) Alternative positioning, popular in many European centers.

puter-assisted image-guided neuronavigational systems for this purpose *(5)*. Such frameless stereotactic systems give the surgeon more information for transsphenoidal surgery and a safe trajectory in both the sagittal *and* the coronal plane. In "reoperations," this is invaluable and minimizes the likelihood of loss of the midline, making the procedure considerably safer. After the nose and face have been cleansed with an aqueous-based antiseptic solution, application of decongestants and submucosal infiltration of the nasal mucosa with a dilute (1:200,000) epinephrine solution significantly reduce bleeding and make submucosal dissection easier.

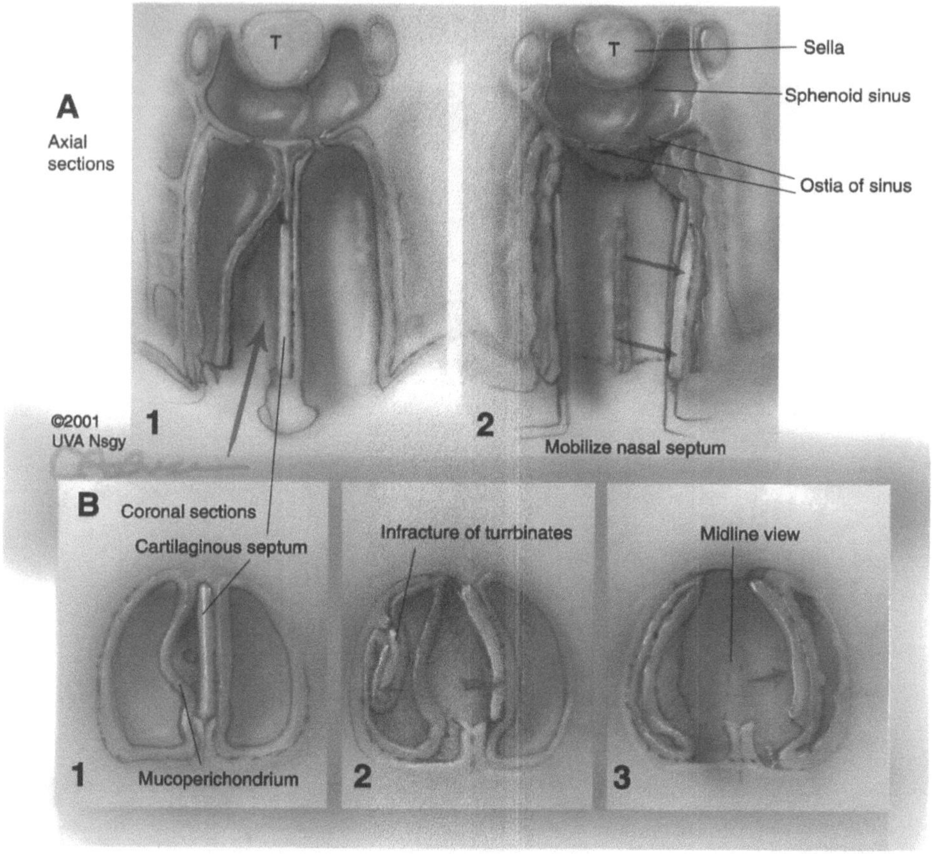

Fig. 3. Septal flaps and nasal dissection. (A) *1*, Right anterior submucosal tunnel. *2*, Nasal septum with adherent left-sided mucosa displaced laterally. (B) *1*, Anterior septal tunnel. *2*, Fracture of turbinate and displacement of septum. *3*, Exposure of the face of sphenoid. T, tumor.

There are three approaches to the sphenoid sinus: the endonasal submucosal approach, the sublabial approach, and the direct transnasal septal pushover approach. Selection of one over the others depends on the size of the nostril, the size of the lesion, the presence of previous nasal surgery, and the surgeon's preference. We tend to favor the basic endonasal approach in most instances. We reserve the sublabial incision for larger and more difficult lesions when a broader corridor of surgical access is required, and tend to use the transnasal septal pushover technique in the setting of previous nasal surgery or among pediatric patients.

Our standard endonasal approach involves a right hemitransfixtion incision over the caudal aspect of the nasal septum, allowing a submucosal plane of dissection to be fashioned on one side of the septum. The dissection continues posteriorly, elevating the nasal mucosa away from the cartilaginous septum back to its junction with the bony septum (Fig. 3). A vertical incision is then made at this junction point, and bilateral posterior submucosal tunnels are created on either side of the perpendicular plate of the ethmoid. The articulation of the cartilaginous septum with the maxilla is then dissected free, and an attempt is made to raise the inferior mucosal tunnel on the opposite side so that the cartilaginous septum can be displaced laterally without creating inferior mucosal tears. A self-retaining nasal speculum can then be introduced to straddle the perpendicular plate of the ethmoid, exposing the face of the sphenoid sinus. A portion of the perpendicular plate is removed and preserved for eventual sellar reconstruction.

Once the anterior face of the sphenoid sinus is reached, videofluoroscopy or neuronavigational image guidance is used to make any necessary adjustments to the final position and trajectory of the retractor blades. The correct orientation is crucial at this stage, with respect not only to the midline but also to the eventual approach window, defined superiorly by the tuberculum and inferiorly by the clivus. Too acute an angle will result in penetration of the anterior fossa floor, whereas too obtuse an angle will direct one toward the midclivus. Identification of the vomer and the sphenoid ostia on either side are useful landmarks, and having them in the center of the field generally prevents misdirection in these early stages of the exposure (Fig. 4). Once the operating microscope has been introduced, the anterior wall of the sphenoid is opened with small-bone rongeurs and Kerrison punches and the sinus is entered.

The mucosa within the sinus is resected, reducing bleeding and decreasing the risk of postoperative mucocele formation. With the internal sphenoid bony landmarks now clearly visible, the surgeon checks orientation with respect to the carotid arteries, the sellar floor, the anterior fossa floor (Fig. 4), and clivus. Correlating the operative anatomy with the neuronavigational data ensures that the trajectory is both midline and within the approach window.

The sellar floor should be clearly visible. With some tumors, the sellar floor is so eroded or thin that it can be fractured with a blunt hook. If the floor of the sella is thick, a small chisel can be used to remove a square of bone. A high-speed drill with diamond burr will gently remove particularly thick fossa bone in safety, a useful maneuver in the underpneumatized fossa and in Cushing's microadenomas. Continuous videofluoroscopic control or image-guidance monitoring ensure safe sellar entry, exposure, and trajectory. Once the sellar floor has been opened, it is widened with a Kerrison punch. Adequate bony exposure is crucial to the success of the transsphenoidal approach, extending from one cavernous sinus to the other in the lateral direction and from just short of the junction of the anterior fossa floor and sella to the clivus in the other, particularly when dealing with large tumors. We advocate wide bony removal in virtually every case.

Exposure within the sella proper is carried out with the operating microscope magnification adjusted so that the sella fills the entire field of vision. An invasive

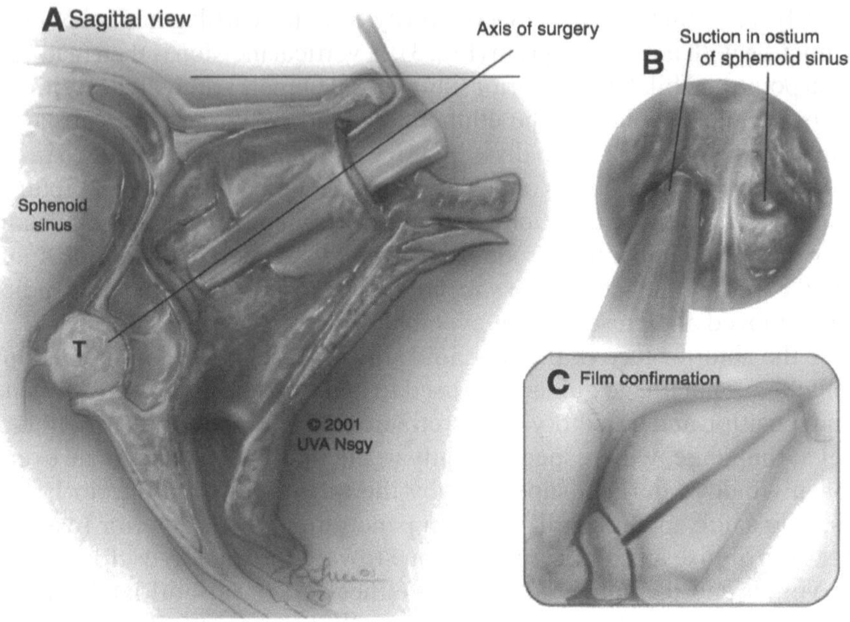

Fig. 4. (A) Trajectory of approach to tumor in sella. (B) Exposure of sphenoid ostium. (C) Lateral radiograph to confirm anatomic position.

tumor may erode through the anterior dura of the sella, but in most cases the dura will be intact. Before the dural incision is made, the position of the carotid arteries should be noted from the imaging and thus avoided (Fig. 5). The site of dural opening is selected, cauterized, and incised either in a cruciate fashion or with the excision of a dural window. A subdural cleavage plane between the pituitary gland or tumor and the underlying dura is then developed.

For the typical macroadenoma, the tumor is entered with a ring curette, loosened, and then removed with a relatively blunt curette and forceps (Fig. 6). Tumor removal should be done in an orderly fashion. Our practice has been to first remove the tumor in the inferior aspect and then proceed laterally, from inferior to superior on both sides, removing tumor along the medial side of the cavernous sinus.

One must resist coring the central and most accessible portion of the tumor first, because this may cause premature descent of the diaphragma and entrapment of more laterally situated tumor, and delay the superior dissection until the lesion is relatively free elsewhere. This minimizes trauma to the pituitary stalk and secondarily transmitted trauma to the hypothalamus. Occasionally it may be necessary to follow the tumor into one cavernous sinus or the other or to deal with a tumor directly involving the diaphragma. In either instance, any maneuver

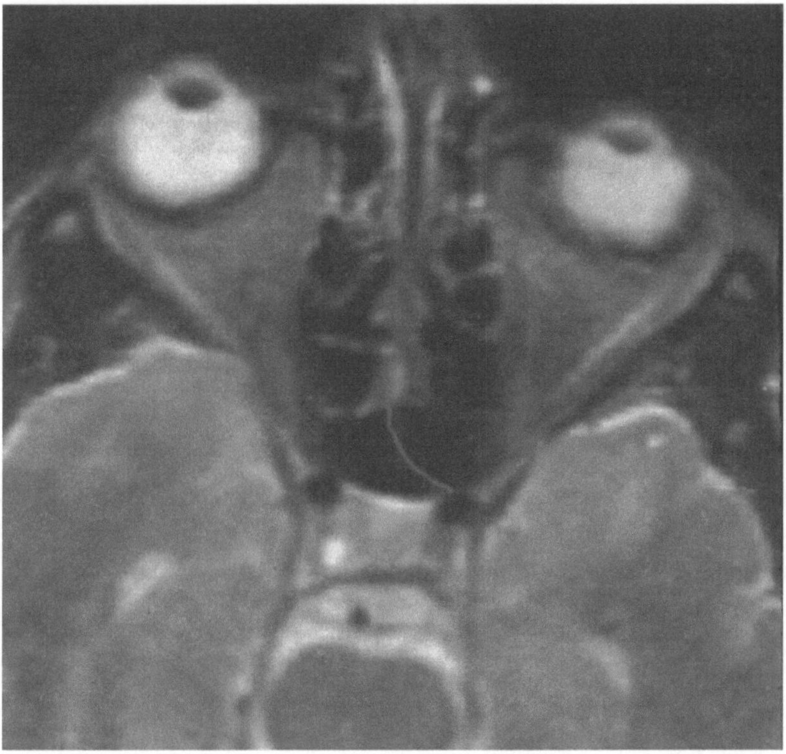

Fig. 5. T2 axial MRI showing classic source of error. The sphenoid septum starts behind the base of the vomer and swings over to lie immediately in front of the left carotid.

more forceful than gentle curetting may be a dangerous move and pulling adherent fragments must be avoided.

Decompression of the intrasellar portion of the tumor frequently permits a suprasellar extension to prolapse into view within the sella. Once this has been resected, the diaphragma subsequently prolapses and generally signifies that the resection is complete. Some surgeons use a temporary increase in intracranial pressure to improve descent of the suprasellar component. The Valsalva maneuver, performed by the anesthetist is popular, although higher and slightly more prolonged pressure increases are achieved with a lumbar drain introduced at the time of the induction of anethesia.

Verification that no residual tumor remains is provided by direct inspection or with the help of dental mirror, a nasopharyngoscope, or a small fiber-optic endoscope. Bleeding from the tumor bed can usually be controlled by tamponade with cotton patties or Gelfoam.

In all cases, a concerted effort is made to preserve normal pituitary tissue. In a large diffuse adenoma, normal glandular tissue usually appears as a thin mem-

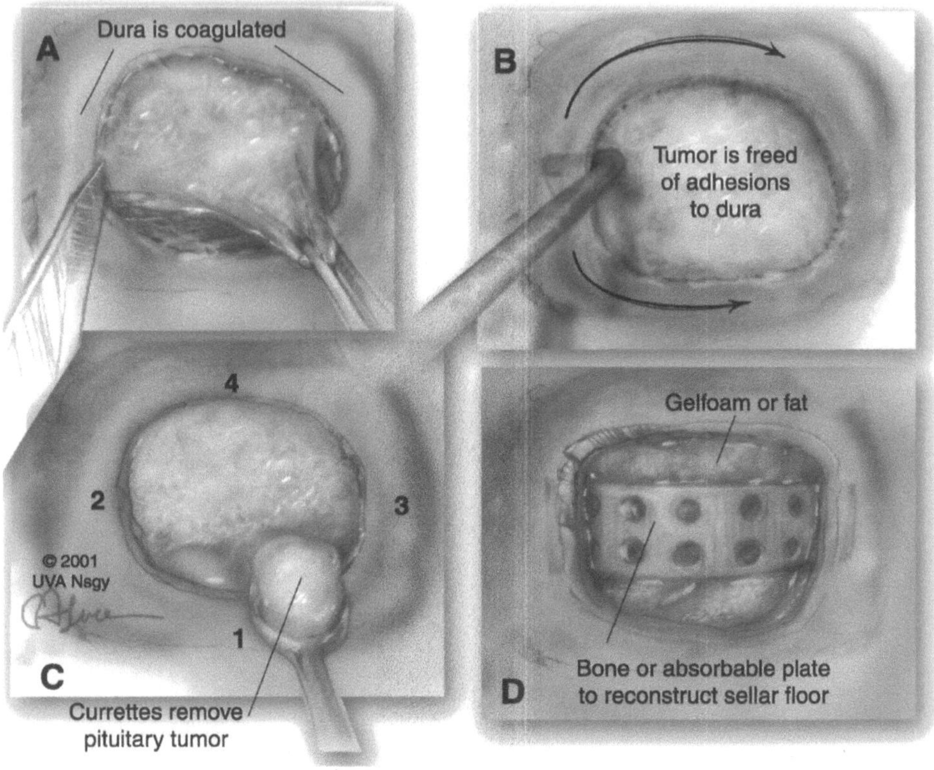

Fig. 6. Sellar dissection. (A) Coagulation and excision of dura of sellar floor. (B) Subdural dissection with right-angled hook. (C) Removal of tumor tissue, sequential steps. (D) Reconstruction of sellar floor.

brane, situated superolaterally against the sellar wall. The orange-yellow color of the gland, together with its firm consistency, distinguishes it from the grayish color and finely granular texture typical of the tumor. A biopsy of the suspected glandular remnant may be taken for confirmation, but the appearance is often so typical that this tissue can be left behind with confidence.

Microadenomas require a different strategy because it is well recognized that many will not be seen upon opening the dura. In these cases, a systematic search through an apparently normal gland is required. We begin with a transverse glandular incision, followed by subdural dissection and mobilization of the lateral wings. If the incision in the gland is deep enough, lateral pressure with a Hardy dissector usually causes the microadenoma to herniate into the operative field. Its location can then be delineated, its cavity entered, and its removal completed by use of a small ring curette and cup forceps. All suspicious tissue is removed, and a biopsy specimen is occasionally obtained from the residual and presumed normal pituitary gland.

Special mention is necessary for the approach to microadenomas in CD. A careful and systematic dissection of the sellar contents is required. If a tumor is not evident upon opening the dura or after examining all glandular surfaces, the gland must be incised and systematically explored. Subtle changes in tissue color, texture, or the contour of the gland will aid in the identification of an adenoma and distinguish it from the normal gland. If no adenoma is found, excisional biopsies from within the substance of the gland are obtained, beginning with the central mucoid wedge. If an adenoma is not evident in the resected material, the lateral wings of the gland are carefully inspected and resected as necessary. Where no obvious tumor is found in the adult for whom fertility is not an issue, a subtotal hypophysectomy may be performed, leaving only a stump of residual anterior lobe tissue attached to the stalk. If careful examination of the resected tissues still fails to reveal the adenoma, both cavernous sinuses and the posterior lobe must be inspected. The latter has, on rare occasion, been known to harbor a minute adenomatous nodule. Failing to see an adenoma raises the possibility of a supradiaphragmatic tumor nodule. Given the additional operative risks of a diaphragmatic breach, one would not ordinarily contemplate transdiaphragmatic exploration without clear imaging evidence pointing to such a possibility.

After the tumor has been removed and hemostasis has been achieved, the sella must be reconstructed and closed. We prefer not to leave dead space in the sella. If no cerebrospinal fluid (CSF) leak has occurred, the sella is loosely packed with Gelfoam. However, if there is a CSF leak, some form of tissue graft becomes mandatory. Reconstruction of the sellar roof can be attempted with a piece of homologous dural graft material or fascia lata; however, this step probably adds little to the security of the seal. Current practice favors simple packing of the sella with fat taken from the right lower quadrant of the abdomen. The fat is soaked in chloramphenicol solution, rolled in Avitene, trimmed to appropriate size, and snugly placed within the sella. In either case, the sellar floor is then carefully reconstructed using a suitably trimmed piece of cartilage or bone. In cases where previous surgery has been performed and no bone is available, alternative materials for closure include banked bone allograft, slowly resorbable polymer stents, or methylmethacrylate.

If an intraoperative CSF leak has occurred, the sphenoid sinus is packed with fat, but in the absence of a leak, it is left free of foreign material. The posterior septal space may be re-implanted with crushed nasal bone and cartilage. The septal flaps are re-approximated, and the nasal septum is returned to its midline insertion. Any accessible mucosal tears are repaired with fine catgut sutures. Bilateral endonasal packs, consisting of gauze packing within the “fingers” of a rubber glove that have been lubricated with petroleum jelly or antibiotic ointment, are placed in the nostrils. The nasal and/or gingival incisions are closed with interrupted 4-0 catgut sutures, and a gauze mustache dressing is applied.

Complications of the Transsphenoidal Approach

The transsphenoidal approach is safe and has a low complication rate. In fact, it is one of the safest procedures in contemporary neurosurgical practice. As determined by several retrospective cumulative series, operative mortality and major morbidity rates are 0.5% and 2.2%, respectively *(6)*. In one of the most recent series of transsphenoidal surgeries performed for CD during the current decade, mortality and permanent morbidity rates were 0.9% and 1.8%, respectively *(7)*.

Operative deaths, though fortunately rare, are usually the result of intracranial hemorrhage, hypothalamic damage, or meningitis related to CSF fistulas. A variety of other complications can also occur with this approach *(8)*.

Hypothalamic Injury

Damage to the hypothalamus may result from direct surgical injury and also from hemorrhage or ischemia provoked by the procedure. Clinical manifestations of hypothalamic damage include death, coma, diabetes insipidus, memory loss, and disturbances of vegetative functions (morbid obesity, uncontrollable hunger or thirst, and disturbances in temperature regulation). Such complications are more frequent in patients with previous craniotomy or radiation *(9)*. A gentle surgical technique and avoidance of traction on the tumor capsule and pituitary stalk will minimize the occurrence of such injuries.

Visual Damage

Damage to the optic nerves and chiasm can also occur from direct surgical trauma, hemorrhage, or ischemia. Fractures of bony structures at the base of the skull can damage optic nerves and can occur from misdirected placement and aggressive opening of transsphenoidal retractors. Many patients have preoperative compromise of visual function, making them more vulnerable to further damage. Assessment of the bony anatomy, careful and gentle technique, confirmation of surgical landmarks, and effective use of navigational guidance to direct the approach are important measures for avoiding these complications. Finally, at the time of sellar reconstruction, overpacking the sella can cause chiasmal compression, whereas under packing can, occasionally, lead to a secondary empty sella with the late onset of visual loss caused by chiasmatic prolapse (a single personal case and three or four further cases from previous surgery elsewhere).

Vascular Complications

Although rare, arterial injury is a well-known complication of transsphenoidal surgery and is one of the main causes of operative mortality of the procedure *(1)*.

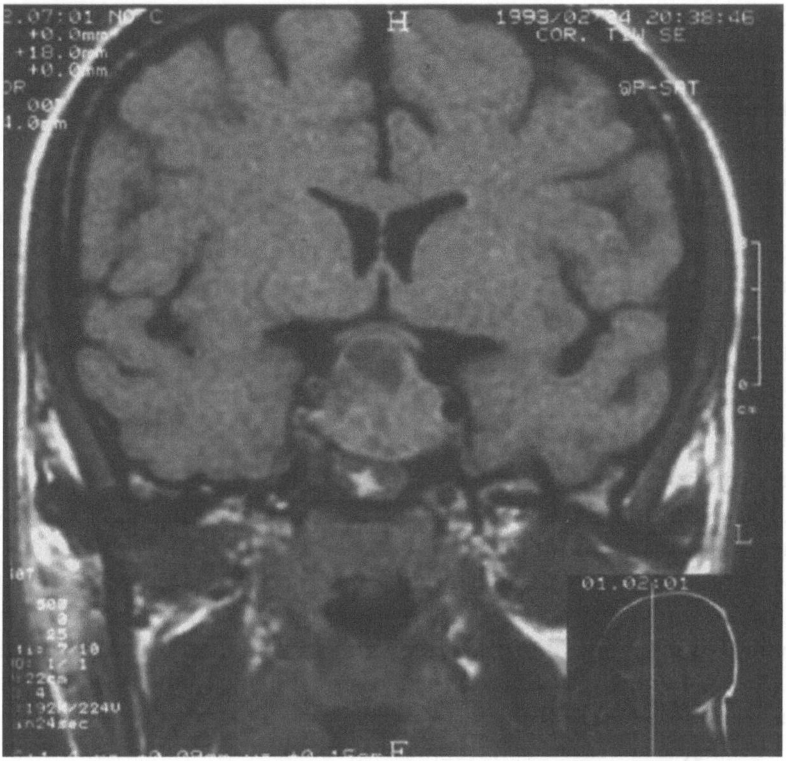

Fig. 7. A traumatic aneurysm compressing the chiasm, seen on top of a GH macroadenoma in a coronal unenhanced T1 MRI scan. The surgeon had missed the midline, damaged the carotid, and abandoned the procedure. The patient survived an intercontinental flight despite arterial nasal hemmorrhage and was managed by endovascular coil occlusion of the aneurysm, transsphenoidal surgery, and radiotherapy.

Virtually every transsphenoidal series includes at least one example of arterial injury, most of which have proven fatal (Fig. 7). The intracavernous portion of the carotid artery tends to be the most vulnerable, followed by other components of the Circle of Willis. Because the tumor may be quite adherent to arterial structures, arteries may be lacerated, perforated, avulsed, or damaged such that they develop spasm or intraluminal thrombosis. Intracranial hemorrhage, thrombotic and embolic stroke, and the development of false aneurysms or carotid-cavernous fistulae are the usual sequelae of such injuries. When vascular injury is suspected, tamponade should be used to control hemorrhage and an immediate postoperative angiogram obtained. If a false aneurysm is seen, it should be obliterated by endovascular means. Again, a gentle technique devoid of aggressive traction on the tumor capsule, not deviating from the midline, and repeated assessment of bony landmarks are the most effective means of avoiding these devastating complications.

Cerebrospinal Fluid Rhinorrhea

CSF rhinorrhea and meningitis are among the more common serious complications associated with transsphenoidal surgery. It is the result of disruption of the sellar diaphragm, which is usually thinned, adherent to tumor, and susceptible to direct or traction injury. In the presence of a leak, careful closure of the sella is crucial. In the postoperative period, close observation for leaks and a high index of suspicion for possible meningitis is crucial. Postoperative leaks are usually obvious at the time the nasal packing is removed and are best managed by prompt transsphenoidal re-exploration, identification of the leak, and resealing.

Cavernous Sinus Injury

Pituitary tumors involve the cavernous sinus with some regularity. In some cases, the tumor may be adherent to the medial wall of the sinus only, whereas in other more invasive tumors, frank invasion of the sinus interstices occurs. Injury to the cavernous sinus and its contents can occur as the surgeon is stripping the tumor from the medial dura, following the tumor into the sinus, or overzealously packing sinus bleeding. The carotid artery and the sixth cranial nerve are most vulnerable to such maneuvers; the third and fourth cranial nerves are damaged less frequently.

Iatrogenic Hypopituitarism

In most instances, existing pituitary function can usually be preserved. Among microadenomas, our recent experience indicates that loss of one or more anterior pituitary functional axis occurs in approx 3% of cases *(10)*. For macroadenomas, we have found that anterior pituitary function can be preserved in more than 95% of cases, provided that pituitary function was normal preoperatively. In contrast, patients with established preoperative endocrine deficits, partial or complete restoration of endocrine function is achieved in only 16%. Although temporary diabetes insipidus occurs in one third of all patients, it is permanent in no more than 3%.

Brainstem Injury

Damage to the brainstem may occur with a misdirected approach that violates the clivus, or more commonly, when a larger tumor erodes the clivus, exposing the underlying dura.

Nasal Complications

Generally less immediate and rarely fatal, complications relating to the nasofacial aspect of the procedure can be annoying and persist for some time after surgery. The use of too much force when spreading the retractor may result in diastasis or fracture of the hard palate or the cribriform plate, the latter being another source of CSF rhinorrhea. In the postoperative period, the mucosa of the sphenoid sinus may become infected, giving rise to a febrile sinusitis and the eventual development of a mucocele. Inadequate hemostasis in the nasal portion of the procedure may lead to superficial would hemorrhage and swelling. Careless handling of the nasal mucosa, the nasal septum, and the nasal spine may result in an external nasal deformity, which may be distressing, both cosmetically and functionally. Loss of smell can also occur, presumably because of damage to nerve endings in the nasal mucosa. Finally, overaggressive enlargement of the basal pyriform aperture can damage distal branches of the alveolar nerves and/or vessels, which may devitalize or desensitize the teeth and gums of the maxilla.

NEW DEVELOPMENTS IN TRANSSPHENOIDAL SURGERY

Endoscopic Approaches

This important development is addressed in Chapter 10.

Neuronavigational Guidance

Some form of guidance has always been an essential component of modern pituitary surgery. Whereas videofluoroscopy has served the purpose extremely well, frameless stereotaxy with archived computed tomography (CT) or magnetic resonance imaging (MRI) exploits the whole concept of neuronavigation to its fullest *(5)*. Frameless stereotaxy allows precise planning of the approach with reference to lesion perimeters, anatomic landmarks such as the carotid arteries, and other potential operative hazards. Again, as mentioned, it is particularly helpful in reoperative pituitary surgery where few normal anatomic landmarks remain. In addition to encouraging early reports, citing low complication rates and good operative outcomes, there is no question that frameless stereotaxy adds greatly to surgeon comfort and confidence during the procedure. However, the surgeon using the technique must always remember that the information used is based on navigation points that are prerecorded and are only as accurate as the system allows in a perfectly set-up state. Minor movement in the pin holders results in a disastrous loss of accuracy.

Image-Guided Pituitary Tumor Resection: **Intraoperative Magnetic Resonance Imaging**

For all tumors, complete tumor resection is advantageous. In hormonally active tumors, endocrine remission requires complete removal, and for nonfunctioning tumors we believe radical resection is of importance in reducing recurrence. One of the most difficult skills to acquire in pituitary surgery is knowing when this has been achieved. Difficulties in assessing completeness occur for several reasons. These include the small operative field, the need to see recesses of the sella beyond limits of direct vision, the reliance upon indirect clues such as alterations in diaphragmatic contour and descent, and perhaps vague fullness evident upon palpation with micro-instruments.

Intraoperative MRI takes away this reliance on experience and should be a major advance in resection control. Surgery is performed with the patient lying directly on the table of the MRI scanner. After the standard transsphenoidal procedure, an intraoperative MRI scan is performed while the operative exposure and sterile field are both maintained so that if residual tumor is seen, further resection is undertaken. Although the precise role of intraoperative MRI in pituitary tumor surgery awaits further definition, it is possible that future developments in this technology will enhance the effectiveness of transsphenoidal surgery.

Other Advances

An important advance during recent years has been the realization that repeat transsphenoidal surgery represents a good option in selected patients with recurrent or persistent disease. In the past, there was a reluctance to undertake reoperations for pituitary tumors because of technical difficulties and higher complication rates *(9)*. Consequently, radiotherapy was usually given as an alternative. Today, when undertaken by a surgeon with well-developed skills, it is a safe and effective option. Our own experience indicates that complication rates are now only minimally higher than those of initial operations. Techniques such as the transnasal septal pushover, which obviates difficult septal dissection and provides safe access through a previously operative field, have contributed to this success *(11)*. Neuronavigational techniques and endoscopic assistance have also added to the safety.

A final innovation has been the development of the extended transsphenoidal approach, which broadens the range of transsphenoidal surgery, to include lesions previously believed accessible only to transcranial approaches. Not only does this include adenomas with unusual configurations but also other mass lesions, particularly craniopharyngiomas with suprasellar, retrosellar, or anterosellar dispositions. This approach, which is as much a conceptual advance as it is technical, involves greater resection of skull base from below and permits removal of genuine intracranial pathology via the transsphenoidal route. In doing so, it pushes the limits of transsphenoidal surgery to a new frontier *(12)*.

REFERENCES

1. Laws ER Jr. Vascular complications of transsphenoidal surgery. Pituitary 1999;2:163–170.
2. Thapar K and Kovacs K. Tumors of the sella region. In: Bigner DD, McLendon RE, Bruner JM, eds. *Russel and Rubinstein's Pathology of Tumors of the Nervous System.* Baltimore: Williams and Wilkins; 1998:561–677.

3. Laws ER Jr, Thapar K. 1995. Surgical management of pituitary adenoma. J Clin Endocrinol Metabol 1995;9:391–406.
4. Elias WJ, Laws ER Jr. Trans-sphenoidal approaches to lesions of the sella. Schmidek HH, ed. *Schmidek and Sweet Operative Neurosurgical Techniques*. Philadelphia: WB Saunders; 2000.
5. Elias W, Chadduck J, Alden T, Laws ER Jr. Frameless stereotaxy for transsphenoidal surgery. Neurosurgery 1999;45:271–277.
6. Zervas NT. Surgical results for pituitary adenomas: results of an international survey. In: Black PM, Zervas NT, Ridgeway EC, Martin J, eds. New York: Raven Press; 1992:377–385.
7. Semple P, Laws E. Complications in a contemporary series of patients who underwent surgery for Cushing's disease. J Neurosurg 1999;91:175–179.
8. Laws ER Jr and Kern EB.Complications of transsphenoidal surgery. Clin Neurosurg 1976;23:401–416.
9. Laws ER Jr, Fode NC, Redmond MJ. Transsphenoidal surgery following unsuccessful prior therapy. J. Neurosurg 1985;63:823–829.
10. Laws ER Jr, Thapar K. Pituitary surgery. Endocrinol Metab Clin North Am 1999;28:119–131.
11. Wilson WR, Laws ER Jr. Transnasal septal displacement approach for secondary transsphenoidal surgery. Laryngoscope 1992;102:951–953.
12. Kaptain GJ, Vincent DA, Sheehan JP, Laws ER Jr. Trans-sphenoidal approaches for the extracapsular resection of midline suprasellar and anterior cranial base lesions. Neurosurgery 2001;49:94–101.

ADDITIONAL READING

Cappabianca P, AlfieriA, deDevitiis E. Endoscopic endonasal transsphenoidal approach to the sella: towards functional endoscopic pituitary surgery (FEPS). Minim Invas Neurosurgery 1998;41:66–73.

Ebersold MJ, Quast LM, Laws ER Jr., Scheithauer B, Randall RV. Long-term results in transsphenoidal removal of nonfunctioning pituitary adenomas. J Neurosurg 1986;64:713–719.

Jho H. Endoscopic pituitary surgery. Pituitary 1999;2:139–154.

Laws ER Jr., Chenelle AG, Thapar K. Recurrence after transsphenoidal surery for pituitary adenomas: clinical and basic science aspects. In: Von Verder K and Fahlbusch R, eds. *Pituitary Adenomas—From Basic Research to Diagnosis and Therapy. Amsterdam: Elsevier; 1996:3–9.*

Laws ER, Vance M. Radiosurgery for pituitary adenomas and craniopharyngiomas. Neurosurg Clin North Am 1999;10:327–336.

Laws ER, Vance M, Thapar K. Pituitary surgery for the management of acromegaly. Horm Res 2000;53:71–75.

Powell MP, Thompson D: The neurosurgical approach to the hypothalamo-hypophyseal tumors. In: Brook CB, ed. *Clinical Paediatric Endocrinology*. Oxford: Blackwell; 1995:349–357.

9 Transcranial Surgery

Michael P. Powell, MB, BS, FRCS
and Jonathan R. Pollock, BM, BCh, FRCS (S/N)

CONTENTS

INTRODUCTION

Although there was once a debate about the merits of transsphenoidal and transcranial surgeries, this argument is now outdated. The introduction of selective microadenomectomy by Hardy has focused the attention of the subsequent generation of neurosurgeons upon the intrasellar aspects of pituitary surgery *(1)*. Removal of a microadenoma is unarguably better performed from below and, therefore, the number of transsphenoidal procedures wordwide has risen up dramatically since the 1960s. With this accumulation of experience, the transsphenoidal operation has been increasingly applied where it was formerly contraindicated, especially to suprasellar tumors *(2–6)*. In our practice, transsphenoidal surgery is the first option for the majority of tumors at first presentation, even for those with a large suprasellar component.

There is also an improving understanding of the behavior of nonfunctioning adenomas, which constitute most of the tumors with a suprasellar component. A transsphenoidal operation for a tumor with suprasellar extension may not provide complete tumor clearance, but because most tumors grow slowly, serial scanning for surveillance of the tumor remnant or timely radiotherapy may be preferable to a craniotomy, especially in high-risk patients.

From: *Management of Pituitary Tumors: The Clinician's Practical Guide, Second Edition*
Edited by: M. P. Powell, S. L. Lightman, and E. R. Laws, Jr. © Humana Press Inc., Totowa, NJ

Craniopharyngiomas deserve special mention. They are among the most difficult tumors to remove. Although they may be found in the intrasellar region and thereby removed relatively easily, when they extend into the third ventricle and hypothalamus they pose both difficult management and technical problems related to their invasiveness. In every pituitary surgeon's series, it is craniopharyngiomas that have the highest rate of complications, recurrence, and mortality. Seemingly successful surgery with a pristine postoperative scan can leave the patient with severe hypothalamic damage. In this chapter, we reference several approaches to craniopharyngiomas. To both the surgical editors, it seems that with increasing experience in specialization in sellar surgery, more and more operations on these tumors will be performed using the transsphenoidal procedure, particularly the extended transsphenoidal route.

Specific indications remain for the transcranial approach in a minority of cases, and these warrant separate discussion.

INDICATIONS FOR TRANSCRANIAL SURGERY

Indications for transcranial surgery are summarized in Table 1 and described under the following subheadings.

Tumors With a Large Suprasellar Component

Hardy's classification, as discussed in Chapter 7, allows a formal description of tumor size that remains helpful in defining likely candidates for a transcranial operation.

The merits of a transcranial operation for a large tumor depend on the clinical indication for surgery. For patients with visual failure, one apparent advantage of the transcranial approach is the direct view of the optic apparatus and the adjacent tumor. One might believe that this allows a better decompression of the optic apparatus than is possible with a transsphenoidal operation. This was the belief of the early exponents of pituitary surgery; Harvey Cushing found that recovery of normal vision occurred in 21% of his transfrontal cases, compared with 9% of those operated on via the transsphendoidal route *(7)*. In the modern era, however, it is clear that excellent visual results have been obtained from transsphenoidal surgery *(8,9)* and visual failure does not normally indicate the need for a transcranial operation.

For treating hormone excess, complete resection of the adenoma, which is required for cure, is most frequently achieved when the tumor is small and is approached transsphenoidally. Large endocrine tumors, on the other hand, are more difficult to cure irrespective of the approach; even an exemplary resection is not necessarily rewarded with a cure. Other characteristics of the tumor, apart from the size, may have a negative influence on endocrine outcome, especially the presence of dural or cavernous sinus invasion. As Laws observed in a

Table 1
Indications for Transcranial Surgery

Tumors with a large suprasellar component
Recurrent tumors with visual failure
Abnormal skull-base anatomy
Tough fibrous tumors
A small or underpneumatized fossa

reviewer's remark: "It is naive to think that one can perform a total removal of an invasive pituitary adenoma" *(10)*. Hence a complex transcranial procedure whose aim is to remove every fragment of tumor is likely to fail. Rather, the aim should be to remove as much tumor as possible in order to optimize the benefits of subsequent drug treatment or radiotherapy.

Recurrent Tumors With Visual Failure

Patients with visual failure form the largest transcranial group in the authors' series of recurrences. In patients with recurrent tumors, complete tumor removal is not a realistic goal if adverse prognostic features, such as cavernous sinus invasion, are present on magnetic resonance imaging (MRI) scan. With a functioning adenoma, a repeat transsphenoidal operation may be indicated. When the main symptom is visual failure and if it is clear that complete resection is not possible, the best approach is often to treat the symptomatic suprasellar component via a craniotomy.

Abnormal Skull-Base Anatomy

In patients who have had previous transsphenoidal or rhinologic surgery, the transsphenoidal approach to the sella is complicated by previous loss of anatomical landmarks. Since identification of the midline is essential for a safe operation that avoids the risk of carotid injury, the transcranial approach may be preferable in revision surgery if the tumor is mainly suprasellar. In our experience, the use of an interactive image-guidance system has greatly improved the degree of confidence with which repeat transsphenoidal surgery may be attempted, thus reducing the number of patients requiring a transcranial operation for this indication.

Firm Fibrous Tumor

Although an important practical problem, firm fibrous tumors have produced relatively little discussion in the literature. They may be difficult and dangerous to access from below, and the transcranial route may be preferred in such cases *(11)* or there may be an argument for leaving them alone. If the capsule of a firm tumor is closely applied to the chiasm, chiasmal vessels, pituitary stalk, or hypothalamus, then the traction required to remove it from below is associated with high morbidity from damage to these structures. The firm nature of the tumor may be discovered during a transsphenoidal operation, or the evidence may be inferred from preoperative radiology. Snow found that 70% of tumors that were isointense with surrounding brain on T2-weighted MRI were of firm consistency at surgery *(12)*.

Bromocriptine treatment is associated with an increased incidence of fibrosis *(13)*, and this may be anticipated in patients who have had a long preoperative course of the drug. It begs the question of the indications for the operation. Increased fibrosis has also been reported in patients with somatotroph adenomas pretreated with somatostatin analogs *(14,15)*, although this is not our experience. Patterson found that previous radiotherapy correlated with an increased incidence of a firm tumor at operation *(16)*. Rather than use a craniotomy in these cases, Abe observed that the tumor remnant descended into the sella during a 2-mo period after transsphenoidal operation *(17)*. He then employed a second transsphenoidal operation to remove the remnant; we have occasionally used this approach.

A Small or Underpneumatized Fossa

A small fossa with a large suprasellar lesion above is always a difficult technical challenge for the transsphenoidal approach. It is often found in conjunction with an underpneumatized sphenoid which we believe may be the cause of the extent of the suprasellar component.

This is a rare indication for transcranial surgery but can present problems even in adults. In children, we have usually operated successfully via the transsphenoidal route with the aid of a high-speed drill to access the sella *(18)*.

PRINCIPLES OF TRANSCRANIAL SURGERY

Conventional microsurgical techniques are applied to approach the sellar region regardless of which transcranial route is used. The operating microscope and micro-instruments are employed, and the approach is performed along anatomic tissue planes using as little retraction as possible.

Most authorities recommend starting high-dose steroids before surgery. In our unit, we give 8 mg dexamethasone intravenously with induction of anesthesia where there are no prior contraindications for its use. Pituitary tumors are usually operated on as elective cases and acutely raised intracranial pressure is not commonly present. Nevertheless, the sella is well concealed beneath the frontotemporal region and a relaxed brain is required, especially in younger patients with small extracerebral cerebrospinal (CSF) spaces. Further relaxation can be achieved by generous removal of CSF. A lumbar drain may be used, but in the authors' experiences, opening the basal cisterns early in the procedure to allow CSF drainage is a satisfactory alternative. Mannitol can be given to produce additional relaxation of the frontal lobes, if required.

The treatment of the optic apparatus requires particular care. The surgeon should resist the temptation to "strip" the tumor from the optic apparatus at craniotomy. The stretched optic nerves are extremely vulnerable, and the compressed vasa vasorum may be damaged, causing optic nerve ischemia *(19)*. Van Alphen went so far as to say: "Touching the optic nerve may cause a permanent visual defect" *(20)*.

We believe that the vulnerability of the optic nerves limits the usefulness of the cavitron ultrasonic surgical aspirator (CUSA), which becomes hot and is a potential cause of optic nerve injury, and also of the laser, which is also best avoided in this region. Piecemeal microsurgical tumor removal is always preferable.

In summary, suprasellar lesions can safely be approached and removed transcranially by careful adherence to microsurgical principles and with minimal technologic assistance.

TRANSCRANIAL APPROACHES

Several transcranial routes have been described for either pituitary adenomas or other tumors of the sellar region, such as craniopharyngiomas. These are summarized in Fig. 1 and Table 2 (p. 154). These approaches reflect the various directions in which the suprasellar component of these lesions may grow. Apart from the region of the optic chiasm, access may be required to the anterior or the middle fossa and sometimes to the third ventricle or the cavernous sinus.

Although each surgical route has its keen exponents and its specific applications, one must not forget that a combination of approaches may be required, either at one operation or in stages. In general, however, the best results are achieved by becoming familiar with one approach that can safely be applied in the majority of cases. We, therefore, carry out most intracranial operations via the oblique subfrontal route as described in the following subheading and reserve other routes for difficult cases. These are the high craniopharyngiomas and similar lesions that involve the third ventricle, particularly when there is a prefixed chiasm that limits access to the tumor from the subfrontal approach.

Subfrontal

The oblique subfrontal operation is of key historical significance because it has been in continuous use since Charles Frazier first described it in 1913 *(21)*. This route was adopted by Harvey Cushing, who used an extradural variant, an operation eloquently described by Henderson *(7)*.

Despite the changing indications for pituitary surgery and various modifications to the flap, the arguments in favor of the oblique subfrontal approach remain entirely relevant in the 21st century. The approach gives excellent bilateral access to the optic nerves and the chiasm. The superior sagittal sinus is not divided, and the falx is left intact. Because the approach is off the midline, it is unnecessary to enter the frontal sinus if it is small. The unilateral nature of the operation limits the retraction that is required, thus minimizing the risk of injury to the olfactory tracts and the frontal lobes.

The patient is positioned supine, with a small degree of head up tilt to aid venous drainage. The head is in slight extension to encourage the brain to relax away from the skull base. The Mayfield pinholder provides rigid fixation and acts as a base for intrancranial retraction, but it is just as safe to use a padded horseshoe. A number of incisions can be used, but in the patient who has a normal hairline, a bicoronal incision is cosmetically acceptable. Midline forehead incisions *(21)* heal almost invisibly, and it is flap resorption and burr holes that are more often the cause of cosmetic problems if rigid flap fixation is not used. Whether titanium plates or other fixation devices improve the cosmetic results in the long-term, only time will tell.

With a high-speed drill, a small entry hole is made in the skull. This is made in the anterosuperior margin of the right temporalis muscle, just below the superior orbital ridge. In making the flap, it is important to take the anterior bone cut as close to the anterior fossa floor as possible. This can be carried to within a centimeter of the midline, before turning the craniotome superiorly.

We use an osteoplastic flap, which is more prevalent in UK practice. The flap is hinged on the temporalis muscle. If the frontal air sinus is entered, the mucosa is stripped from the flap and a formal repair is made with temporalis fascia and tissue glue at the end of the procedure. The dura is opened in a Y-shaped fashion. It should be noted that at the frontal tip, a large dural draining vein can easily be damaged if the incision is too bold.

Gentle retraction can now be applied under the frontal lobe. If the bone flap incision is made correctly, little elevation of the brain is required—and the less the better. It is most accurately done using the microscope, which is brought in at this stage. Care should be given to preserving the olfactory tract by mobilizing this as much as possible. If done without due care, a small artery bleeds persistently, which can obscure all further attempts at fine dissection, and the patient may well be rendered anosmic.

Space is created by gently advancing the brain retractor tip toward the right optic nerve. Once this structure is seen, its covering of arachnoid is sharply incised to allow the release of CSF. As CSF is drained away, the brain slackens and further gentle retraction can be used.

The characteristic bony anatomy of the anterior fossa floor and the sphenoid wing is extremely helpful in guiding the operator to the optic nerves. We have, therefore, found interactive image guidance of limited use during this particular operation.

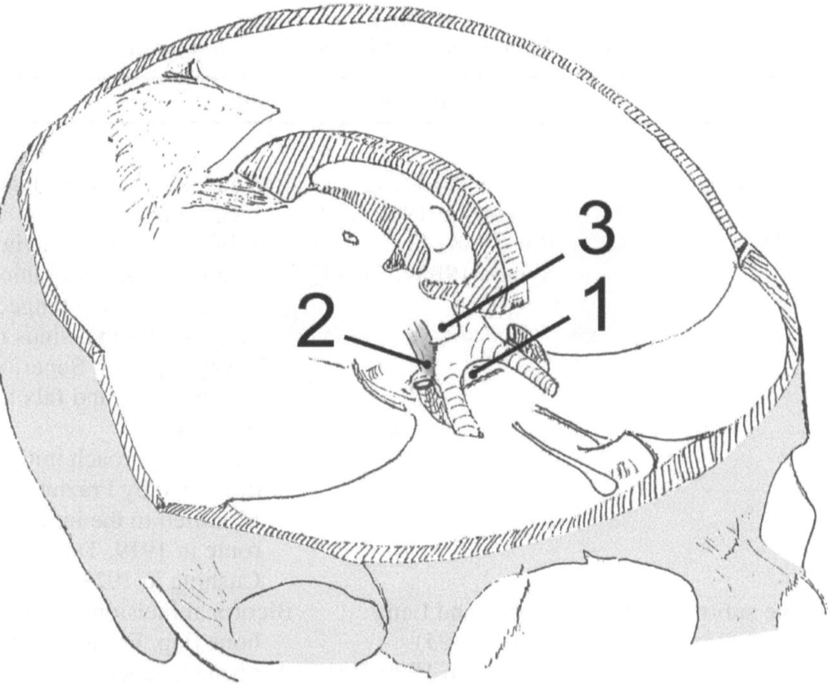

Fig. 1. The schematic view from the right anterior oblique approach of the skull and parasellar regions. The view includes olfactory tracts, optic nerves and chiasm, internal carotids, anterior and posterior margins of the sella, pituitary stalk, and top of gland. The corpus callosum, roof of the third ventricle with Monro's foramen, and the mouth of the aqueduct are also shown. Not that the right optic tract and part of the upper right chiasm have been removed at the broken line to show the stalk behind. Lesions at 1 are relatively straightforward and are approached either by the subfrontal or pterional routes. Lesions at 2 require more planning but can be approached from subfrontal (particularly if the chiasm is not prefixed) or infratemporal/orbito-zygomatic routes, or by extended transsphenoidal approach. Lesions at 3, in the third ventricle are probably best approached through the lamina terminals or even by the transcallosal route.

The lesion is next identified between the optic nerves, although the left nerve is often not visible at this stage. The capsule of the tumor is gently freed from the right optic nerve, and any further adhesions between it and the frontal lobe surface are freed with sharp and blunt dissection. As we have emphasized, every effort should be made to minimize manipulation of the optic nerve. Luckily, adenomas usually do separate easily, although meningiomas often have a close pial involvement. Caution is the watchword here.

Working between the optic nerves, the tumor can be entered. Gentle bipolar coagulation is applied, followed by a horizontal incision just above the planum.

Table 2
Transcranial Approaches to Pituitary Region Tumors

Approach	*Selected references*	*Features*
Subfrontal		
Oblique subfrontal	Frazier 1913 *(21)* Henderson 1939 Ray 1968 *(23)* Symon 1988 *(22)*	Various skin incisions, including bicoronal. Low subfrontal approach via a small osteoplastic craniotomy. Osteoplastic flap hinged laterally. Frontal sinus not always opened. Superior sagittal sinus and falx not divided. Extradural approach initially described by Frazier. Modified to the intradural route in 1919. Taken up by Cushing in 1929.
Midline subfrontal	Choux and Lena 1998 *(25)* Fahlbusch 1999 *(26)*	Bicoronal incision and bicoronal bone flap. Frontal sinus opened. Superior sagittal sinus and falx divided. Risks of bilateral frontal lobe retraction and olfactory tract retraction.
Transglabellar	Perneczky 1999 *(27)*	Spectacle incision within eyebrows. Anterior wall of frontal sinus removed as free flap. Access to intradural compartment via posterior wall of frontal sinus.
Pterional		
Pterional or frontolateral	Dandy 1932 Van Alphen 1975 *(20)* Fahlbusch 1999 *(26)*	Frontolateral craniotomy. Sylvian fissure split to expose retrochiasmal tumor. Adopted by Dandy in 1920. Limitations imposed by the intervening internal carotid and its branches.
Lateral		
Transcranial epidural	Dolenc 1997 *(10)*	Pterional craniotomy; extradural bone removal and reflection of the outer layer of the cavernous dura. Microsurgical dissection of cavernous sinus.

Table 2
(continued)

Approach	*Selected references*	*Features*
Subtemporal	Cushing 1914 *(29)*	Temporal craniectomy. Developed in dogs by Horsley to reach the gasserian ganglion. two-stage operation. High morbidity from temporal lobe retraction and cranial nerve deficits. Found impractical by Cushing. Now obsolete.
Transtemporal	Symon and Sprich 1985 *(30)*	Frontotemporal craniotomy. 2-cm anterior temporal lobectomy. Access to interpeduncular fossa. Employed for craniopharyngiomas.
Third ventricle		
Trans-lamina terminalis	King 1979 *(33)* Bhagwati 1990 *(34)* Suzuki 1998 *(35)*	An addition to the subfrontal approach. Useful with a prefixed chiasm to access a third ventricular component
Transcallosal	Ture 1997 *(36)*	Parasagittal bone flap. Callosal incision.

The tumor is then gutted. With adenomas, this is often easy with a sucker and small tissue rongeurs. The Angell-James are favored by the authors but are sadly no longer made. Meningiomas may need more robust dissection, and craniopharyngiomas can usually be emptied before the membrane is removed.

With the tumor gutted, it is often simple to peel the capsule out of the back of the cavity, preserving the pituitary stalk. The left optic nerve and both carotid arteries have been seen by this time and treated with due respect. Usually there is little bleeding; what there is can be controlled with patties and bipolar coagulation.

One source of potential difficulty during the subfrontal approach is the prefixed chiasm. When the optic nerves are short, the chiasm lies directly between the surgeon and the tumor. In this case, access below the chiasm can be improved by drilling through the tuberculum sellae to enter the sphenoid sinus *(23)*. An alternative is to reach the intraventricular tumor above the chiasm via the lamina terminalis (*see* the following section). The sacrifice of an already-blind optic nerve to improve access, a maneuver described by Walter Dandy, is an absolute last resort and better consigned to the past *(24)*.

Midline Subfrontal

A symmetric midline flap with division of the superior saggital sinus and the falx is an option, but for the reasons stated, the author prefers the unilateral approach, especially for pituitary adenoma. The operation has been applied to craniopharyngiomas *(25,26)* and is also useful for tumors sited more anteriorly, such as certain planum sphenoidale meningiomas. It may also be used if a translamina terminalis approach is planned. The view of the third ventricle is then obtained in the midline.

Transglabellar

In patients with a large frontal sinus, we have found the transglabellar route to be useful. This employs the frontal sinus as an entry point. A spectacle-type incision is sited within the eyebrow on each side, with a short horizontal component crossing the bridge of the nose; this incision heals without sign. The scalp flap is retracted upward to expose the glabella. A minicraniotomy free flap is fashioned from the anterior wall of the frontal sinus using the high-speed craniotome. The posterior wall of the sinus is then opened, and the superior sagittal sinus is coagulated or tied at its origin before being divided. On opening the dura, the operator can proceed along the floor of the anterior fossa toward the chiasm and the related tumor, which are dealt with as described in the preceding section *(27)*. Again, care is required to protect the olfactory nerves.

Pterional

A pterional flap provides access to the tumor along the sphenoid wing. This may be useful when there is a significant retrochiasmal component, especially where a prefixed chiasm limits the access from the subfrontal direction. The Sylvian fissure is split at its medial aspect to improve access. Unfortunately, despite these maneuvers, access to the pituitary tumor is still limited by the carotid artery and its branches.

Van Alphen termed this the frontotemporal approach and cited the protection of the olfactory tract as a reason for employing it *(20)*. Snow and Patterson have suggested that when pterional access is required, the subfrontal operation may be extended to provide this. A large flap is fashioned to allow access to the subfrontal corridor and also to include the pterion, which is then removed with the high-speed drill *(28)*.

Lateral Approaches

Transcranial Epidural

Dolenc has applied his extensive experience of the cavernous sinus to a transcavernous approach to the sella *(10)*.

The operation involves the exposure of the lateral wall of the cavernous sinus via a pterional craniotomy with extensive bone removal of the lesser sphenoid wing and the anterior clinoid process. Direct visualization is made of the cranial nerves in the lateral wall of the cavernous sinus, and the approach to the sella is made between these structures *(11)*.

For the reasons stated in the previous section, a careful assessment of the benefits of this approach must be made before applying it to a case of pituitary adenoma. In particular, the operator must be sure that the morbidity of the operation will not outweigh any benefits gained by an attempt at radical resection.

Subtemporal and Transtemporal

The subtemporal route to the pituitary gland was the first transcranial route employed by Victor Horsley and Harvey Cushing. It was done via a subtemporal decompressive craniectomy and had the advantage of a short trajectory but the disadvantage of incurring morbidity from temporal lobe retraction. Cushing applied the approach in 100 dogs, and both he and Horsley were probably falsely encouraged in attempting this route by the shallow canine middle fossa. After eight attempts at the approach in humans, Cushing concluded that it was impractical *(29)*. The intradural subtemporal approach is now effectively obsolete.

Symon has used a transtemporal operation to approach craniopharyngiomas *(30)* and also a giant pituitary adenoma *(31,32)*. In this procedure 2 cm of the temporal pole was removed to permit access to the interpeduncular fossa and to allow radical removal of the tumor.

Third Ventricle

Numerous approaches via the third ventricle have been described. For suprasellar tumors, the most common indication for these approaches is to remove a craniopharyngioma.

With a pituitary adenoma, if it is possible to debulk the suprasellar component from below, this removes the need to access the tumor in the third ventricle directly.

The two most useful approaches are the transcallosal and the translaminal terminalis. These routes allow access to the anterior part of the ventricle into which suprasellar lesions most commonly extend. We do not provide a detailed description in this chapter.

Translamina Terminalis

First described by King *(33)*, the translaminal terminalis approach may be used in conjunction with the subfrontal operation, especially when the optic nerves are short and the chiasm, therefore, lies immediately in front of the tumor *(34)*. A bifrontal flap may be used to approach the lamina along the midline, which gives symmetric visualization of the third ventricle. The lamina terminalis is identified superior to the chiasm and incised. Additional maneuvers have been described to enhance access, including division of the anterior communicating artery or the chiasm *(35)*.

Transcallosal

This is applicable to the superior component of a suprasellar tumor, which cannot be brought down and accessed by an inferior approach. It has rarely been used by the authors for tumors of suprasellar origin, but is mentioned here for completeness. Transforaminal, interforniceal, or transchoroidal routes into the third ventricle may be used *(36)*.

REFERENCES

1. Hardy J. Transsphenoidal microsurgery of the normal and pathological pituitary gland. In: *Microsurgery as Applied to Neurosurgery*. Germany: Thieme Verlag Co; 1969; 180–194.
2. Couldwell WT, Weiss MH. The transnasal transsphenoidal approach. In: Apuzzo MLJ, ed. *Surgery of the Third Ventricle*. 2nd ed. Baltimore: Williams and Wilkins; 1998.
3. Fahlbusch R, Honegger J. Extended transsphenoidal approach to the pituitary region and upper clivus. In: *Operative Skull Base Surgery*. Torrens M, Al-Mefty O, Kobayashi S, eds. Edinburgh, UK: Churchill Livingstone; 1997.
4. Kouri JG, Chen MY, Watson JC, Oldfield EH. Resection of suprasellar tumors by using a modified transsphenoidal approach: report of four cases. J Neurosurg 2000;92:1028–1035.
5. Kitano M, Taneda M. Extended transsphenoidal approach with submucosal posterior ethmoidectomy for parasellar tumors. J Neurosurg 2001;94(6): 999–1004.
6. Kaptain GJ, Vinvent DA, Sheehan JP, Laws ER. Trans-sphenoidal approaches for the extracapsular resection of midline suprasellar and anterior cranial base lesions. Neurosurgery 2001;49:94–101.
7. Henderson WR. The pituitary adenomata. A follow-up study of the surgical results in 338 cases (Dr Harvey Cushing's series). Br J Surg 1939;26:811–921.
8. Laws ER, Jr, Trautmann JC, Hollenhorst RW, Jr. Trans-sphenoidal decompression of the optic nerve and chiasm. Visual results in 62 patients. J Neurosurg 1977;46:717–722.
9. Cohen AR, Cooper PR, Kupersmith MJ, Flamm ES, Ransohoff J. Visual recovery after transsphenoidal removal of pituitary adenomas. Neurosurgery 1985;17:446–452.
10. Dolenc VV. Transcranial epidural approach to pituitary tumors extending beyond the sella. Neurosurgery 1997;41(3):542–550.
11. Adams CBT. *A Neurosurgeon's Notebook*. Oxford: Blackwell Science; 1999; 147.
12. Snow RB, Johnson CE, Morgello S, Lavyne MH, Patterson RH. Is magnetic resonance imaging useful in guiding the operative approach to large pituitary tumors? Neurosurgery 1990;26(5):801–803.
13. Esiri M, Bevan JS, Burke CW, Adams CB. Effect of bromocriptine treatment on the fibrous tissue content of prolactin-secreting and nonfunctioning macroadenomas of the pituitary gland. J Clin Endocrinol Metab 1986;63(2):383–388.
14. Barkan AL, Lloyd RV, Chandler WF, et al. Preoperative treatment of acromegaly with long-acting somatostatin analog SMS 201–995: shrinkage of invasive pituitary macroadenomas and improved surgical remission rate. J Clin Endocrinol Metab 1988;67:1040–1048.
15. Ezzat S, Horvath E, Harris AG, Kovacs K. Morphological effects of octreotide on growth hormone-producing pituitary adenomas J Clin Endoc and Metab 1994;79:113–118.
16. Patterson RH. The role of transcranial surgery in the management of pituitary adenoma. Acta Neurochir 1996;(Suppl 65):16–17.
17. Abe T, Iwata T, Kawamura N, Izumiyama H, Ikeda H, Matsumoto K. Staged transsphenoidal surgery for fibrous nonfunctioning pituitary adenomas with suprasellar extension. Neurol Med Chir (Tokyo) 1997;37(11):830–835; discussion 835–837.
18. Massoud AF, Powell M, Williams RA, Hindmarsh PC, Brook CG. Transsphenoidal surgery for pituitary tumors. Arch Dis Child 1997;76(5):398–404.

19. Dawson BH. The blood vessels of the human optic chiasma and their relation to those of the hypophysis and thalamus. Brain 1958;81:207–217.
20. Van Alphen HAM. Microsurgical fronto-temporal approach to pituitary adenomas with extrasellar extension Clin Neurol Neurosurg 1975;4:246–256.
21. Frazier CH. Lesions of the hypophysis from the viewpoint of the surgeon. Surg Gynecol Obstet 1913;17:724–736.
22. Symon L. Intracranial approaches to tumors in the area of the sella turcica. In: *Rob and Smith's Operative Surgery: Neurosurgery*. 4th ed. Symon L, Thomas DGT, Clark K, eds., London: Chapman and Hall Medical; 1988.
23. Ray BS. Intracranial hypophysectomy. J Neurosurg 1968;28:180–186.
24. Dandy W. The brain. In: *Dean Lewis's Practice of Surgery. Birmingham, AL. Classics of Neurology Library*. Reprinted 1987; 591.
25. Choux M, Lena G. Craniopharyngioma. In: Apuzzo MJ, ed. *Surgery of the Third Ventricle*. Baltimore: Williams and Wilkins 1998;1143–1181.
26. Fahlbusch R , Honnegger J, Paulus W, Buchfelder M. Surgical treatment of craniopharyngiomas: experience with 168 patients. J Neurosurg 1999;90(2):237–250.
27. Perneczky A. *Keyhole Concept in Neurosurgery*. Stuttgart, Germany: Thieme; 1999.
28. Snow RB, Patterson RH. Craniotomy for pituitary tumors. In: Kaye AH, Black P, eds. *Brain Tumors*. 2nd ed. Stuttgart, Germany: Thieme; 1999.
29. Cushing H. Surgical experiences with pituitary disorders. JAMA 1914;63:1515.
30. Symon L, Sprich W. Radical excision of craniopharyngioma: results in 20 patients. J Neurosurg 1985;62:174–181.
31. Symon L, Jackubowski J, Kendall B. Surgical treatment of giant pituitary adenomas. J Neurol Neurosurg Psychiatry 1979;42:973–982.
32. Symon L, Jakubowski J. Transcranial management of pituitary tumors with suprasellar extension. J Neurol Neurosurg Psychiatry 1979;42:123–133.
33. King TT. Removal of intraventricular craniopharyngiomas throught the lamina terminali. Acta Neurochir (Wien) 1979;45:277–286.
34. Bhagwati SN, Deopujari CE, Parulekar GD. Lamina terminalis approach for retrochiasmal craniopharyngiomas. Childs Nerv Syst 1990;6:425–429.
35. Suzuki J. The bifrontal anterior interhemispheric approach. In: Apuzzo MLJ, ed. *Surgery of the Third Ventricle*. 2nd ed. Baltimore: Williams and Wilkins; 1998.
36. Ture U, Yasargil MG, Al-Mefty O. The transcallosal-transforaminal approach to the third ventricle with regard to the venous variations in this region. J Neurosurg 1997;87:706–715.

10 Endoscopic Endonasal Transsphenoidal Surgery

Paolo Cappabianca, MD,
and Enrico de Divitiis, MD

CONTENTS

THE EVOLUTION OF THE TECHNIQUE

The existence of a route through the nose to the brain that avoided disfiguring the face was well known to the Egyptians (2600 BC), who used to insert special hooked instruments up through the nostril and the sphenoid sinus to extract the brain in the mummification process.

In the early 1900s, the same route was revived by Hirsch for the treatment of sella turcica lesions. He performed his first operation in a patient with a sellar lesion by means of a five-step procedure under local anesthesia. Despite the success of the operation, which required the removal of the left middle turbinate and of the ipsilateral ethmoid sinus without damaging the nasal septum, he changed his technique to Kocher's technique, a submucosal resection of the septum to reach the sphenoid sinus using a transrhinoseptal approach. A few years later in 1914, Cushing standardized the sublabial transeptal transsphenoidal approach that was, until recently, the most common approach used by neurosurgeons to treat sellar lesions. This procedure was adapted and modern-

From: *Management of Pituitary Tumors: The Clinician's Practical Guide, Second Edition*
Edited by: M. P. Powell, S. L. Lightman, and E. R. Laws, Jr. © Humana Press Inc., Totowa, NJ

ized by Guiot (1958), Hardy (1969), Laws (1977), Post (1980), Tindall and Barrow (1986), and many others, improving the technique, thus making it safe and effective and with a low complication rate *(1)*.

Guiot, in 1963 *(2)*, was the first to propose the use of the endoscope within the transnasorhinoseptal microsurgical approach to explore the sellar contents, but his idea was not used. It would be 30 yr before advances in optical technology permitted the development of adequate instrumentation that has allowed the widespread use of endoscopes in nasal and paranasal sinus surgery (FESS) by otolaryngologists *(3–5)*. After a brief period in which some authors *(6,7)* employed an endoscope-assisted technique, Jho, in 1993 *(8)*, started to perform a *"pure" endoscopic endonasal transsphenoidal surgery* through the nasal cavity, as Hirsch 80 yr before had proposed and attempted in a primitive form.

SURGICAL PROCEDURE

The Endoscope in Pure Transsphenoidal Surgery

The procedure is performed with an endoscope as the only optical tool throughout the operation, i.e., *pure endoscopic surgery*, and not using the microscope with the endoscope, i.e., endoscope-assisted microsurgery.

Only *rigid endoscopes* without a working channel, 4 mm in diameter; 0°, 30°, and 45° angled lenses; and 18–30 cm in length are employed. They must be inserted into an outer sleeve that, when connected to an irrigation system, clears the lens. Surgical instruments are introduced through the same nostril alongside the endoscope. The endoscope is connected to a monitor and a video recording unit by means of a video camera and is illuminated through an optical fiber cable using a xenon light source. The majority of the operation is performed with a 0° endoscope using the angled lenses (30°, 45°) for further exploration of the intrasellar cavity and the suprasellar region. During the procedure, the endoscope is held by the surgeon's non dominant hand until the sphenoid sinus is entered, then an adjustable endoscope holder is fixed to the surgical table, providing a fixed image of the operating field and freeing both of the surgeon's hands.

Neurosurgeons who are experienced in microscopic transsphenoidal surgery still require practice to overcome the steep learning curve, caused mainly by the absence of the standard nasal speculum. Despite a wider working angle enabling more structures to be seen simultaneously, the narrow working space is difficult to get used to. With the loss of the speculum, which provides a sense of surgical scale, the surgeon must be careful to avoid quick movements close to the surgical target, because the endoscopic image is two dimensional. It is possible to lose depth perception inside the nasal cavity and the sphenoid sinus, increasing the risk of serious damage. Careful in-and-out movements with the endoscope give the surgeon set points at different depth levels of the surgical route and recover the three-dimensional sense of depth.

Surgical Steps

The technical description of the transsphenoidal surgical procedure has been described elsewhere in detail *(9,16)*. The main steps are reported here.

After general anesthesia, the patient is placed supine, with the legs slightly flexed, the trunk tilted 10°–20°, and the head turned 10° toward the surgeon and fixed in a Mayfield headrest without pins.

The endoscopic equipment (monitor, light source, video camera, video recorder) is positioned behind the head of the patient and in front of the operator who stands facing the chin in the position shown in diagram in Fig. 2A in Chapter 8. The fluoroscope C-arm or neuronavigation system are used as normal.

The nasal cavities are packed with gauze pledgets soaked in a diluted solution of 5% chlorohexidine gluconate, the face and the nose are prepared in the same way, and the patient draped.

The Nasal Step

The endoscope is introduced into the chosen nostril and cottonoids soaked with diluted adrenaline (1:100,000) or with xilomethazoline hydrochloride are placed between the middle turbinate and the nasal septum. These nasal decongestants, together with the controlled hypotension, minimize mucosal bleeding. After removing the cottonoids, the space between the septum and middle turbinate, if narrow, can be increased by gently mobilizing the head of the middle turbinate laterally.

The *sphenoid ostium* is the crucial anatomical point of the procedure because it is the entrance to the sphenoid sinus. It is extremely variable in shape, size, and position. It can be reached in several ways. The endoscope can be (1) introduced between the nasal septum and the middle turbinate, with a 30° angle with respect to the floor of the nasal cavity, or (2) inserted in the angle between the nasal septum and the floor of the nasal cavity until it reaches the choana. When the superior edge of the choana is identified, the endoscope follows the spheno-ethmoid recess for about 1.5 cm, between the superior turbinate and the nasal septum, until the natural sphenoid sinus ostium is identified. When reached, an *endoscope holder* is used to fix the instrument during the anterior sphenoidotomy and the next steps.

The Sphenoid Step

Once identified, the sphenoid sinus natural ostium is enlarged all around, using Kerrison's rongeurs or a microdrill, particularly in a downward and lateral direction, where bleeding from branches of the sphenopalatine artery can occur. The enlargement is completed with the removal of the sphenoid rostrum up to the contralateral ostium. Once the anterior wall of the sphenoid sinus is opened, the sphenoid septae can be identified and removed. The anterior wall of the sellar floor should now be recognizable, with the spheno-ethmoid planum above and

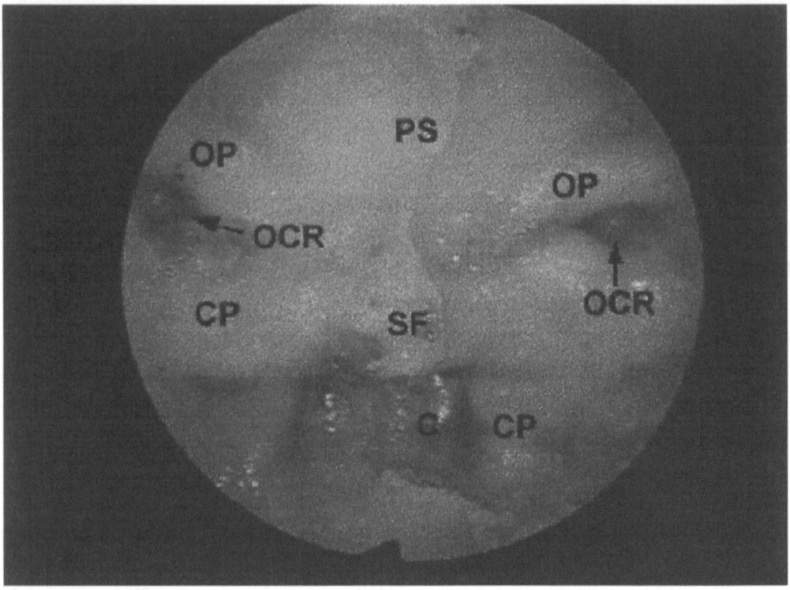

Fig. 1. Panoramic view of the sphenoid cavity (cadaver study). C, clivus; CP, carotid prominence; OCR, opto-carotid recess; OP, optic prominence; PS, planum sphenoidale; SF, sellar floor.

the clival indentation below. Lateral to the sellar floor the bony prominences of the intracavernous carotid artery and the optic nerve can be seen and between them the opto-carotid recess, shaped by the pneumatization of the anterior clinoid process (Fig. 1).

The Sellar Step

The sellar floor, like the whole sphenoid cavity, is covered by mucosa, which is only displaced laterally if normal. It may be removed if abnormal or if infiltrated by the sellar lesion. How the sellar floor is opened depends on its thickness: if it is intact, entry is made by a microdrill with diamond burr; if it is eroded or thinned, it can be entered simply by means of a dissector. Once an opening has been made, it is enlarged with Kerrison's rongeurs and/or Stammberger circular cutting punch (Karl Storz, www.karlstorz.com).

The opening of the sellar floor must be extended as required, reaching, if necessary, the sphenoid planum above, the clivus below, and the carotid protrusions bilaterally.

The dura is incised in a linear or cross fashion. Curets and suction with slow and circular movements are used to remove large tumor fragments initially. The endoscope is then advanced into the tumor cavity for complete removal, followed by the dissection of the capsule, if possible. The Valsalva maneuver by

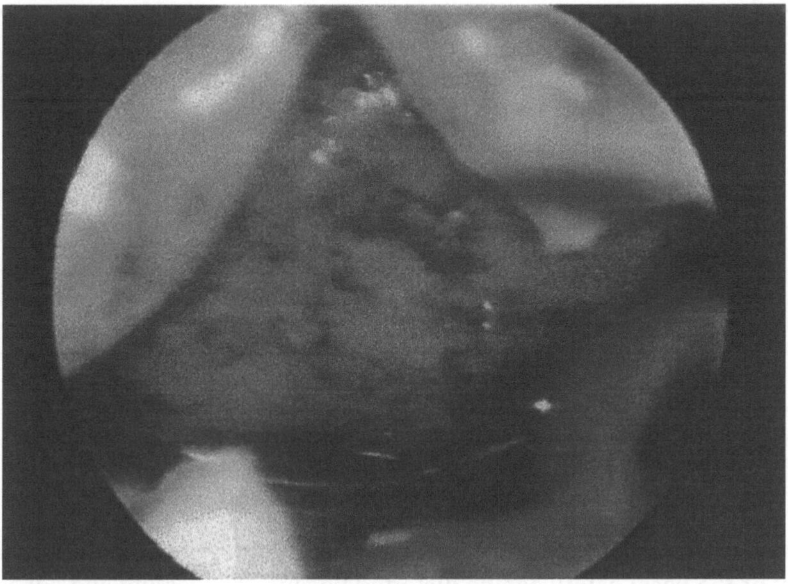

Fig. 2. A close-up view of the suprasellar cistern after the removal of an intrasuprasellar macroadenoma (0° endoscope).

temporarily increasing intracranial pressure may be helpful in producing the descent of the residual tissue into view in cases of suprasellar expansion. The descent of the cistern is often seen at this stage of the procedure (Fig. 2), and a view of the optic chiasm or of the anterior part of the Circle of Willis can be obtained if the arachnoid is opened *(11)*.

After tumor removal, if there is evidence or risk of a cerebrospinal fluid (CSF) leak, closure of the sella may be performed using a polyester-silicone dural substitute and fibrin glue (Fig. 3) *(12)* as described *(13)*. This provides a barrier to the sphenoid sinus, reduces empty space, and prevents the descent of the chiasm into the sellar. If there is no leak, no repair is required.

The Adaptability of the Procedure

The whole procedure commonly involves one nostril, through which the endoscope (fixed to its holder) plus one or two instruments are inserted. Two important variants determine a deviation from the standard procedure:

The Anatomy of the Nasal and Paranasal Cavity

The nasal and paranasal anatomy can be distorted by (1)hypertrophy of the turbinates on both sides from various nasal pathologies, (2) by the presence of a concha bullosa of the middle turbinate, and (3) by other anatomic variations that, narrowing the nostrils, can cause difficulties in reaching and working safely in

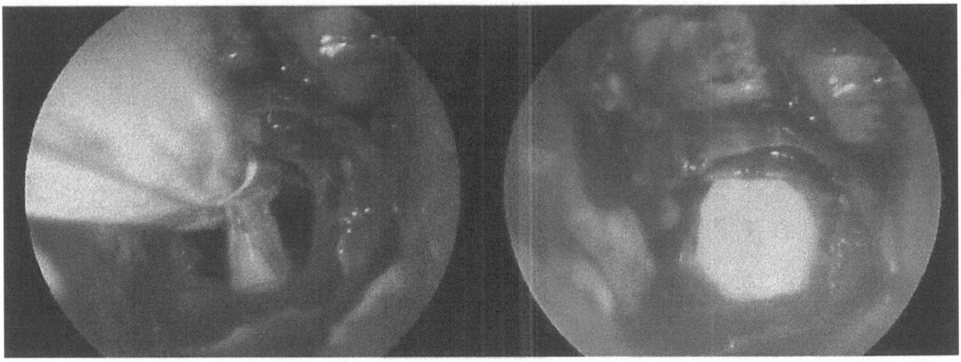

Fig. 3. Reconstruction of the sellar floor using a polyester-silicone dural substitute, which is introduced with the forceps in a bent fashion and is placed intradurally and/or extradurally, according to the necessity.

the sellar region. Also, in recurrence after a previous transsphenoidal approach, the anatomy of the nasal cavity can be distorted because of scarring and adhesions.

Extension of the Sellar Lesion

The surgical procedure is not strictly median because of the nasal septum and the prominence of the nasal turbinates (especially the middle and the superior) that can prevent the endoscope and other instruments from being angled sufficiently laterally to the limit of the lesion. When access to the sellar lesion extends beyond the angle of maneuver of the instruments, even if the endoscope allows the surgeon to see the lesion, it may not be possible to remove it.

The endoscopic endonasal procedure can be adapted to different patterns of extension of the sellar lesion, allowing adequate surgical access. These modifications include hemisphenoidotomy, the enlarged approach with the removal of superior and/or supreme turbinate, and the bilateral nostril approach.

PRESENT SERIES

From January 1997 *(14)* to December 2000, 150 consecutive patients with pituitary tumors and other related lesions underwent endoscopic endonasal transsphenoidal surgery.

There were 93 women and 57 men, with an age range of 16 to 75 yr (median 45.4 yr). The majority (125 patients) had pituitary adenomas; 105 of which were macroadenomas and 20 were microadenomas. Macroadenomas were totally removed in 60 cases, near totally in 28, (>80%) and only a partial removal was achieved in 17. Of the 20 microadenomas, 17 patients had total removal of the lesion. The patient population, case distribution, and tumor removal are listed in detail in Table 1.

Table 1
Patient Population and Case Distribution of the Present Series

Pathology	*No. of cases*	*Surgical removal*				
		Total	*Subtotal*	*Partial*	*Biopsy*	*Other*
Pituitary adenoma						
NF	69	38	19	12	–	–
PRL	9	7	1	1	–	–
GH	30	18	9	3	–	–
ACTH	13	11	2	–	–	–
GH-PRL	3	2	–	1	–	–
GH-TSH	1	1	–	–	–	–
Craniopharyngioma	6	3	2	–	1	–
Rathke's cleft cyst	3	3	–	–	–	–
Arachnoid cyst	2	–	–	–	–	2 Marsupialized
Sellar theratoma	1	–	–	1	–	–
Clivus chordoma	3	–	–	–	3	–
Olfactory neuroblastoma	1	–	–	–	1	–
Sphenoid metastasis	1	–	–	–	1	–
Sphenoid mucocele	2	–	–	–	–	2 Cured
Residual nasal meningocele	1	1	–	–	–	–
CSF leak	5	–	–	–	–	5 Sealed
Total	150	84	33	18	6	9

NF, nonfunctioning; PRL, prolactin; GH, growth hormone; ACTH, adenocorticotropic homrone; TSH, thyroid-stimulating hormone.

Endoscopic endonasal surgery allows a significantly shorter post-operative stay compared with conventional microsurgical transsphenoidal surgery. In our series, 63 out of the 150 patients were discharged within 2 d of surgery and 109 within 4 d (Table 2). Longer postoperative stay was usually caused by diabetes insipidus, CSF leak, or other major complications or social reasons.

Surgical complications are few (Table 2) and show a significant *reduction* compared with the many series of conventional microsurgical transsphenoidal surgery *(15)*.

ADVANTAGES OF THE PROCEDURE

The main advantages of the endoscopic procedure are the absence of the nasal speculum, which creates a fixed tunnel, and the near coaxially control of the micro-instruments.

Without the nasal speculum:

- The endoscopic operation starts from the natural ostium of the sphenoid sinus and *avoids the submucosal nasal phase and orodental complications* caused by the incision in the bucco-gingival junction (if used), septal perforations, nasal scars, and damage to the nasal spine, making it a *minimally traumatic procedure*.

Table 2
Postoperative Hospitalization and Surgical Complications of the Present Series

			No. of cases	%
Postoperative hospitalization	1–2 d		63/150	42
	3–4 d		46/150	31
	5–6 d		27/150	18
	7–9 d		14/150	9
Complications	Nasofacial	Epistaxis	2/150	1,3
	Sphenoid sinus	Sphenoid sinusitis	3/150	2
	Sella turcica	CSF leak	4/150	2,6
	Intracranial	Thalamic ischemia	1/150	0,6
		Swelling of the residual tumor	1/142 [a]	0,7
		Meningitis	1/150	0,6
	Visual	Intrasuprasellar haematoma	1/150	0,6
	Carotid artery	ICA injury—pseudoaneurysm	1/150	0,6
	Cavernous sinus	Transient VI cranial nerve palsy	1/150	0,6
Endocrine complications	Permanent post-operative diabetes insipidus		5/140 [b]	3,5
	Postoperative anterior pituitary insufficiency	Worsening of 1 axis	14/140 [b]	10
		Worsening of 2 axis	7/140 [b]	5

[a]Have been excluded: 5 cases of CSF leak, 2 cases of sphenoid mucocele, and 1 case of residual nasal meningocele.

[b]Have been excluded: 5 cases of CSF leak, 2 cases of sphenoid mucocele, 1 case of olfactory neuroblastoma, 1 case of sphenoid metastasis, and 1 case of residual nasal meningocele.

- There is no fixed tunnel, and the surgeon can, therefore, make significantly wider movements with the instruments, especially laterally.
- There is no postoperative facial swelling or nasal pain caused by spreading of the blades of the nasal speculum.
- *Nasal packing* is not used because the procedure is endonasal and there is no need to approximate the dissected septal mucosa to the septal cartilage at the end of the procedure. As a consequence, postoperative breathing difficulties are avoided.

- The recovery is *quick*, often with a single postoperative overnight stay, especially in nonfunctioning macroadenomas.

The other advantages arise from the use of the endoscope itself:

- The endoscope, like the microscope, is still simply a surgical tool for seeing but, unlike it, offers a *wider surgical field*, even with the 0° lens, a field that can be further enlarged by using angled lenses (30°, 45°). Being able to work in a wider surgical field is safer and, moreover, the angled-lens endoscope enables the surgeon to operate on tumors in the suprasellar region under direct visual control.
- The endoscope magnifies a part of the central surgical field. This close-up view helps contrast the tumor from the surrounding structures, permitting a much clearer and safer removal of the lesion.

Surgical indications for endoscopic pituitary surgery are the same as those for conventional microscopic transsphenoidal procedures. An added bonus is that the treatment of recurrences is easier *(16)*. Often, a second conventional operation is more difficult and has more risks. The distorted anatomy, adhesions, scars, and septal perforation may lead to the loss of the midline and potential injury to structures in and around the sella. With the endoscopic procedure, avoiding the submucosal nasal phase of the conventional operation, the real beginning of the operation is in the sphenoid sinus. The endoscope provides better anatomic orientation in the nasal cavity, and in the sphenoid sinus the panoramic view permits the distinction of the borders of the previous approach from the surrounding structures.

PROBLEMS RELATED TO THE PROCEDURE

The endoscopic technique has a *steep learning curve*. Because of this, longer operating times are encountered initially, but with adequate experience become shorter, especially in recurrences.

A major criticism of the endoscope is the lack of three-dimensional vision. The video monitor does not give a sense of depth, and the image is slightly distorted at the periphery (barrel effect).

New instruments are required. The instruments designed for microsurgical transsphenoidal surgery are not ideal for the endoscope. The bayonet shape of conventional instruments keeps the surgeon's hands from blocking the operative field as happens with the microscope *(17)*. The endoscope has the "eye" at its tip and needs straight instruments inserted close to it.

Last but not least is the controversial bleeding control problem during the procedure. Two types of bleeding can occur. First, a slight but continuous venous ooze from the nasal mucosa, particularly during the first part of the procedure, may necessitate continuous irrigation and movement of the endoscope. Second, significant arterial bleeding, from either branches of the sphenopalatine artery or, much more seriously, the internal carotid artery, is a major problem. During the initial series when this occured, the standard speculum and the microscope had to quickly be used. However, currently, with training, the bleeding can be controlled using the endoscope alone.

THE FUTURE

The endoscope, particularly in a well-pneumatized sphenoid sinus, allows the surgeon to see an astonishing amount of anatomic detail, such as the planum sphenoidale, the clivus, the carotid, and optic bony protuberances. Pathologies arising or extending in these regions are obvious candidates for endoscopic surgical removal. These include suprasellar craniopharyngiomas, tuberculum sellae meningiomata, macroadenomas involving the cavernous sinus, and upper clival chordomas *(18)*.

To be effective and safe, these procedures need:

- Adequate endoscopic skill;
- A detailed knowledge of the anatomy of different pathologies of these regions to avoid major injuries;
- Dedicated instruments to perform the operation under the best conditions with both the 0° or angled endoscopes;
- Adequate materials and techniques of reconstruction for the planum sphenoidale and the clivus, to prevent CSF leaks.

Knowledge of anatomy, the improvement of surgical equipment, and the development of intraoperative ultrasonography and intraoperative magnetic resonance imaging could extend what is possible in the sella to these parasellar pathologies.

REFERENCES

1. Landolt AM. History of pituitary surgery; transsphenoidal approach. In: Landolt AM, Vance ML, Reilly PR, eds. *Pituitary Adenomas.* New York: Churchill Livingstone;1996:307–314.
2. Guiot G, Rougerie J, Fourestier M, et al. Explorations endoscopiques intracrannienes. Presse Med 1963;71:1225–1228.
3. Kennedy DW. Functional endoscopic sinus surgery. Technique. Arch Otolaryngol 1985;111:643–649.
4. Messerklinger W. Background and evolution of endoscopic sinus surgery. Ear Nose Throat J 1994;73:449–450.
5. Stammberger H, Posawetz W. Functional endoscopic sinus surgery. Concepts, indications and results of the Messerklinger technique. Eur Arch Otorhinolaryngol 1990;247:63–76.
6. Jankowski R, Auque J, Simon C, Marchal JC, Hepner H, Wayoff M. Endoscopic pituitary tumor surgery. Laryngoscope 1992;102:198–202.
7. Liston SL, Siegel LG, Thienprasit P, Gregory R. Nasal endoscopes in hypophysectomy [letter]. J Neurosurg 1987;66:155.
8. Jho Carrau RL, Ko Y: Endoscopic pituitary surgery. Vol 5. In: Wilkins RH, Rengachary SS, eds. *Neurosurgical Operative Atlas.* Park Ridge, IL: American Association of Neurological Surgeons;1996:1–12.

9. de Divitiis E, Cappabianca P. Endoscopic endonasal transsphenoidal surgery. Vol 27. In: Pickard JD, ed. *Advances and Technical Standards in Neurosurgery*. New York: Springer Verlag;2002:137–177.
10. Jho HD, Jho HD. Endoscopic transsphenoidal surgery. Vol 1. In: Schmidek HH, ed. *Schmidek and Sweet Operative Neurosurgical Techniques. Indications, Methods and Results*. Philadelphia: WB Saunders;2000:385–397.
11. Cappabianca P, Alfieri A, de Divitiis E, Tschabitscher M. *Atlas of Endoscopic Anatomy for Endonasal Intracranial Surgery*. New York: Springer Verlag;2001: p. 134.
12. Cappabianca P, Cavallo LM, Mariniello G, de Divitiis O, Becerra Romero ADC, de Divitiis E. Easy sellar reconstruction in endoscopic endonasal transsphenoidal surgery with polyester-silicone dural substitute and fibrin glue: technical note. Neurosurgery 2001;49:475–476.
13. Spaziante R, de Divitiis E, Cappabianca P. Repair of the sella after transsphenoidal surgery. Vol 1. In: Schmidek HH, Sweet WH, eds. *Operative Neurosurgical Techniques. Indications, Methods, and Results*. Philadelphia; WB Saunders; 2000:398–416.
14. Cappabianca P, Alfieri A, de Divitiis E. Endoscopic endonasal transsphenoidal approach to the sella: towards Functional Endoscopic Pituitary Surgery (FEPS). Minim Invas Neurosurg 1998;41:66–73.
15. Ciric I, Ragin A, Baumgartner C, Pierce D. Complications of transsphenoidal surgery: results of a national survey, review of the literature, and personal experience. Neurosurgery 1997;40:225–237.
16. Cappabianca P, Alfieri A, Colao A, et al. Endoscopic endonasal transsphenoidal surgery in recurrent and residual pituitary adenomas: technical note. Minim Invas Neurosurg 2000;43:38–43.
17. Cappabianca P, Alfieri A, Thermes S, Buonamassa S, de Divitiis E. Instruments for endoscopic endonasal transsphenoidal surgery. Neurosurgery 1999;45:392–396.
18. Jho HD, Carrau RL, McLaughlin ML, Somaza SC. Endoscopic transsphenoidal resection of a large chordoma in the posterior fossa. Neurosurg Focus 1996;1(3):1–7.

11 Early Postoperative Management

Michael P. Powell, MB, BS, FRCS,
Jonathan R. Pollock, BM, BCh, FRCS (A/N),
Stefanie Baldeweg, MD, MRCP, and
Stafford L. Lightman, MB, BChir, PhD, FRCP, FMedSci

Contents

INTRODUCTION

When the patient emerges from the operating room, there are three main interests at play. The first are those of the patient who has a major desire to get rid of the significant discomfort in his or her nose and would like to have it unblocked as well so as to be able to breathe normally. He or she is also thirsty.

The second interest is that of the surgeon. His or her major concern is that the operation has been done properly, no worsening of the condition has occurred, and any endocrine condition for which the operation has been done has been cured.

From: *Management of Pituitary Tumors: The Clinician's Practical Guide, Second Edition*
Edited by: M. P. Powell, S. L. Lightman, and E. R. Laws, Jr.

The third interested party is the endocrinologist. His or her wish is to ensure the continuing normal function of the remainder of the pituitary gland and to check that the surgeon has done his work adequately.

These interests can be dealt with in the following categories:

(1) Pain management.
(2) Fluid balance.
(3) Perioperative endocrine management.
(4) Nonendocrine complications.
(5) Discharge planning.

Where to manage the patient postoperatively is also a matter of debate. In our unit, the patient recovers in a recovery area for approx 1 h and then returns to the ward for routine postoperative monitoring and general nursing care. However, in many units, the patient is managed in an intensive care unit. Whereas this strategy is admirable for absolute safety, it is almost certainly unnecessary overtreatment. Invasive monitoring and multiple observations in the context of recovery from a relatively simple transsphenoidal procedure are probably unwarranted, unless there are questions of nursing quality.

PAIN MANAGEMENT

Transsphenoidal surgery is unquestionably painful. The majority of patients find the initial postoperative pain and blocked nose distressing. As a consequence, it is routine to give the patients morphine for pain. It will be interesting to see if endoscopic surgery will reduce this need, because our initial observations suggest that this is a much less painful procedure. Patients who have undergone a craniotomy are also given morphine for pain. Codeine, when given as an alternative, is idiosyncratic in effectiveness and pain control more haphazard.

FLUID BALANCE

The combination of mouth breathing after transsphenoidal surgery and the lack of oral intake preoperatively means that the pituitary patient commonly experiences early postoperative thirst. Furthermore, anesthetists normally keep their patients well hydrated during surgery, and excretion of this fluid load can result in an episode of polyuria. It is, therefore, important to recognize that neither the thirst nor the polyuria are necessarily a sign of diabetes insipidus (DI).

Although it is essential to monitor fluid balance in patients, 4-h urine outputs and specific gravity measurement are an inadequate way to keep abreast of fluid management. Nevertheless, they are still sometimes misguidedly used by the inexperienced, and the authors have previously seen transient hypotonic polyuria during the first 12 h misdiagnosed and treated with synthetic vasopressin (dDAVP). The unfortunate patient who has been misdiagnosed has by then had a 12-h iatrogenic water retention and may be hyponatremic. He or she then has a second period of a normal physiologic attempt at correction with a second period of high urine output. If truly unfortunate, this, too, will be treated by zealous junior medical staff and a second bolus of dDAVP given. To avoid such problems, a simple and consistent management regimen should be followed:

Patients should be allowed to drink freely. Until they do so, iv fluids can be given according to standard postoperative protocols. One liter of normal saline in 12 h is sufficient.

Once normal drinking has commenced, the rate of saline infusion can be slowed. A careful record of input and output must be kept. Urinary specific gravity, although commonly recorded, is only a vague pointer to posterior pituitary well-being and should be interpreted with caution. A formal diagnosis of DI should only be made after urine and serum osmolarity measurements. It is confirmed in the presence of raised plasma osmolarity >287 mosM/kg and urine osmolarity <200 mosM/kg, giving a ratio of urine to plasma of <1.2. If plasma osmolarity is normal, another cause of the polyuria should be sought. Plasma sodium is a useful parameter to review because it can be estimated rapidly . Sodium >146 mmol/L suggests the possibility of DI.

Diagnostic confusion may occur when treatment of hypertension with diuretics is continued perioperatively. These patients need careful assessment by the endocrinologist.

Once established, DI is treated with dDAVP. The correct dose is the smallest required to abolish the polyuria. In the presence of nasal packs, 1–2 μg as an intramuscular injection up to 12 h is usually sufficient. Once the packs are out, it is easier to give as a nasal spray as the nasal mucosa absorbs from the moment it is free of the packs. Each "puff" is 10 μg, and one to two puffs every 12 h is usually sufficient. Some patients prefer the oral preparation for long-term maintenance, often because they have been misinformed that the spray must be refrigerated. The only disadvantages are variable absorption and higher cost.

SYNDROME OF INAPPROPRIATE ANTIDIURETIC HORMONE SECRETION

Hyponatremia as a complication after pituitary surgery is a symptomatic problem in 1 in 25 cases in our unit. In a prospective study, it was found more frequently, being observed in 3 out of 25 patients reported by Whitaker et al. *(1)*, and 25% of 61 patients observed by Olson et al. *(2)* during a 2-wk period after surgery. Most patients are discharged before that time, so it is not practical to monitor them. Our practice is to monitor urine output and serum sodium during the hospital stay and to be wary if the patient complains of an unexplained sense of "lack of well-being" at the time of discharge. If unwell, the patient is not discharged until serum sodium is checked.

Left untreated, hyponatremia may cause seizures and, ultimately, coma. Treatment consists of fluid restriction to <1.5 L of free fluid daily until the sodium returns to normal. The symptoms of confusion and drowsiness may persist beyond the time that the biochemistry returns to normal. Second-line treatment involves the administration of hypertonic saline. This is seldom necessary and should only be given under endocrine supervision with extreme care because of the rare but dangerous complication of central pontine myelinolysis.

PERIOPERATIVE ENDOCRINE MANAGEMENT

The first concern in endocrine management is to ensure that the hypothalamic-pituitary-adrenal axis is functioning satisfactorily. The easiest way to ensure that sufficient cortisol is present to cover the stress of the operation is to give a bolus of hydrocortisone with induction of anesthesia. Postoperatively, the hydrocortisone can be continued, tapering the replacement level to physiologic replacement levels. Standard replacement is either hydrocortisone 15 mg on rising and 5 mg in the late afternoon or, alternatively, 10 mg on rising, 5 mg at midday, and 5 mg in the late afternoon. Levels should be retested with either a Synacthen test or an insulin stress test at some time after discharge, usually in 2 mo.

Using this regimen, although safe, will be unnecessary in a proportion of patients. In patients with microadenomas, both somatotroph and prolactinomas, replacing cortisol is often unnecessary and it is safe to check a single postoperative 9 AM level, and if more than 350 mmol/L (12.8 μg/dL), the surgeon should have no further concern. This is the policy we have followed for at least our last 500 transsphenoidal patients without problems.

For large tumors, it is safer to rely on some type of replacement. However, if normal cortisol levels existed preoperatively, as they frequently do, postoperative cortisol levels have an 84% chance of being normal as well. Most units would place patients on standard replacement therapy until they can have formal testing of adrenal function (synacthen test or insulin test) in the outpatient department. In some cases, however, a single 9 AM cortisol level of >350 mmol/L (12.8 μg/dL) following no replacement for >24 h can be considered adequate.

SPECIAL ENDOCRINE INVESTIGATIONS

Although early postoperative measurements are helpful for management, they are only indicators of the success or failure of surgery. All should be repeated in the early postdischarge period at approx 2 mo.

Prolactinomas

Prolactin (PRL) has a short half-life of hours, and a single postoperative level in the normal range can be considered indicative of a cure. If the level is in the 700–1000 mU/L range, this may represent a cure, because PRL levels can be increased by the stress of the procedure and by perioperative antiemetics. It is worth repeating: If the level remains high, when surgery was expected to be successful and particularly if the tissue taken at surgery was histologically confirmed, then reoperation is strongly advised.

Growth Hormone-Secreting Tumors

Most surgeons rely on a postoperative glucose tolerance test with growth hormone (GH) levels. Unless special arrangements exist most laboratories do not run GH assays every day. As a consequence, the patient has usually been discharged before the results return, because most patients with acromegaly have short in-patient stays. The initial reduction in GH levels to cure or semicure levels (<10 ng/mL, 20 mU/L) often lead to early and significant improvement in the symptoms they had, particularly sweating and carpal tunnel. Even obstructive airway symptoms can ameliorate. Some experts recommend that no decision should be made before the standard 6-wk period has elapsed and the patient retested (Fahlbusch, personal communication).

The decision to reoperate is a tricky one. Clearly, in absolute failure to cure, reoperation is worthwhile, but things are seldom so black and white. Postoperative scanning in a near cure is not usually helpful *(3,4)*. The surgeon often has a feel for whether active tissue is left. When this is not the case, do not operate but reduce GH with somatostatin analogs.

Cushing's Tumors

The early postoperative assessment is probably the most difficult area of management in the spectrum of this fascinating and complex disease. Cured patients, unlike those with acromegaly and patients with visual loss, seldom feel well. In fact, it is almost a truism to say that a patient with Cushing's who has been cured feels "rotten" for a while. The patient may lose his or her red color and may regain his or her normal blood pressure, but many feel "washed out" and their skin becomes dry, itchy, and flaky.

Biochemically, profound suppression of normal adrenal secretion has occurred because of long-term steroid-induced inhibition of the hypothalamic-pituitary axis. The early morning postoperative cortisol should be low, below 50 nmol/L (1.8 μg/dL) being considered a cure *(5)*.

In our practice, we withhold replacement until this level has been achieved. Alternatively, the patient can be replaced until an early formal check, off hydrocortisone for >24 h, has been carried out. If the level fails to fall within 72 h, re-exploration is advised. If the result is equivocal, 24 h urine free cortisols (UFCs) may be carried out to further clarify the issue.

When cortisols fail to suppress and the surgical findings, particularly with histologic confirmation, strongly suggest the presence of tumor, re-exploration is strongly indicated.

NONENDOCRINE COMPLICATIONS

The Nasal Airway

We employ dehydrated sponges as nasal packs (Merocel®, Xomed Surgical Products, Jacksonville, FL) and find these are much better tolerated than yards of ribbon gauze, which was previously used. The nasal packs provide a relatively gentle tamponade of the battered nasal mucosa. Ribbon inserted into the finger of a surgical glove is a good alternative and may be less unpleasant to remove. However, the extraction of any form of nasal pack is unpleasant, and the difference in discomfort is only a matter of degree.

We remove the packs as soon as we reasonably can. This is usually on the first postoperative day. Leaving them in for a longer period makes them increasingly more difficult to remove because of organized clot and may even require significant analgesia or even anesthesia at removal. We use a single tampon in the operated nostril, unless the mucosa is torn. Interestingly, a confused patient sometimes removes the packs within minutes of waking up in the recovery room. Complications from this have yet to be observed. Occasionally we have managed with no packs in patients with asthma with long-standing airway obstruction with no problem. Perhaps it is time to re-evaluate the need for packs, especially because the endoscopists do without them altogether.

Visual Problems

Most patients notice an improvement in their vision within hours of surgery, often as soon as consciousness returns in the recovery room. Many studies have shown that this occurs in more than 80% of patients *(6,7)*. Equally fortunately, visual deterioration is rare, occurring in less than 3% in a survey by Ciric *(8)*. If vision deteriorates postoperatively, early rescanning is mandatory. However, the scan, particularly the standard emergency computed tomography (CT) series may be difficult to interpret. Intracavity hematomas of some sort are sometimes seen even in "normal" recovering patients, and residual tumor is also a distinct possibility that can look surprisingly similar to clot. For the majority of us without an interventional magnetic resonance (MR) scanner, urgent re-exploration is the best option when there is any question of a significant clot.

A formal visual check after surgery should be carried out within the first few postoperative weeks. Ophthalmology departments find it difficult to get patients to concentrate adequately for the complexities of the Humphrey test or a Goldman field in the first 24–48 h, and prefer a longer delay to give a meaningful assessment. Vision can go on improving for many months, if not years, after surgery.

Cerebrospinal Fluid Rhinorrhea

Although a small leak of cerebrospinal fluid (CSF) is seen at operations, it can usually be managed without any problems, even for those of us who do not formally repair the fossa floor. Combinations of repair material or even judicious bipolar coagulation of the dura as practiced by de Tribolet (personal communication) are usually sufficient to contain the leak (*see also* Chapter 8). Persistent postoperative rhinorrhea, on the other hand, demands reoperation and repair.

The authors have abandoned temporary lumbar drainage, even though it has worked occasionally in the past. The complications of air encephalopathy and late meningitis, which we have all seen, means that we repair all late leaks at formal reoperation as soon as possible.

There is no evidence to support the use of prophylactic antibiotics when a CSF leak is diagnosed, but any symptoms or signs of meningitis require prompt lumbar puncture with CSF microscopy and appropriate antibiotic therapy.

DISCHARGE

The time required to accomplish the goals stated can be extremely variable, but in uncomplicated cases, our patients remain in hospital for approx 4 d. Earlier discharge times are quoted by some authors *(9)*. An important factor is the need to rule out endocrine complications before discharge, especially if, as in our unit, the patient population is not drawn entirely from the immediate locality.

The dosage of discharge medications, especially steroids, and their purpose, should be clearly explained to the patient. It is especially important to advise patients who are discharged on hydrocortisone replacement of the need to double the daily dose of steroid in case of an accident or severe illness. A steroid card is issued with written instructions. The drug regimen and the plans for continuation of therapy or retesting are communicated to the patient's family practitioner.

At discharge plans can be made for the timing of formal endocrine assessment as an outpatient and for postoperative imaging, which is usually undertaken at 3 mo.

REFERENCES

1. Whitaker SJ, Meanock CI, Turner GF, et al. Fluid balance and secretion of antidiuretic hormone following transsphenoidal pituitary surgery. A preliminary series. J Neurosurg 1985;63:404–412.
2. Olson BR, Gumowski J, Rubino D, Oldfield EH. Pathophysiology of hyponatremia after transsphenoidal pituitary surgery. J Neurosurg 1997;87:499–507.
3. Rajaraman V, Schulder M. Postoperative MRI appearance after transsphenoidal pituitary tumor resection. Surg Neurol 1999;52:592–598; discussion 598–599.
4. Yoon PH, Kim DI, Jeon P, Lee SI, Lee SK, Kim SH. Pituitary adenomas: early postoperative MR imaging after transsphenoidal resection. Am J Neuroradiol 2001;22:1097–1104.
5. McCance DR, Besser M, Atkinson AB. Assessment of cure after transsphenoidal surgery for Cushing's disease. Clin Endocrinol (Oxf) 1996;44:1–6.
6. Cohen AR, Cooper PR, Kupersmith MJ, Flamm ES, Ransohoff J. Visual recovery after transsphenoidal removal of pituitary adenomas. Neurosurgery 1985;17:446–452.
7. Powell MP. Recovery of vision following transsphenoidal surgery for pituitary adenoma. Br J Neurosurg 1995;9:367–373.

8. Ciric I, Ragin A, Baumgartner C, Pierce D. Complications of transsphenoidal surgery: results of a national survey, review of the literature, and personal experience. Neurosurgery 1997;40:225–236; discussion 236–237.
9. Jho H-D. Endoscopic endonasal pituitary surgery: evolution of surgical technique and equipment in 150 operations Min Invas Neurosurg 2001;44:1–12.

12 Long-Term Postoperative Management

Paul V. Carroll, MD, MRCP,
and Ashley B. Grossman, MD, FRCP, FMedSci

Contents

INTRODUCTION

Long-term surveillance with periodic assessment is mandatory for all patients with a history of a pituitary operation. The frequency and intensity of surveillance is determined by several factors, including the histologic nature, location, size, and hormone secretion of the original tumor and the use of radiotherapy. Those with residual disease require specially structured monitoring, including assessment of remaining pituitary function, determination of hormone secretion by the tumor, and imaging of the pituitary fossa and surrounding structures. This chapter addresses these issues with respect to individual pituitary tumor types.

From: *Management of Pituitary Tumors: The Clinician's Practical Guide, Second Edition*
Edited by: M. P. Powell, S. L. Lightman, and E. R. Laws, Jr.

PROLACTIN-SECRETING PITUITARY ADENOMA (PROLACTINOMA)

Prolactin (PRL)-secreting tumors are the most common form of functioning pituitary tumor. Most are microadenomas (<1 cm in size) and usually present with galactorrhea, disturbance of menstrual regularity, infertility, and, in the male, decreased sexual function *(1,2)*. Diagnosis is made by measurement of circulating PRL and pituitary imaging. Spurious hyperprolactinemia may result from measurement of complexed but bioinactive macroprolactin, and an extraction assay should be considered in all patients who have elevated serum PRL on conventional testing, especially where the level is discordant with the clinical presentation. In general, preservation of normal anterior and posterior pituitary function is the rule in patients with PRL-secreting microadenomas, but assessment of basal hormone levels is recommended in all patients.

The initial treatment of prolactinomas involves the use of oral dopamine agonist therapy. Rapid reduction in PRL levels and shrinkage of both micro adenomas and macroadenomas occur in the majority of patients *(3)*. In general, pituitary function is unaffected, but infarction has been described, which may result in loss of adenocorticotropic hormone (ACTH), thyroid-stimulating hormone (TSH), growth hormone (GH) and gonadotropins. Monitoring of basal levels and performance of dynamic testing, as outlined in Appendix 1 (*see* p. 197 *et seq.*), is recommended, particularly in macroadenomas.

In rare cases, dopamine agonist therapy is unsuccessful, often related to noncompliance, poor tolerance, or adverse effects. However, before diagnosing intolerance or resistance, a second agent, such as cabergoline or quinagolide, should be tried. When true resistance is diagnosed, pituitary surgery and/or external beam irradiation may be considered. Larger more invasive tumors are less likely to be cured by surgery, as are those patients with the highest preoperative prolactin levels *(4)*. After a surgical procedure, assessment of ACTH reserve, water balance, TSH, GH, and gonadotrophin reserve should be performed before discharge, as outlined in the next subheading. Long-term surveillance of anterior pituitary function is necessary after irradiation to assess the reserve of GH and other pituitary hormones. Surveillance of the pituitary fossa and endocrine assessment should follow the model outlined for the treatment of acromegaly (next subheading).

ACROMEGALY (GROWTH HORMONE-SECRETING PITUITARY ADENOMA)

The majority of patients with acromegaly have a pituitary macroadenoma, which frequently extends outside the sella and may result in compression of the optic apparatus and visual failure *(5)*. Most tumors secrete GH alone, but up to a third result in hyperprolactinemia *(6)*. This may result from tumoral cosecretion or stalk compression. GH-secreting adenomas occur either spontaneously or in the context of genetic conditions, such as multiple endocrine neoplasia (MEN)-1, McCune-Albright syndrome, and Carney complex syndrome. Once the diagnosis of acromegaly is established, surgery is the primary treatment of choice, resulting in a rapid reduction in circulating GH levels and reduction in the size of the abnormal pituitary gland. The majority of lesions are approached by the transsphenoidal route, but larger tumors extending above the sella may require transcranial operation *(7)*. Microadenomas are frequently "cured," but this is seen in less than 50% of macroadenomas.

After pituitary surgery, both residual pituitary function and the GH secretory status should be evaluated. Basal endocrine testing for 9 AM cortisol, thyroxine, TSH, follicle-stimulating hormone (FSH), luteinizing hormone (LH), testosterone/estrogen, PRL, and serum and urinary osmolality should be performed before discharge. When there is doubt, assessment of ACTH reserve should be performed as outlined subsequently.

GH secretory status can be assessed using a five-point GH day curve (Appendix 1, *see* pp. 200–201). In acromegaly, GH secretion loses its normal pulsatile pattern, and values do not vary widely throughout the day. Serum insulin-like growth factor-I (IGF-I) is a marker of hepatic GH responsiveness and correlates well with GH levels *(8)*, but age- and sex-normalized ranges are required. Recent evidence suggests that assessment as early as 1 wk postoperatively will allow for prediction of outcome. Because prolonged GH excess contributes to major morbidity and more than a doubling in cardiovascular and cerebrovascular mortality, efforts should be taken to ensure safe levels of GH in the circulation *(9,10)*. In difficult cases, an oral glucose tolerance test may be necessary. Current evidence indicates that average serum GH concentrations ≤5 mU/L (2 μg/L) reduce morbidity/mortality to that of a background population when associated with normalization of the serum total IGF-I concentration *(11)*. A recent consensus statement defined cure as a nadir GH after an oral glucose load <1 μg/L (approx 2 mU/L), provided the total IGF-I was within the age-matched normal reference range *(12)*. However, many would use assessment of mean GH levels to <5 mU/L (2 μg/L) as a more clearly established criterion. Most endocrine centers treat patients with acromegaly with the intention of achieving this level. After pituitary surgery, an early GH day curve combined with serum total IGF-I measurement will indicate whether surgery alone has been sufficient *(13)*.

Current evidence suggests that in patients with acromegaly secondary to a GH-secreting microadenoma, surgery alone will result in cure in approx 70%–90% of patients. This figure falls when a macroadenoma (<50%) or a giant adenoma (<20%) is present. Those with the highest preoperative GH concentrations are least likely to be cured by surgery alone *(13,14)*. In those with continuing GH excess, further treatment is indicated, and the majority of patients will undergo conventional fractionated three-field external beam irradiation. A second surgical procedure will result in safe GH levels in only 20% of patients *(14)*.

Recognizing that radiotherapy does not result in an instant lowering of GH levels, medical treatment is commonly used, especially in the short-term. On average, 2 yr after external beam irradiation, GH levels have decreased by approx 50%, with a further fall resulting in 75% reduction at 5 yr *(15)*. Newer stereotactic techniques, when used appropriately, may effect a more rapid reduction in GH levels. However, because the tumor in such cases is usually a macroadenoma, we would only use radiosurgery as "salvage therapy" in the face of poor control of tumor secretion or regrowth after conventional radiotherapy.

Additional available medical therapies include the use of dopamine agonists and somatostatin analogs *(16)*. Bromocriptine will normalize GH levels in only 10% of patients, although this may rise to 30% with the newer agent cabergoline. Octreotide and lanreotide, particularly in their depot formulations, which last 4–6 wk, will normalize mean GH levels in 70%–80% of patients and are, therefore, highly effective, albeit expensive. The recently developed GH receptor antagonist, pegvisomant, may be used in patients resistant to these agents, when it eventually becomes available *(17)*. Periodic assessment with IGF-I measurement and GH day curve testing should be performed at regular intervals to facilitate titration of doses and determine response to radiotherapy. After irradiation it is reasonable to assess GH status after appropriate discontinuation of medical therapies at 6-mo intervals for 2 yr and yearly thereafter.

CUSHING'S DISEASE (ACTH-SECRETING PITUITARY ADENOMA)

Endogenous glucocorticoid excess (Cushing's syndrome [CS]) most commonly results from an ACTH-producing pituitary adenoma. The majority are small microadenomas, and are difficult to define on magnetic resonance imaging (MRI) imaging: the mean size of an ACTH-secreting pituitary adenoma is 6 mm. Adenomectomy is the treatment of choice to control Cushing's disease (CD), and it is recommended that surgery be performed by a specialist surgeon. In this setting, approx 90% of patients with CD will undergo successful cure, i.e., a lowering of cortisol production to within the normal range *(18)*. However, this figure falls to 50–65% (in three recent British audits; Oxford, Newcastle, and the National Hospital, London) if cure implies removal of all tumor tissue such that the residual cortisol from the normal corticotrophs is suppressed to below the detectable range.

Removal of the ACTH-secreting adenoma results in an immediate reduction in circulating ACTH levels, with consequent lowering of serum cortisol concentrations. The remaining corticotrophs require a variable period of recovery before restoration to normal ACTH secretion and feedback control. A stricter definition of surgical cure is based on measurement of postoperative early morning serum cortisol concentration, with a value <50 nmol/L (1.8 μg/dL) indicative of a successful outcome. Occasionally, low but detectable values decrease with time to normal or subnormal levels, but immediate postoperative values >100 nmol/L

(3.6 μg/dL) in general indicate residual corticotroph adenoma. Management of patients after pituitary surgery for CD can be subdivided into patients with continuing glucocorticoid excess and those with successful cure.

Long-Term Management of Patients After Successful Pituitary Surgery for Cushing's Disease

Many patients will have undetectable (<50 nmol/L or 1.8 μg/dL) early morning cortisol concentrations after pituitary surgery. Once cure has been established, replacement glucocorticoids should be initiated and titrated to ensure satisfactory clinical response and biochemical levels. Many centers favor the use of hydrocortisone or cortisone acetate, facilitating measurement of cortisol concentrations to monitor therapy. Most patients receive divided doses, typically three times a day, taken before rising in the morning, at midday and in the early evening, allowing for circadian dynamics close to those seen in the healthy population. A hydrocortisone day curve (HCDC) allows measurement of this pattern (*see* "Endocrine Protocols", Appendix 1, p. 201). All patients should receive a "steroid card" and instruction on management of glucocorticoid replacement during periods of illness, while specialist centers may also provide an "emergency pack" for parenteral (usually intramuscular) hydrocortisone administration during severe illness.

Spontaneous recovery of preserved corticotrophs usually occurs within 2 yr in most cases of successful cure of CD, but recovery may be delayed considerably beyond this time *(19)*. After assessment of pituitary function and establishment of glucocorticoid replacement, patients should be periodically reassessed to determine recovery of the ACTH-adrenal axis. We favor re-admission for assessment initially after a 3- to 6-month interval, with subsequent reassessments at 6- to 12 month intervals. The reassessment after successful cure of CD includes successive daily measurements of early morning serum cortisol concentrations for 72 h after discontinuation of glucocorticoid. If values remain undetectable, replacement is reinitiated and the patient discharged to be evaluated at a later date. In those with detectable cortisol concentrations, particularly >100 nmol/L (3.6 μg/dL), a provocative test of ACTH reserve is performed, either in the form of the insulin-hypoglycemia test or a glucagon stimulation test (*see* "Endocrine Protocols", Appendix 1, pp. 197–198). Other centers may perform outpatient assessment of hypothalamic-pituitary-adrenal axis activity.

In those patients achieving satisfactory responses, glucocorticoid replacement can be discontinued. An intermediary response (>200 nmol/L [7.3 μg/dL] and <550 nmol/L [20 μg/dL]) is frequently observed and in such a case a clinical judgment is made whether glucocorticoid replacement is necessary and at what dosing regimen.

Periodic reassessment should be continued, and generally the lowest dose considered clinically safe is chosen, with the availability of an emergency supply. In those with reemerging ACTH-adrenal secretion, identification of normal circadian dynamics and exclusion of recurrence of CD is undertaken during these assessments. Once measurable serum cortisol levels are evident, the circadian pattern may be evaluated during 48 h with measurement of cortisol levels at 9 AM, 6 PM, and 12 AM, the last value ideally with the patient asleep for the most accurate interpretation. The low dose dexamethasone suppression test (*see* Appendix 1, p. 200) should be performed to further exclude recurrent CD.

All patients with CD require life-long endocrine surveillance, and attention should be paid to body composition, psychologic health, blood pressure, carbohydrate tolerance, lipid status, and bone mineral density (BMD). At least yearly clinic attendances are required, with periodic assessment to exclude recurrence of disease. Established associated conditions should be aggressively treated, and BMD measured using dual-energy X-ray absorptiometry (DXA). BMD will increase in time with cure of CD; however, if there is a severe persistent deficiency, bisphosphonates may be used; however, the effects of the agents in human pregnancy are not yet established. Recent evidence indicates that reversible GH-deficiency (GHD) may persist for as long as 2 yr after successful treatment of CD. It has been recommended that definitive assessment of GH status in adults with cured CD be delayed for this period *(20)*. In addition, the possibility of delayed hypopituitarism should be considered and measurement of basal pituitary function performed. If necessary, a provocative test of ACTH and GH reserve can be carried out and occasionally, a water deprivation test if cranial diabetes insipidus (DI) persists after surgery (*see* Appendix 1, pp. 198–199).

Cushing's Disease Persisting After Pituitary Surgery

A significant proportion of patients with CD continue to have measurable cortisol levels after pituitary surgery, indicating total or partial failure in removing the adenoma. They may have invasive macroadenomas, and surgery was mandatory to reduce tumor bulk and correct visual failure from compression of the optic chiasm. After noncurative surgery, an immediate decision should be made as to whether a second surgical intervention is indicated. This may involve reexploration of the pituitary fossa or a full removal (total hypophysectomy) of remaining pituitary tissue. If a second procedure results in undetectable early morning cortisol concentrations, subsequent management is as outlined earlier.

In those with evidence of continuing ACTH hypersecretion, further measures to control cortisol levels are necessary. In most cases, medical management with adrenolytic drugs is indicated, with metyrapone, ketoconazole, and mitotane being the most widely used. When initiating metyrapone, a test dose (usually 750 mg by mouth) may be given as a metyrapone "sensitivity test" (*see* Appendix 1, p. 201). Maintenance treatment is then started with equal divided doses taken every 8 h. In the case of all adrenolytics, the response to treament may be assessed using a Cushing's "day-curve" (*see* Appendix 1, pp. 199–200), with doses titrated to achieve mean cortisol concentrations between 150 and 300 nmol/L (equivalent to the normal daily production rate).

The majority of patients with unsuccessful surgery for CD are considered for pituitary irradiation. Conventionally, this is delivered in fractions during a 5- to 7-wk period in the form of three-field external beam irradiation. Newer radiotherapy techniques include the Gamma Knife and X-knife (*see* Chapter 14), but we do not recommend these as initial treatment. In all cases, the ACTH time course response to treatment is variable, with 6 to 12 mo typically passing before significant benefits are seen. Patients may achieve remission within 1 yr after radiotherapy *(21)*, particularly in childhood, but usually many years are required before medical therapy can be terminated. Periodic remeasurement of the CDC is required with careful titration of adrenolytic drugs.

In resistant cases where the combination of pituitary surgery and irradiation have failed to control CD and/or medical therapy is poorly tolerated, bilateral adrenalectomy should be considered. Provided all adrenal tissue is removed, satisfactory reduction in the circulating cortisol level is seen. This procedure is frequently performed by minimally invasive surgery or laparoscopy, but care is required because the adrenal glands are often large, vascular, and friable in CD. The presence of continuing cortisol excess after adrenalectomy raises the possibility of the presence of adrenal rests.

After bilateral adrenalectomy, all patients require both corticosteroid and mineralocorticoid replacement. Pituitary surveillance is mandatory in patients with CD who have undergone adrenalectomy. Nelson's syndrome of pituitary tumor enlargement in this situation results in marked elevation of circulating ACTH concentrations with resultant pigmentation of the skin *(22)*. Regular imaging, combined with measurement of ACTH before and after the morning dose of glucocorticoids, facilitates monitoring for the development of Nelson's syndrome. It remains unclear whether and to what extent pituitary radiotherapy lessens this complication, but in general, advances in surgery have rendered early bilateral adrenalectomy less common.

GLYCOPROTEIN-SECRETING PITUITARY ADENOMAS

Thyrotrophs and gonadotrophs produce the glycoproteins TSH, LH, and FSH, repectively. Each of these consists of an α- and a β-subunit. The α-subunit shares a common structure, with the different β moieties responsible for differing hormonal action.

Gonadotropin Tumors

Although believed to be rare, many nonfunctioning pituitary adenoma (NFPA) may stain for LH and or FSH and are gonadotrophin-producing *(23)*. Most patients present with a macroadenoma and/or features of hypopituitarism *(24)*.

Tumors may produce FSH, LH, and α-subunit, alone or in combination *(25)*. Preoperative recognition of the pattern of hormone production is important for accurate diagnosis and for monitoring response to treatment. Initial management for these tumors is surgery, with the transsphenoidal approach used in the majority *(26)*. Little data are available regarding the success of surgery, but it is likely that surgery alone is rarely curative. Measurement of hormone levels may act as a guide to surgical response, with later elevations suggestive of regrowth *(27)*. Pituitary irradiation has a central role in the management of these tumors and is recognized to reduce recurrence rates. Medical therapies include the use of dopamine agonists, somatostatin analogs and gonadotropin-releasing hormone (GnRH) analogs, although success rates are generally low. Long-term surveillance with careful visual field and MRI assessment is mandatory in such patients, because tumor regrowth may occur. Measurement of gonadotropin levels and serum concentrations of α-subunit may sometimes be useful.

Thyroid-Stimulating Hormone-Secreting Tumors

These are rare tumors, representing approx 2 % of all pituitary adenomas *(28)*. Typically, the presentation is with features of hyperthyroidism, often a mass lesion is present, and these tumors may cosecrete GH or prolactin *(29)*. Most TSH-secreting adenomas produce an excess of the α-subunit, and an elevated molar ratio of α-subunit to intact TSH is present in the serum. Treatment of TSH-secreting tumors is directed at both correction of hyperthyroidism and therapy for the tumor. Antithyroid drugs are usually indicated before surgery. The initial management should be surgical, but data regarding the usefulness of operation are scanty. Success, defined as normalization of thyroid function, has been reported to be approx 40% *(30)*; therefore, postsurgical follow-up is essential. If TSH/α-subunit levels remain elevated, radiation therapy should be considered. Dopamine agonist drugs and somatostatin analogs have also been used, with particularly positive reports after octreotide use *(29)*.

CLINICALLY NONFUNCTIONING PITUITARY ADENOMA

The most common pituitary macroadenomas seen in adults are classified as clinically nonfunctioning pituitary adenoma (NFPA). Although termed nonfunctioning, many display positive immunostaining for gonadotropins LH and FSH, whereas "silent" corticotroph and somatotroph tumors may also occur. Presentation may be incidental when neuroimaging has been performed for reasons other than pituitary assessment. Alternatively, a macroadenoma causes mass effects including headache and visual failure. In general, pituitary function is preserved in early cases, although hyperprolactinemia related to disinhibition related to stalk compression is frequently present. As the tumor enlarges, progressive loss of GH, the gonadotropins, and eventually ACTH and TSH axes will occur.

In macroadenomas, surgical treatment is indicated, with the transsphenoidal route favored. In those patients with preoperative hypopituitarism, recovery of hormone secretion may occur *(31)*. The recurrence rate of NFPA treated by surgery alone is considerable *(26)*, and many centers advocate the use of radiotherapy in most patients after surgery. However, improvements in neurosurveillance, largely MRI, may allow patients to be followed closely in the absence of radiotherapy. Review of pituitary function and replacement of pituitary hormones should follow the protocol set out for acromegaly earlier. Periodic rescanning should be performed because recurrences may occur years after primary treatment. With standard radiotherapy (as detailed in Chapter 13), recurrence will be less, probably considerably less than 5%.

MALIGNANT PITUITARY TUMORS

The majority of pituitary tumors are histologically benign. However, local dural invasion is not uncommon *(31)*. Occasionally such tumors are more aggressive, and rarely, central nervous system (CNS) or more distant metastases are present, indicating pituitary carcinoma in 0.2% of all primary pituitary tumors *(32)*. Such malignant tumors are frequently functional, and treatment of the primary is directed toward local excision, radiotherapy, and, where appropriate, medical therapy such as dopamine agonists or octreotide.

Recurrent disease after previous radiotherapy presents a difficult management problem with progressive visual loss and neurologic disability proceeding to rapid death in many cases. Careful surveillance with neuroimaging and hormonal assessment is required, particularly to facilitate planning of further intervention and to assess responses to treatment. Commonly, standard three-field external beam irradiation has been delivered, making further treatment of this type limited because of toxicity to the optic chiasm. "Salvage" stereotactic radiotherapy with the Gamma Knife or sterotactic multi-arc radiotherapy (SMART) may be considered in individual patients. Although no controlled trials have been performed, cytotoxic chemotherapy has also been used in select cases. The response rate is variable, and progressive disease has been observed in most reports *(33)*. Targeted radioisotope treatment, such as ^{90}Y-labelled somatostatin analogs, may have a role in this rare condition in the future.

CRANIOPHARYNGIOMA

Craniopharyngiomas originate from squamous rest cells in the remnant of Rathke's pouch located between the adenohypophysis and the neurohypophysis. These neoplasms may be entirely intrasellar (25%), solely extrasellar, or found in both areas. Commonly, these tumors present with nonendocrine symptoms, but anterior pituitary failure is frequent. GH deficiency and hypogonadotropic hypogonadism are the usual findings, but with diabetes insipidus (DI) occurring more commonly than in tumors of the anterior pituitary *(34,35)*.

Surgery is the treatment of choice, transsphenoidally where possible; however, because most tumors have an extrasellar component, recurrence following surgery alone is common *(36)*. The majority of patients require radiotherapy after surgery for craniopharyngioma. The consequences of treatment vary with the extent and location of the tumor and whether radical resection is undertaken. As complete an excision as possible, but with avoidance of damage to the carotid vessels, optic apparatus, and hypothalamus, offers the best long-term prognosis *(37)*. DI and anterior pituitary failure are common after surgery, and these deficiencies may be permanent (38). Careful evaluation of ACTH and TSH status and water balance should be performed before discharge after any surgical procedure.

In those patients with recurrent tumors, further surgery may be necessary with marsupialization of cystic components, internal or external shunting, and occasionally cystic insertion of radionuclide. Clearly, long-term follow-up is central to the management of these patients, and most will require full pituitary hormone replacement, including desmopressin and growth hormone (*see* the following subheading).

LONG-TERM MANAGEMENT OF THE PATIENT FOLLOWING PITUITARY RADIOTHERAPY

Pituitary irradiation is used to decrease the rates of tumor recurrence and to reduce the excess hormone secretion of functioning pituitary adenomas. There is some debate regarding the case selection of patients best treated by this modality. Conventional irradiation of the pituitary fossa is three-field external beam irradiation. This stereotactic technique delivers charged particle beams that can be targeted to deposit ionizing radiation at a specific depth. Radiotherapy of this type is delivered in fractions (usually less than 200 cGy/d) designed to reduce damage to the optic chiasm, that is believed to be largely mediated through effects on the blood vessels supplying this structure.

Alternative methods of radiation delivery include the use of photon techniques. Examples include the design of the Swedish γ unit, termed the Gamma Knife, and linear accelerator methodology, termed the X-knife (*see* Chapter 14).

The main adverse consequence of pituitary irradiation is hypopituitarism, the incidence of which is greater the more compromised the function before radiation delivery. The somatotroph is most sensitive to radiation damage, followed by gonadotrophs and corticotrophs. The TSH axis is relatively insensitive, and DI as a result of loss of posterior pituitary function is exceedingly rare. Rates of hypopituitarism vary from series to series, but in patients who are irradiated for acromegaly, 25% required new endocrine replacement after 5 yr, with this figure rising with further passage of time *(39)*. When assessed 10 yr after fractionated radiotherapy, 47% of patients were hypogonadal, 30% hypoadrenal, and 16% hypothyroid in another series *(40)*. The rate of GH deficiency is likely to be significantly greater than 50%.

Recurrence of functioning tumors and regrowth of primary tumors after pituitary irradiation have also been the subject of debate. Ten-year recurrences for acromegaly (8%), CD (12%), NFPA (17%), and prolactinoma (24%) have been reported *(41)*. In addition, regrowth of tumors has been reported varying from 21% to 32% during roughly a 10-yr period, significantly lower rates than observed in the nonirradiated population *(42)*. As noted, our own recurrence rates appear to be considerably less than these figures.

After irradiation of pituitary tissue, regular surveillance is mandatory to detect development of hypopituitarism, particularly GH deficiency. Basal pituitary profiles, including measurement of IGF-1 and assessment for the clinical features of GH deficiency, should be performed regularly. Dynamic testing should be performed in cases of clinical doubt. In addition, regular imaging is required to assess tumor response to radiotherapy and to facilitate early detection of recurrence. Initial MRI/computed tomography (CT) imaging may be performed 6 mo after surgery (less than this and perioperative changes are likely to obscure the assessment), and regularly thereafter with increasing time interval depending on clinical response. Accurate assessment of visual fields is a useful adjunct. The response of functioning tumors to irradiation should also be regularly assessed, as outlined in the previous subheadings. The responses in CD and acromegaly need especially vigilant monitoring, because typically these patients are on medical treatment (e.g., adrenolytic drugs, somatostatin analogs), which must be titrated to response.

HORMONE REPLACEMENT AFTER PITUITARY SURGERY

Strategies to determine deficiencies in both anterior and posterior pituitary function are outlined in the previous subheadings. Protocols for the performance of basal and dynamic testing are detailed in Appendix 1 and are summarized in Table 1.

Until recently, conventional replacement therapy for the hypopituitary adult has focused on the use of glucocorticoid, thyroxine, and sex steroid replacement. dDAVP is used to treat DI related to hypothalamic/posterior pituitary dysfunction. It is now established that GH is essential for health in the adult, and GH replacement is dealt with in the next subheading. Although traditionally thyroid and vasopressin deficiencies were treated with oral thyroxine and intranasal desmopressin, various preparations of glucocorticoid and sex steroid are available for use in hypopituitarism. These formulations are summarized in Appendix 2.

We advocate the use of hydrocortisone as replacement glucocorticoid, because this preparation lends itself to monitoring serum levels, and in general administration three times daily leads to optimal subjective feelings of good

Table 1
Determination of Pituitary Hormone Status and Summary of Replacement Hormones

Hormone	*Test*	*Replacement*	*Forms*
ACTH	IHT/glucagon	Glucocorticoid	Oral
TSH	T4/TSH	Thyroxine	Oral
GH	IHT/glucagon	GH	Subcutaneous
FSH/LH	FSH/LH/ Testosterone/ estradiol	Testosterone/estrogen	Oral, implant, transdermal, intramuscular
ADH	Water deprivation test/smolalities /U&E	dDAVP	Oral, subcutaneous, intranasal

ACTH, adrenocorticotrophic hormone; IHT, insulin-hypoglycemia test; TSH, thyroid-stimulating hormone; GH, growth hormone; FSH, follicle-stimulating hormone; LH, leutinizing hormone; ADH, anti-diuretic hormone; U & E, urea and electrolytes.

health. The first dose should be at or just before rising, and the latest in the late afternoon or early evening. The dose should be doubled during any intercurrent pyrexial illness, and an emergency pack of intramuscular hydrocortisone 100 mg can be available for use during severe vomiting or diarrhea. As noted, a "steroid card" should be held by the patient and, ideally, a Medic-Alert bracelet worn in countries where this is available. Recent data suggest that previous dose regimens were too high, and generally 15–20 mg daily should be adequate.

Thyroid hormone replacement is relatively straightforward, with a usual daily dose of 0.1 mg levothyroxine being sufficient. TSH monitoring is unhelpful in this situation.

For the sex steroids, there is no consensus as to the optimal form of estrogen and progesterone, and this should be given as standard hormone replacement therapy. For the younger patient, the oral contraceptive preparations are slightly unorthodox, but we can see no reason why they should not be used, especially because they may allow the patient to feel more "normal" in relation to her peers. For men, there are several testosterone treatments, attesting to the belief that none is perfect. The cheapest and most popular form is injectable testosterone enanthate, 100 mg weekly, 250 two or three weekly, or 500 mg three or four weekly; however, the injections may be uncomfortable, and the pharmacokinetics are far from ideal, especially with the larger doses. In some UK centers, implants are favored and may last for up to 6 mo. Of the patches, currently the only one still available in the UK has a high incidence of skin sensitivity problems. The oral preparation, testosterone undecanoate, must be given two or three times daily, and dosing is difficult because blood levels of testosterone are unreliable indicators of its efficacy (it is mainly metabolized to dihydrotestosterone). A "buccal" slow-release

Table 2
Clinical Features of Growth Hormone Deficiency in Adults

Background
Known pituitary pathology ± previous treatment
Full conventional pituitary hormone replacement
Need for growth hormone (GH) treatment as a child
Symptoms
Abnormal body composition
Reduced lean body mass
Increased abdominal adiposity
Reduced strength and exercise capacity
Impaired psychological well-being
Depressed mood
Reduced vitality and energy
Emotional lability
Signs
Overweight, with predominantly central (abdominal) adiposity
Thin, dry skin; cool peripheries; poor venous access
Reduced muscle strength
Reduction exercise performance
Depressed affect, labile emotions
Investigations
Stimulated GH level below 9 mU/L (3.5 μg/L)
Low or low-normal serum insulin-like growth factor (IGF)-I
Elevated serum lipids, particularly low-density lipoprotein cholesterol
Reduced lean body mass/increased fat mass
Reduced bone mineral density

preparation may become available with in the next year or two, while in the United States a gel formulation looks promising and will soon be available in Europe. In the end, the choice of replacement sex steroid should be decided upon after discussion between patient and physician.

GROWTH HORMONE REPLACEMENT

Over the past 15 yr it has been established that circulating GH continues to have important biologic functions in regulating body composition, psychologic health, exercise performance, and aspects of intermediary metabolism in the adult. Many well-designed studies have shown that GH deficiency results in adverse effects on these variables, and that these abnormalities can be largely corrected by GH replacement *(43)*. Although expensive, most Western countries have now approved recombinant human GH for use in the adult with severe hypopituitarism.

Not all subjects with GH deficiency have significant symptoms. In treated pituitary tumor patients, those with complaints relating to poor quality of life, altered body composition, with documented dyslipidemia or reduced bone mineral density, should undergo assessment for GH deficiency (Table 2). Severe GH deficiency has been defined as a peak GH response on provocative testing <9 mU/L (3.5 μg/L) and GH has a license for use in this group. The insulin-hypoglycemia test (*see* Appendix 1, p. 197) is the gold standard. In most patients, two tests of GH reserve are required and a dynamic test is usually combined with a GH day-curve and measurement of serum total IGF-1. Recombinant GH is manufactured by several companies and is often in the form of a powder for reconstitution before injection using a multidose pen device. A ready-to-use liquid form has recently been developed. Patients are taught to self-administer subcutaneous injections, usually at bedtime. Most centers advocate initiation of a small dose with regular clinical assessments and measurement of IGF-1 to ensure individual dose titration to minimize adverse effects *(44)*.

REFERENCES

1. Wilson C, Dempsey L. Trans-sphenoidal microsurgical removal of 250 pituitary adenomas. J Neurosurg 1978;48:13–22.
2. Schlechte J, Sherman B, Halmi N, et al. Prolactin-secreting pituitary tumors in amenorrheic women: a comprehensive study. Endocr Rev 1980;1:295–308.
3. Thorner MO, Schran HF, Evans WS, Rogol AD, Morris JL, MacLeod RM. A broad spectrum of prolactin suppression by bromocriptine in hyperprolactinaemic women: a study of serum prolactin and bromocriptine levels after a cure and chronic administration of bromocriptine. J Clin Endocrinol Metab 1980;50:1026–1033.
4. Laws ER Jr, Ebersold MJ, Piepgras DG, et al. The role of surgery in the management of prolactinomas. In: MacLeod RM, Thorner MO, Scapagnini U, eds. *Prolactin, Basic and Clinical Correlates.* New York: Springer-Verlag; 1985: 849–853..
5. Nabarro JD. Acromegaly. Clin Endocrinol 1987;26:481–512.
6. De Pablo F, Eastman RC, Roth J, Gorden P. Plasma prolactin in acromegaly before and after treatment. J Clin Endocrinol Metab 1981;53:344–352.
7. Melmed S. Acromegaly. NEngl J Med 1990;322:966–977.
8. Barkan AL, Beitins IZ, Kelch RP. Plasma insulin-like growth factor/somatomedin C in acromegaly: correlation with the degree of growth hormone secretion. J Clin Endocrinol Metab 1988;67:69–73.
9. Bates AS, van't Hoff W, Jones JM, Clayton RN. An audit of outcome of treatment in acromegaly. Q J Med 1993;86:293–299.
10. Orme SM, McNally RJQ, Cartwright RA, Belchetz PE. Mortality and cancer incidence in acromegaly: a retrospective cohort study. J Clin Endocrinol Metab 1998;83:2730–2734.
11. Swearingen B, Barker FG, Katznelson L, et al. Long-term mortality after trans-sphenoidal surgery and adjunctive therapy for acromegaly. J Clin Endocrinol Metab 1998;83:3419–3426.
12. Giustina A, Barkan A, Casanueva FF, et al. Criteria for cure of acromegaly: A consensus statement. J Clin Endocrinol Metab 1999;85:526–529.
13. Kaltsas GA, Isidori AM, Florakis D, et al. Predictors of the outcome of surgical treatment in acromegaly and the value of the mean growth hormone day curve in assessing postoperative disease activity. J Clin Endocrinol Metab 2001;86:1645–1652.

14. Fahlbusch R, Honneger J, Buchfelder M. Surgical management of acromegaly. Endocrinol Metab Clin North Am. Ed (Melmed S, ed.) 1992;21:669–692.
15. Eastman RC, Gorden P, Roth J. Conventional supervoltage irradiation is an effective treatment for acromegaly. J Clin Endocrinol Metab 1979;48:931–940.
16. Jenkins PJ, Akker S, Chew SL, Besser GM, Monson JP, Grossman AB. Optimal dosage interval for depot somatostatin analogue therapy in acromegaly requires individual titration. Clin Endocrinol 2000;53:719–724.
17. Trainer PJ, Drake WM, Katznelson L, et al. Treatment of acromegaly with the growth hormone-receptor antagonist pegvisomant. N Engl J Med 2000;342:1171–1177.
18. Mampalam TJ, Tyrrell JB, Wilson CB. Trans-sphenoidal microsurgery for Cushing's disease. A report of 216 cases. Ann Intern Med 1998;109:487–493.
19. Lindholm J, Kehlet H. Re-evaluation of the 30-min ACTH test in assessing hypothalamic-pituitary-adrenocortical function. Clin Endocrinol 1987;26:53–59.
20. Hughes NR, Lissett CA, Shalet SM. Growth hormone status following treatment for Cushing's syndrome. Clin Endocrinol 1999;51:61–66.
21. Schteingart DE, Tsao HS, Taylor CI. Sustained remission in Cushing's disease with mitotane and pituitary irradiation. Ann Intern Med 1980;92:613–618.
22. Nelson DH, Meakin JW, Thorn GW. ACTH-producing pituitary tumors following adrenalectomy for Cushing's syndrome. Ann Intern Med 1960;52:560–569.
23. Klibanski A, Deutsch PJ, Jameson JL, et al. Luteinizing hormone-secreting pituitary tumor: biosynthetic characterization and clinical studies. J Clin Endocrinol Metab 1987;64:536–542.
24. Katznelson L, Alexander JM, Klibanski A. Clinically nonfunctioning pituitary adenomas. J ClinEndocrinol Metab 1993;76:1089–1094.
25. Snyder PJ. Gonadotroph cell adenomas of the pituitary. Endocr Rev 1985;6:552–563.
26. Ebersold MJ, Quast LM, Laws ER Jr, Scheithauer B, Randall RV. Long-term results in trans-sphenoidal removal of nonfunctioning pituitary adenomas. J Neurosurg 1986;64:713–719.
27. Harris RI, Schatz NJ, Gennarelli T, Savino PJ, Cobbs WH, Snyder PJ. Follicle-stimulating hormone-secreting pituitary adenomas: correlation of reduction of adenoma size with reduction of hormonal hypersecretion after trans-sphenoidal surgery. J Clin Endocrinol Metab 1983;6:1288–1293.
28. Mindermann T, Wilson CB. Thyrotropin-producing pituitary adenomas. J Neurosurg 1993;79:521–527.
29. Smallridge RC. Thyrotropin-secreting pituitary tumors. Endocrinol Metab Clin North Am 1987;16:765–792.
30. McCutcheon IE, Weintraub BD, Oldfield EH. Surgical treatment of thyrotropin-secreting pituitary adenomas. J Neurosurg 1990;73:674–683.
31. Selman WR, Laws ER, Scheithauer BW, Carpenter SM. The occurrence of dural invasion in pituitary adenomas. J Neurosurg 1986;64:402–407.
32. Doniach I. Pituitary carcinoma. Clin Endocrinol 1992;37:194–195.
33. Kaltsas GA, Grossman AB. Malignant pituitary tumors. Pituitary 1998;1:69–81.
34. Bunin GR, Surawicz TS, Witman PA, Preston-Martin S, Davis F, Bruner JM. The descriptive epidemiology of craniopharyngioma. J Neurosurg 1998;89:547–551.
35. Sklar CA. Craniopharyngioma: endocrine abnormalities at presentation. Pediatr Neurosurg 1994;21(suppl 1):18–20.
36. Fahlbusch R, Honegger J, Paulus W, Huk W, Buchfelder M. Surgical treatment of craniopharyngiomas: experience with 168 patients. J Neurosurg 1999;90:237–250.
37. Scott RM, Hetelekidis S, Barnes PD, Goumnerova L, Tarbell NJ. Surgery, radiation, and combination therapy in the treatment of childhood craniopharyngioma- a 20-year experience. Pediatr Neurosurg 1994;21(suppl 1):75–81.
38. Sklar CA. Craniopharyngioma: endocrine sequelae of treatment. Pediatr Neurosurg 1994;21(suppl 1):120–123.

39. Wass JAH, Plowman PN, Jones AE, Besser GM. The treatment of acromegaly by external pituitary irradiation and drugs. In: *International Symposium: Challenges in Hypersecretion. Human Growth Hormone*. New York: Raven Press; 1985:199–206.
40. Feek CM, McLelland J, Seth J, et al. How effective is external pituitary irradiation for growth hormone-secreting pituitary tumors? Clin Endocrinol 1984;20:401–408.
41. Laws ER, Thapar K. Surgical management of pituitary adenomas. In: *Pituitary Tumors. Baillieres Clinical Endocrinology and Metabolism.* 1985:391–406.
42. Turner HE, Stratton IM, Byrne JV, Adams CBT, Wass JAH. Audit of selected patients with nonfunctioning pituitary adenomas treated without irradiation. A follow-up study. Clin Endocrinol 1999;51:281–284.
43. Carroll PV, Christ ER, Bengtsson BA, et al. Growth hormone deficiency in adulthood and the effects of growth hormone replacement: a review. J Clin Endocrinol Metab 1998;83:382–395.
44. Drake WM, Coyte D, Camacho-Hubner C, et al. Optimizing growth hormone replacement therapy by dose titration in hypopituitary adults. J Clin Endocrinol Metab 1998;83:379–381.
45. Trainer PJ, Besser GM. *The Bart's Endocrine Protocols*. Edinburgh: Churchill Livingstone; 1995.

APPENDIX 1
PROTOCOLS FOR BASAL ASSESSMENT AND DYNAMIC TESTING OF ANTERIOR AND POSTERIOR PITUITARY FUNCTION

Cortisol (09.00 h)
Free thyroxine (FT4), thyroid-stimulating hormone (TSH)
Prolactin
Growth hormone, insulin like-growth factor-I (IGF-I)
Follicle stimulating hormone (FSH), leutenizing hormone (LH), testosterone, estradiol
Urea and electrolytes, paired serum and urine osmolalities

INSULIN HYPOGLYCEMIA TEST

Procedure

Perform after an overnight fast omitting morning medication
Weigh patient
Insulin iv bolus at 09.00 h
- usual dose 0.15 U/kg
- Cushing's syndrome and acromegaly 0.3 U/kg

Observe for signs of hypoglycemia, correlate with glucometer recording
If hypoglycemia not evident at 45 min, consider repeating full dose
Administer 50% dextrose if severe hypoglycemia occurs
Follow test with lunch containing carbohydrate and hydrocortisone if indicated

Sampling

Laboratory samples for glucose, growth hormone, cortisol at –15, 0, 30, 45, 60, 90, 120, and 150 min.
Glucometer reading at 0, 15, 30, 45, 60, 90, and 120 min.

Normal response

Nadir plasma glucose falls beneath 2.2 mmol/L (40 mg/100 ml). Serum cortisol rises by more than 170 nmol/L (6.0 μg/dL) to above 550 nmol/L (20 μg/dL). GH peak greater than 20 mU/L (8.0 μg/L) in adults.

Note: This test is contraindicated in those with ischemic heart disease, epilepsy, or an unexplained history of loss of conciousness. Hypoadrenalism should be treated before performance of the test with omission of replacement corticosteroid the morning of the test. Prepubertal subjects undergoing testing of GH status should have androgen priming before testing.

---

* These endocrine-testing protocols have been developed over many years; a detailed summary of these and more tests is available in Trainer PJ, Besser GM. The Bart's Endocrine Protocols. Edinburgh, UK: Churchill Livingstone; 1995.[45]

GLUCAGON TEST

Procedure

Perform after an overnight fast omitting morning mediation
Weigh patient
Glucagon subcutaneous bolus at 09.00 h
 1 mg <90 kg
 1.5 mg >90 kg

Sampling

Plasma glucose, serum cortisol, and GH at –15, 0, 90, 120, 150, 180, 210, and 240 min.

Normal response

Plasma glucose rises to peak at 90 min.
Cortisol rises by more than 180 nmol/L (6.5 μg/dL) to peak at greater than 550 nmol/L (20 μg/dL).
Growth hormone rises to more than 20 mU/L (8.0 μg/L).

Note: the test is contraindicated after a prolonged fast and in those with untreated hypoadrenalism.

WATER DEPRIVATION TEST (WDT)

Procedure

Continue usual medications up to the morning of the test with the omission of desmopressin (dDAVP, Ferring) for 24 h. Fluids may be taken as normal until 07.30 h the day of testing with a light breakfast at 06.30 h. Caffeine and smoking should be discontinued from midnight.

Fluid intake and urine output from midnight should be recorded.

The WDT should be performed under direct observation. No fluid should be available in the room—taps should be removed from sinks.

The basal weight is recorded and no oral intake permitted after 07.30 h. The patient is reweighed at 4, 6, 7, and 8 h into the test. If >3% initial body weight is lost, the serum osmolality should be urgently measured.

After 8 h, the osmolalities should be reviewed and a decision made as to whether the test should continue for a further period. Once serum osmolality has reached a plateau, and/or the urine output has not decreased, dDAVP 2.0 μg intramusculary should be administered with permission to drink free fluids. Urine samples should be collected for a further 4 h.

Sampling

All urinary voidings should be measured and recorded as detailed in the accompanying table.

Time (h)	*Hr*	*Urine sample*	*Weigh*	*Time*	*Hr*	*Plasma sample*
0730	0	Discard	Yes			
				0800	0.5	P1
0830	1	U1				
1030	3	Discard				
				1100	3.5	P2
1130	4	U2	Yes			
1330	6	Discard	Yes			
				1400	6.5	P3
1430	7	U3	Yes			
1530	8	U4	Yes	1530	8	P4
1630	9	U5	Yes	1630	9	P5

After dDAVP, collect urine for osmolality hourly for 4 h.

Interpretation

Normal Response

Urinary osmolality rises and urine volume decreases with water deprivation. The U:P should be 2.0 or greater at completion of the test. The rise in plasma osmolality does not exceed 295 mosM/kg.

Cranial Diabetes Insipidus

The urinary osmolality fails to rise appropriately and urine volumes do not show the normal decrease. U:P is less than 2.0. In general the plasma osmolality exceeds 295 mosM/kg. The urinary osmolality rises swiftly after exogenous dDAVP administration.

Primary Polydipsia

The urinary osmolality rises and a U:P >2.0 is achieved, provided there is adequate dehydration. A prolonged WDT is necessary if sufficient dehydration is not achieved.

Nephrogenic Diabetes Insipidus

The urinary osmolalities fail to rise and the urine volumes fail to decrease. The plasma osmolality may rise to greater than 295 mosM/kg. dDAVP administration does not result in a rise in urinary osmolality.

Note: In cases of mild diabetes insipidus, a prolonged WDT may be necessary.

CUSHING'S DAY CURVE

This provides an assessment of biochemical control of Cushing's syndrome, particularly when adrenolytic drugs are being used. It is performed in the nonfasting state beginning after usual medication. A mean serum cortisol between 150 and 300 nmol/L indicates good biochemical control.

Sampling

Serum cortisol in all, ACTH and glucose, if required, at 09.00, 12.00, 15.00, 18.00, 21.00, and 00.00 h (in in-patients).

Note: Metyrapone results in a rise in 11-deoxycortisol, which may crossreact with some cortisol assay.

LOW-DOSE DEXAMETHASONE SUPPRESSION TEST

Procedure

In the nonfasting patient, a basal blood sample should be taken at 09.00 h on day 0. Oral dexamethasone 0.5 mg to be taken strictly every 6-h for 48 h should be commenced immediately after the basal sample. A further blood test should be taken at 48 h (6 h after the last tablet).

Sampling

Serum cortisol should be measured in all cases.

Interpretation

In healthy individuals, the basal 09.00 h serum cortisol ranges between 170 and 700 nmol/L (6-25 μg/dL). Following dexamethasone the 48 hour sample should be <50 nmol/L (1.8 μg/dL). Reasons for failure of suppression include Cushing's syndrome, noncompliance, glucocorticoid resistance, alcoholic pseudo-Cushing's, severe physical or psychiatric illness, and hepatic enzyme induction. Elevated cortisol-binding globulin as occurs in hyperestrogenemic states, such as pregnancy or in those taking the combined oral contraceptive pill, may result in elevated total cortisol, which fails to suppress.

FIVE-POINT DAY CURVE FOR ASSESSMENT OF GROWTH HORMONE STATUS

Procedure

The patient may eat and drink freely. An indwelling cannula is inserted before testing, and medications can be taken as usual.

Sampling

Serum GH and plasma glucose are recorded at 08.30, 11.00, 13.00, 17.00, and 19.00 h.

Interpretation

In normal subjects, the serum GH is usually <0.5 mU/L (0.2 ng/mL) on at least two occasions. In acromegaly, all values are measurable with loss of pulsatility.

HYDROCORTISONE DAY CURVE

Indications

Establishment of the correct dose of hydrocortisone replacement in hypopituitary or hypoadrenal patients.

Procedure

The morning dose of hydrocortisone is omitted, and the patient presents fasting from midnight at 08.00 h. An iv cannula is inserted and the first dose of hydrocortisone is taken after the initial sample.

Sampling

Serum cortisol at time 0, followed by morning dose of hydrocortisone, sampling at 30 and 60 min. Breakfast is then taken, followed by sampling at 2, 3, and 5 h. Lunchtime hydrocortisone is taken, followed by sampling at 7 and 9 h. Evening hydrocortisone is then given, with further samples obtained at 9.5, 10, and 11 h.

Interpretation

The aim is to have adequate circulating cortisol throughout the day, avoiding excessive peaks after each dose. Usually the basal sample indicates a value <50 nmol/L (1.8 μg/dL).

Note: Estrogen should be discontinued for at least 4 wk before the test.

METYRAPONE SENSITIVITY TEST

Procedure

A 750-mg tablet of metyrapone is given to the nonfasting patient at 09.00 h.

Sampling

Serum cortisol at 0, 1, 2, 3, and 4 h.

Interpretation

The nadir value of serum cortisol after a single dose of metyrapone gives some indication of the regular therapeutic dose required.

APPENDIX 2
HORMONE REPLACEMENT THERAPY:
DRUGS, DOSES, AND MONITORING
HYPOTHALAMO-PITUITARY-ADRENAL AXIS

Glucocorticoid Replacement

First-line drug: Hydrocortisone—usually given 2 or 3 times/d.
Monitoring: Hydrocortisone day curve.
Note: The morning dose must be taken on waking, ideally before leaving bed. The evening dose should be taken before 19.00 h. Extra replacement may be necessary during periods of illness/stress. All patients should carry a steroid card and a Medic-Alert pendant/bracelet. An emergency pack, with a parenteral supply (with instructions), should be supplied.
Alternative Drugs: Dexamethasone, Prednisolone, Cortisone acetate.

Mineralocorticoid Replacement (for Adrenalectomy)

Fludrocortisone—usually taken once or twice daily.
Monitoring: Plasma renin activity, aiming for neither marked elevation nor full suppression.

THYROID AXIS

First-line drug: Thyroxine (T4)
Monitoring: Serum FT4. Serum SHBG may useful if hyperthyroidism is suspected.
Alternative drug: Liothyronine (T3)
Monitoring: T4 (T3 can be used to assess overtreatment).

GONADAL AXIS

Male

Lifelong testosterone replacement is indicated unless there is a specific contraindication (e.g., prostate cancer).

Available preparations

- Intramuscular
  - Primoteston depot (testosterone enanthate)
  - Testosterone undecanoate (under trial)
- Oral
  - Testosterone undecanoate
- Topical
  - Transdermal preparations
  - Andropatch/Androderm
- Implant
  - Testosterone pellet

Newer preparations
- Androgel (topical)
- Buccal testosterone
- Long-acting (3 mo) depot injections

Monitoring

Clinical assessment, potency, nadir (trough) testosterone concentraton for intramuscular preparations, steady-state concentration for other forms. Dihydrotestosterone should be measured for those taking oral preparations.

Fertility Induction in the Patient with Hypopituitarism

A combination of Pergonal hMG and hCG are traditionally used with self-administered multiple injections. Recombinant FSH/ LH are now available. Consider using LHRH pump.

Female

Estrogen replacement should be continued on average to at least the age of 50 yr, provided there is no contraindication. Consideration should be given to an extension of treatment at this time based on patient wishes, symptoms, and generated data relating to bone mineral health, lipid status, and breast cancer risk.

Available Preparations

- Implant
- Oral
- Topical

Note: In women with a uterus, estrogen replacement should be combined with progestogen to ensure menstruation.

Monitoring

Clinical response and menstruation, in those taking estradiol by mouth or implant. Serum estradiol is a useful measure in those taking estradiol valerate.

GROWTH HORMONE

Available preparations

rhGH for sc injection.

Alternative preparations: Oral GH secretagogs are currently undergoing trial and may be suitable for patients with hypothalamic lesions but intact somatotrophic function.

Monitoring

Clinical response, quality of life, serum IGF-I concentration.

CRANIAL DIABETES INSIPIDUS

First-line drug: Desmopressin (dDAVP)

Preparations

Oral
Subcutaneous
Intranasal
  Desmospray
  Rhinyl

Monitoring

Serum urea and electrolytes, serum and urinary osmolalities.
Alternative preparations: Carbamazepine, thiazide diuretics, chlorpropamide

13 Conventional Radiotherapy for Pituitary Adenomas

Michael Brada, MD, FRCP, FRCR

CONTENTS

The aim of radiotherapy is to inhibit the growth of pituitary tumor mass and to decrease hormone production in secreting tumors. Despite routine use of radiotherapy for the last four decades, there has not been a single randomized study assessing its efficacy and toxicity in comparison to other management strategies. Nevertheless there is considerable information on patient and disease outcome after radiation. The lack of comparative data, however, makes it difficult to separate the effects of the various therapeutic interventions and those of the disease itself. Radiotherapy is generally given after surgery, and the individual contribution of each treatment modality, particularly to long-term morbidity, is also difficult to distinguish. Despite the uncertainties, radiotherapy is an important component of treatment, and a large proportion of patients with pituitary adenoma receive it sometime during the course of their illness.

From: *Management of Pituitary Tumors: The Clinician's Practical Guide, Second Edition*
Edited by: M. P. Powell, S. L. Lightman, and E. R. Laws, Jr.

BIOLOGIC EFFECTS OF RADIATION

Radiotherapy uses electromagnetic radiation to produce cell damage, which leads to arrest of proliferation and, ultimately, destruction of tumors. The damaging effect of radiation occurs via a cascade of ionization of events. Genomic DNA is currently considered the most important cellular target for radiation damage. Ionization at this site causes a spectrum of damage, including interstrand and intrastrand crosslinks, strand breaks, and damage to nucleotide bases.

The majority of DNA lesions are repaired by normal cellular DNA processes. The repair of some lesions, such as double strand breaks, is either incorrect (leading to mutation) or not possible, and the lesions may become lethal, with cells dying when attempting mitosis. Apoptotic death may also be induced by radiation in some tissues.

Although the processes of radiation-induced damage and repair are common to tumor and normal tissues, there are differences that can be exploited to maximize damage to the tumor with the least damage to normal tissue. This is achieved through fractionation (giving radiation dose in small divided doses) usually on a daily basis. Fractionation and the physical ability to localize radiation to tumors with less dose to surrounding normal tissue are the underlying principles of the effectiveness of radiotherapy for the treatment of tumors, including pituitary adenomas. Despite the limited proliferative potential of most pituitary adenomas, it is likely that the arrest of tumor growth after radiotherapy is attributable to the antiproliferative effect of ionizing radiation. The mechanism underlying the lowering of excess hormone production is poorly understood but is also most likely caused by the depletion of secreting tumor cells.

RADIATION TOLERANCE OF THE CENTRAL NERVOUS SYSTEM

The limitation on the delivery of radiation to the central nervous system (CNS) is the radiation tolerance of the normal brain and spinal cord. Radiation doses beyond conventional tolerance are associated with complications, and these are described as acute, early delayed and delayed reactions based on the time of appearance after treatment completion.

Acute reactions during radiotherapy for pituitary adenoma in the form of acute edema are extremely rare and reversible. Early delayed reactions in the brain are characterized by a transient period of exhaustion, drowsiness, and anorexia, and this is described as the somnolence syndrome *(1)*. The severity relates to the intensity of radiotherapy and the volume irradiated. Apart from tiredness, the full somnolence syndrome after small-volume pituitary irradiation is relatively uncommon.

Delayed normal tissue reaction is attributable to the damage to target cell lineages, which include the oligodendroglia and vascular endothelium. Late delayed damage to the brain from the combination of oligodendroglia loss and endothelial damage leads to demyelination and vascular occlusion, causing necrosis. Lower radiation doses may cause diffuse injury to the white matter with atrophy. Wide field irradiation to the developing brain of children can be associated with cognitive impairment, and this is of particular relevance in children under 5 yr of age. There are no data to suggest that such effect occurs in adults receiving small-volume irradiation to the pituitary.

The estimates of dose fractionation limits for brain necrosis are in the region of 60–62 Gy in 30 fractions *(2–4)*. The risk of brain necrosis after a dose of 64 Gy in 32 fractions to normal temporal lobes as part of curative radiotherapy for nasopharyngeal carcinoma is 5% *(5)*. The risk is highly dependent on fraction size, with most reported cases of damage to the optic apparatus developing after radiation fraction sizes of >2 Gy *(6–8)*. After conventional external beam radiotherapy for pituitary adenoma, there should be negligible or no risk of necrosis or white matter damage.

The CNS is particularly vulnerable to single large doses of irradiation. After single-fraction radiosurgery to parasellar region lesions, including pituitary adenoma, the risk of optic neuropathy has been reported as 27% after doses of 10–15 Gy and 78% after doses of more than 15 Gy to the optic nerve and chiasm *(9)*. Similar risk (24%) has been reported after a single dose of 8 Gy or more *(10)*. Although there is no clear dose response relationship for nerves in the cavernous sinus, single doses between 10–40 Gy have been associated with an 11% risk of neuropathy *(10)*. Single fraction radiosurgery for pituitary adenoma has also been associated with a 25% risk of temporal lobe necrosis *(11)* not seen after conventional fractionated irradiation.

TECHNICAL ASPECTS OF CONVENTIONAL PITUITARY RADIOTHERAPY

Conventional radiotherapy for pituitary adenoma is given with photons by external beam irradiation using a linear accelerator. Interstitial irradiation with insertion of radioactive sources (gold or yttrium) was practiced more than 20 yr ago and is no longer routinely employed. The practical steps in the planning and delivery of conventional external beam radiotherapy include immobilization, computed tomography (CT) and magnetic resonance imaging (MRI) scans for accurate localization of the tumor and computerized 3D planning for localized treatment delivery.

The precision of the entire treatment planning and delivery process is aided by the use of immobilization devices. The most frequently employed is an individually molded closely fitting plastic mask, which can be relocated with an accuracy of 2–5 mm. Increased precision can be achieved with relocatable frames with a relocation accuracy of 0.5–1 mm based on operator skill.

Treatment is given with the patient lying supine. Imaging to define the site of irradiation is performed in the same position, usually in the immobilization device used for treatment. During the planning process, the CT or MRI visible mass is delineated on individual CT/MRI slices on the planning computer, and this is defined as the gross tumor volume (GTV). Pituitary adenoma is best viewed with MRI either alone or combined with CT particularly to delineate cavernous sinus involvement. The margins of the volume (GTV) must also consider information about possible residual disease after surgery. Preoperative images and details of the operative procedure provide important additional information to aid the treatment planning process, particularly to distinguish postoperative changes from residual tumor. Based on the known technical uncertainty of planning, immobilization, and treatment delivery, a 3D margin is added to the GTV and, in conventional radiotherapy, this varies between 5 and 10 mm. The margin should be based on the actual measurement of uncertainty of the whole planning and treatment process specific to a radiotherapy center. GTV with a margin is defined as the planning target volume (PTV). The aim of conventional radiotherapy is to deliver homogeneous dose to the PTV and least dose to surrounding normal tissue.

Conventional radiotherapy uses three fixed radiation fields—an anterior oblique field aimed at the pituitary through the forehead and two lateral opposing beams aimed at the pituitary through the temporal regions. Individually shaped shielding blocks or leaves of a multileaf collimator are increasingly used to shield out normal structures to minimize irradiation of normal brain, and this is described as conformal radiotherapy.

DOSE AND FRACTIONATION SCHEMES

Radiotherapy is usually delivered to the pituitary adenoma using daily fractionation (5 d/wk) to a dose of 45 Gy in 25–30 fractions. Higher doses of irradiation are no more effective in either of tumor control or survival because they carry higher morbidity. To avoid radiation toxicity, particularly to the optic chiasm and nerves, it is important to maintain a daily radiation dose of less than 2 Gy per fraction. Some centers have employed unconventional fractionations usually given in less than 5 wk to a lower dose assumed to be biologically equivalent to conventional daily irradiation. The long-term efficacy and toxicity of this approach compared with conventional radiotherapy is less well defined.

NEW TREATMENT TECHNIQUES (*SEE ALSO* CHAPTER 14)

Radiation can be delivered to the pituitary adenoma with higher precision using stereotactic techniques. These require firm immobilization usually using a relocatable stereotactic frame, high-precision localization of the lesion on CT/MRI using a fiducial coordinate system such as that employed in stereotactic neurosurgery, and a more focused delivery of radiation to a smaller PTV (using

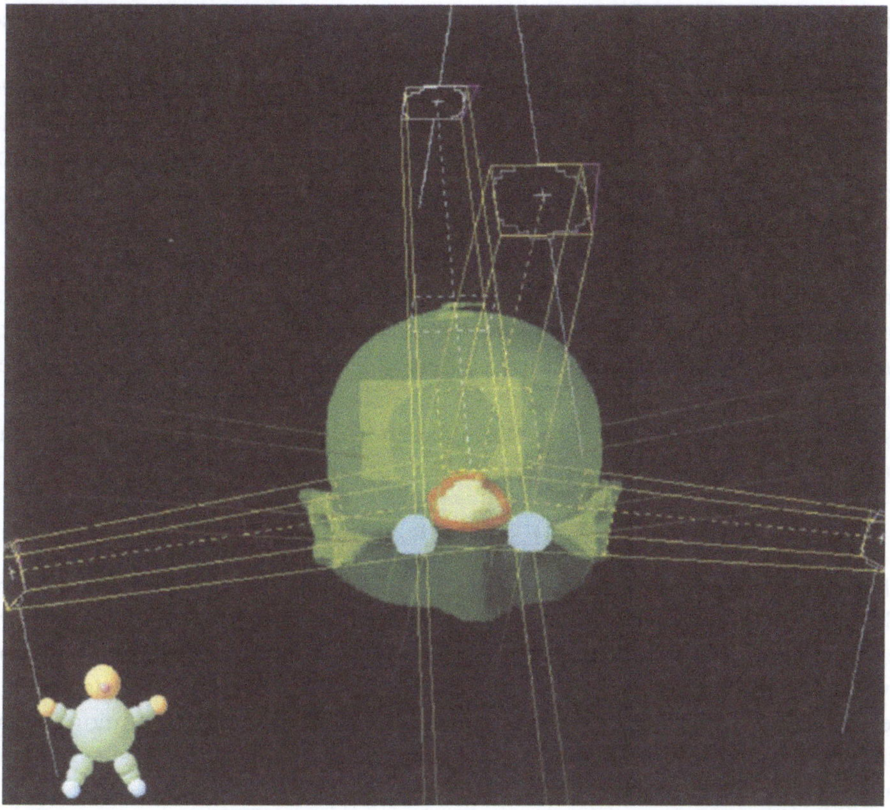

Fig. 1. Stereotactic conformal radiotherapy of pituitary adenoma with four fixed beams shaped using a small-leaf multileaf collimator (figure on the left indicates the direction of 3D view). The central structure is the pituitary tumor with cavernous sinus extension and a margin for inaccuracy.

a smaller margin). More localized irradiation is achieved using multiple fixed individually shaped radiation beams (usually 4–6) distributed in space *(12,13)*, and this is called stereotactic conformal radiotherapy (*see* Figs. 1 and 2). Previously, multiple arc techniques to treat single or multiple isocenters result in nonhomogeneous-dose distribution, and these techniques are not appropriate, particularly in proximity to critical structures. Their use in the treatment of pituitary adenoma is questionable.

High-precision focal irradiation given in multiple doses is described as fractionated stereotactic conformal radiotherapy (SCRT). The dose fractionation schemes for SCRT are usually identical to those described for conventional radiotherapy. High-precision radiation given in a single large dose is described as radiosurgery, regardless of the machine used to deliver it.

A new potentially useful technique of conformation is intensity-modulated radiotherapy (IMRT), which also delivers defined doses to specific regions within and outside the tumor. Although the overall role of IMRT in pituitary radiotherapy is not yet defined, studies using the Peacock system demonstrate inferior dose distribution compared with SCRT *(14)*.

High-energy proton beams deposit energy at the end of their paths within a Bragg peak. Proton irradiation is theoretically considered a superior method of conformal radiotherapy, sparing more normal tissue than could be achieved with conventional photon radiotherapy. There are only a few proton facilities worldwide, and the costs of such installations are not matched by a sufficient magnitude of measurable or even potential benefit. The biologic principles of the damaging effect of protons are identical to photon irradiation.

EFFECTIVENESS OF RADIOTHERAPY

The effectiveness of treatment aimed at tumor eradication is defined in terms of long-term tumor control, survival, and quality of life. Although pituitary adenoma tumor control is well documented, there is limited information on survival and little data on quality of life with treatment toxicity used as a surrogate endpoint. The primary endpoint in patients with secreting tumors is the normalization of elevated hormones. There is a need for additional survival and quality-of-life/toxicity data.

Tumor Control

There are no randomized studies comparing the outcome of surgery with surgery and radiotherapy. Nevertheless, there is considerable information on the recurrence rate of pituitary adenomas that have been incompletely excised. In retrospective comparative studies, the 10-yr progression-free survival of patients receiving radiotherapy is more than 90%, compared with less than 50% after surgery alone *(15)*. After apparent complete excision, the 5-yr progression-free survival is approx 90% in small patient cohorts *(16,17)*. Radiotherapy is usually employed in patients with residual tumor after debulking surgery, where surgery is considered risky, and following failure after surgery. The long-term tumor control reported as progression-free survival is 90–95% at 10 yr and 85–90% at 20 yr *(18–20)*. The antiproliferative effect of radiotherapy is seen equally in nonfunctioning and secreting tumors.

After radiotherapy, tumors remain *in situ* with minimal or no decrease in the size of the tumor mass and tumor control is measured as lack of growth. This is equated with no further risk of compression of surrounding structures and no further need for surgery and its consequent morbidity.

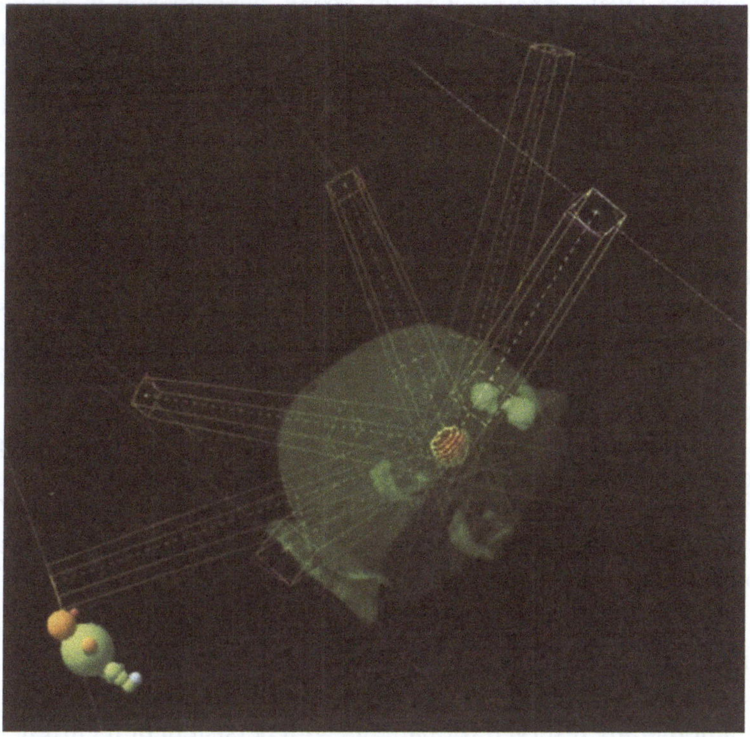

Fig. 2. Stereotactic conformal radiotherapy of a small pituitary adenoma with six fixed beams shaped using a small-leaf multileaf collimator (figure on the left indicates the direction of 3D view). Wire diagram represents high-dose envelope conforming to the shape of the tumor.

Hormonal Control in Secretory Tumors

Primary therapy of secreting pituitary adenoma is surgical removal of the tumor, which results in biochemical cure in 40–70% of patients. Radiotherapy has been used to reduce hormone levels in patients with elevated hormones after surgical excision. After conventional radiotherapy, the majority of elevated hormones return to normal, particularly in acromegaly, with less success reported in Cushing's disease and prolactinoma. There is considerable delay in the normalization of hormones, which is largely related to the pretreatment hormone level. The time to normalization for an individual hormone level ranges from less than 1 to more than 10 yr.

Acromegaly

Despite radical surgery, 50–70% of patients continue to have elevated growth hormone (GH) levels *(21–23)* (both better and worse results have been quoted recently; *see* Introduction), and radiotherapy has been successfully used to reduce the hormone levels. The mechanism of this phenomenon is not known but is presumed to be caused by the depletion of secreting tumor cells. Decrease in GH is slow, with considerable delay before reaching normal GH and insulin-like growth factor (IGF-1) levels. An estimate of the rate of reduction is 50% after an average of 27 (+/–5 mo) *(24)*. This has also been measured as a drop in mean GH level in a population of patients with acromegaly and has been described as halving in approx 2 yr *(25)*.

The rate of reduction of GH is frequently defined as the median time to normalization for a population of patients with acromegaly. The reported median time ranges from 2–7 yr *(24,26,27)*. As the pretreatment GH level is a determinant of delay *(26,28)*, such cohort figures are not a reflection of the rate of decline of individual GH level for a specific patient but are determined by the GH levels in the population with acromegaly studied.

In summary, patients achieve normal GH levels, with delay ranging from 6 mo to more than 10 yr, and the timing is largely dependent on the preradiotherapy GH. This, to some extent, is also related to the size of the adenoma. The current policy is to offer radiotherapy to all patients with persistent GH elevation. In the period before permanent normalization with radiation, somatostatin analogs are used to lower the effective GH level (*see* Chapter 3).

Cushing's Disease

As in acromegaly, primary treatment for Cushing's disease (CD) is surgical, with radiotherapy reserved for patients with persistent or recurrent disease (*see also* Chapter 4). The results reported in retrospective studies suggest that only 50–60% patients achieve normalization of plasma and urinary-free cortisol (UFC) with a delay in the normalization of hormone levels *(29)*. However, a detailed prospective evaluation of 30 adults *(30)* demonstrated remission in all patients 6–60 mo after radiotherapy, with the majority achieving remission in the first 2 yr of treatment. The reason for the discrepancy in reported result is not clear, but low-dose radiation used in some studies may provide part of the explanation.

Nelson's syndrome as a consequence of bilateral adrenalectomy is treated by external beam radiotherapy, and the reported success rate is 30–60%, with worse results after low radiation doses. Prophylactic pituitary irradiation is associated with lower incidence of Nelson's syndrome after adrenalectomy *(31)*.

A reasonable policy is to offer radiotherapy to all patients with residual or recurrent CD, usually in combination with medical treatment. Patients should also be offered prophylactic pituitary irradiation either before or after bilateral adrenalectomy.

Prolactinoma

Primary treatment of prolactinoma is with dopamine agonists (*see* Chapter 2). Radiotherapy is no longer used as initial therapy and is reserved alongside surgery for patients who are intolerant or resistant to dopamine agonists.

Initial studies of radiotherapy as primary treatment documented gradual reduction in prolactin (PRL) levels, with a delay in normalization ranging from 2 to more than 10 yr *(32,33)*. Although radiotherapy is highly effective in preventing regrowth of the tumor mass, recurrence of PRL hypersecretion after conventional radiotherapy is more frequent than in acromegaly or Cushing's syndrome (CS) *(18)*. The apparent difficulty in establishing complete normalization of PRL level is distinguishing the results of radiation-induced hypothalamic injury from poor response to treatment.

Patients with prolactinoma are frequently destined for long-term dopamine agonist therapy. Radiotherapy to the pituitary adenoma can be added to allow discontinuation of medical treatment, although this is not common practice. The advisability of offering treatment also depends on the perceived need to preserve normal pituitary function, and this is an important consideration particularly in women of reproductive age.

Survival

Despite control of excess hormone secretion and a high tumor control rate, the effect of individual treatments on survival of patients with pituitary adenoma is not clear. Poor control of acromegaly has been associated with increased mortality from cardiovascular disease, with a suggestion of reduced mortality when GH levels return to normal *(34–36)*. Large cohort studies of patients with pituitary adenoma, including both secreting and nonfunctioning tumors, have reported excess mortality *(37–42)*, predominantly owing to cardiovascular and cerebrovascular causes. A cohort of patients with pituitary adenoma treated at the Royal Marsden Hospital followed during a 30-yr period had a relative risk of death of 1.58 (95% confidence interval [CI]: 1.32–1.90) compared to an age- and sex-matched normal population. There was excess mortality from pituitary tumors and consequent endocrine disorders, from second brain tumors *(43)*, and from cerebrovascular deaths. Mortality from cerebrovascular disorders accounted for 25% of deaths, with an estimated relative risk of death from cerebrovascular causes of 4.11 (95% CI: 2.84–5.75) compared with the normal population *(61)*. Hypopituitarism has been postulated to contribute to the increased mortality. However, the influence of individual treatment modalities and the specific contribution of radiation to long-term survival remain poorly defined.

SIDE EFFECTS OF PITUITARY IRRADIATION

The damaging effects of radiation can result in neurologic damage, pituitary endocrine failure, second malignancy, and potential vascular effects.

Radiation damage to the optic nerves and optic chiasm in the form of radiation-induced optic neuropathy (delayed normal tissue damage) leads to impairment in visual acuity. After conventional fractionated external beam radiotherapy, the risk of optic radiation neuropathy is 0–2% *(18,20,44)*. The largest series reported a 1.5% risk of visual impairment not attributable to other recognized ophthalmologic causes *(18)*, and most modern series report risk <1% *(44)*.

Although there is fear of temporal lobe damage from radiation passing through normal tissues, where 3-field technique is routine, radiation doses to the temporal lobes are small and no cases of temporal lobe necrosis have been described in modern series. Studies using positron emission tomography (PET) imaging have also failed to demonstrate reduced uptake of fluor-2-deoxy-glucose (FDG) in the temporal lobes *(45)*. Previously reported cases of temporal lobe damage are most likely owing to older radiation techniques using two opposing radiation beams.

There is anecdotal information on the potential damaging effect of pituitary irradiation on cognitive function. However, published cross-sectional data on patients with pituitary adenoma suggest mild dysfunction after surgery with or without radiotherapy, and the contribution to long-term cognitive impairment from radiation alone is not clear *(46–48)*.

The most frequent complication of pituitary irradiation is pituitary endocrine deficiency. The reported sequence of deficiency after radiotherapy is GH deficiency followed by luteinizing hormone (LH)/follicle-stimulating hormone (FSH), adenocorticotropin hormone (ACTH), and thyroid-stimulating hormone (TSH) *(49,50)*. Other authors report no clear difference in the timing of onset of endocrine deficiencies *(51)*. The mechanism of endocrine dysfunction is considered to be hypothalamic damage, and this is largely based on evidence from patients who receive whole-brain irradiation *(52)*. Deficiency in the release of pituitary hormones resulting from cellular depletion or other local injury within the pituitary gland may also play a role, because hypopituitarism has been reported after localized irradiation in the form of interstitial radiotherapy and radiosurgery. The risk of posterior pituitary failure after irradiation is negligible.

The likelihood of developing radiation-induced pituitary deficiency is partly determined by latent or preexisting pituitary dysfunction. In patients not requiring replacement therapy in the immediate postradiotherapy period, the actuarial cumulative probability of requiring hydrocortisone and thyroxine replacement therapy is 10–30% at 10 yr and 30–50% at 20 yr (after doses of 40–50 Gy in 25–30 fractions) (*51* unpublished personal data). Other studies report rates of deficiency at 10 yr of approx 80% for ACTH and 30% for TSH, with a suggestion of faster decline in hormone levels after higher radiation doses *(50)*. From a clinical perspective, regular assessment of pituitary function after radiotherapy is the primary medical activity in the posttreatment period.

Therapeutic radiation is a well-recognized predisposing factor to the development of second brain tumor. Radiation-induced brain tumors have been described after low-dose scalp irradiation for tinea capitis *(53)* and after prophylactic cranial irradiation in acute lymphocytic leukemia (ALL) in children *(54,55)*. The risk of radiation-induced second brain tumor in patients with pituitary adenoma is 1–2% at 10 yr and 2–3% at 20 yr and may be in the form of radiation-induced meningioma, sarcoma, or a malignant glioma *(43,56)*. The relative risk compared with the normal population is 10, with wide CIs because of the relatively small size of the patient populations studied. An unresolved issue is the individual contributions of radiation and potential predisposition to potential malignancy in patients with pituitary adenoma *(57)*.

Patients with pituitary adenoma are at increased risk of cardiovascular and cerebrovascular events *(37,42,58)*. Although this is partly caused by the metabolic consequences of hypopituitarism, it is likely that radiation-induced and possibly surgically induced vascular damage is a contributing factor *(58)*. The magnitude of contribution to the overall risk from radiation is not defined.

RESULTS OF NEW TECHNIQUES OF RADIATION

Fractionated radiotherapy can be delivered with high precision with SCRT. Early results of fractionated SCRT suggest similar outcome in tumor and hormonal control as reported for conventional radiotherapy *(13,59)*. Although it is hoped that the reduction of radiation doses to normal brain and reduction in the amount of normal brain receiving high radiation doses will reduce long-term side effects, the evidence to substantiate it is not yet available.

Radiation delivered to pituitary adenoma with radiosurgery (using single large doses with a high-precision stereotactic technique) is only safely possible for small tumors, ≥5 mm away from the optic apparatus. It is suggested that radiosurgery is associated with faster decline of elevated hormone levels in secreting tumors (*see* Chapter). The published data are currently not conclusive because radiosurgery is reserved for small tumors with only mildly elevated hormone levels and single doses are relatively modest. The efficacy of radiosurgery in long-term tumor control, particularly in nonfunctioning pituitary adenomas (NFPA), is not defined.

TIMING OF RADIOTHERAPY

There is considerable debate about the appropriate timing of radiotherapy in patients with residual nonfunctioning adenoma after surgery. Although postoperative radiotherapy is effective with a low risk of subsequent recurrence, the indolent natural history of pituitary adenoma means that a proportion of patients remain with a static tumor for long periods and some may avoid the need for irradiation. However, a policy of observation requires close surveillance with regular imaging and ophthalmologic assessments and, occasionally, a need for a second surgical intervention with consequent morbidity. Currently, there are no hard data to define the most appropriate timing of radiotherapy (immediate vs delayed), and a randomized study comparing the two policies is required. Such a study should particularly concentrate on the endpoints of long-term effects of the tumor and therapy in terms of functional outcome and survival.

In the absence of data that can identify the preferred policy, there are several factors to consider when deciding on the appropriate timing of radiotherapy. Age and performance status give an indication of tolerance and morbidity of further surgery, and age is an important consideration in the likelihood and the potential duration of hypopituitarism. Older patients and those with poor performance status could therefore be offered radiation earlier rather than later. Established pituitary dysfunction avoids the concern of radiation-induced hypopituitarism and in this situation, radiotherapy can also be given earlier. Tumor size and its proximity to the optic apparatus would favor earlier treatment to reduce the risk of optic chiasm compression and a further potential need for decompressive surgery. Conversely, a small amount of residual tumor after radical surgery or patients with initially small adenomas do not require immediate postsurgical treatment with irradiation.

An important factor, which helps to decide on the timing of radiotherapy, is the biologic behavior of the residual tumor. Although some information can be obtained from proliferation indices *(60)* and apparent tumor invasiveness, the rate of tumor growth can currently only be assessed with some certainty by interval imaging. The rate of change in the size of the residual tumor indicates how urgently irradiation should be started.

Patients with excess hormone secretion after primary therapy are considered for early radiotherapy to shorten the duration of elevated hormone levels.

CONCLUSIONS AND RECOMMENDATIONS

Surgery remains the most appropriate treatment to relieve chiasmal and optic nerve compression and to reduce hormone hypersecretion. Patients with residual or recurrent NFPA may be offered conventional or high-precision external beam radiotherapy delivered in a fractionated manner using multiple fields to a dose of 45 Gy in 25 fractions. The most appropriate timing of radiotherapy after surgery is not defined. The morbidity of treatment is low, with the requirement for hormone replacement therapy the most frequent consequence. Persistent hormone elevation is successfully treated with radiotherapy, particularly in acromegaly and CD although the normalization of hormone levels occurs with delay. In the treatment of prolactinomas, radiotherapy is appropriate for patients who do not tolerate medical treatment and where dopamine agonists have failed. Patients with CD treated with bilateral adrenalectomy are at risk of developing Nelson's syndrome and prophylactic pituitary radiation reduces the risk of tumor growth.

Although radiotherapy is an effective and relatively nontoxic treatment, its role has become accepted without evidence from prospective randomized trials. As a result, many questions, particularly about its long-term effects, remain unanswered. New technological developments in radiation delivery are generally equated with progress and are believed to represent improvement in patient outcome. However, the issues of radiation and its long-term consequences persist and early results, equivalent to those for conventional radiotherapy, are no proof of benefit. In addition, the uncritical acceptance of novel techniques and technologies may yet have unforeseen disadvantages, such as presumed but unproven accuracy of tumor delineation, that may lead to inferior treatment results. Prospective randomized trials evaluating the role of radiotherapy, particularly the critical endpoint of survival, are therefore urgently needed and studies should include not only conventional radiotherapy technology but also all apparently innovative radiotherapy techniques.

REFERENCES

1. Faithfull S, Brada M. Somnolence syndrome in adults following cranial irradiation for primary brain tumors. Clin Oncol 1998;10:250–254.
2. Marks JE, Baglan RJ, Prassad SC, et al. Cerebral radionecrosis: incidence and risk in relation to dose, time, fractionation and volume. Int J Radiat Oncol Biol Phys 1981;7:243–252.
3. Pezner RD, Archambeau JO. Brain tolerance unit: a method to estimate risk of radiation brain injury for various dose schedules. Int J Radiat Oncol Biol Phys 1981;7:397–402.
4. Leibel S, Sheline G. Tolerance of the brain and spinal cord to conventional irradiation. In: Gutin PH, Leibel SA, Sheline GE, eds. *Radiation Injury to the Nervous System.* New York: Raven; 1991:239–256.
5. Lee AW, Foo W, Chappell R, et al. Effect of time, dose, and fractionation on temporal lobe necrosis following radiotherapy for nasopharyngeal carcinoma. Int J Radiat Oncol Biol Phys 1998;40:35–42.
6. Aristizabal S, Caldwell WL, Avila J. The relationship of time-dose fractionation factors to complications in the treatment of pituitary tumors by irradiation. Int J Radiat Oncol Biol Phys 1977;2:667–673.
7. Aristizabal S, Caldwell WL, Avila J, et al. Relationship of time dose factors to tumor control and complications in the treatment of Cushing's disease by irradiation. Int J Radiat Oncol Biol Phys 1977;2:47–54.
8. Harris JR, Levene MB. Visual complications following irradiation for pituitary adenomas and craniopharyngiomas. Radiology 1976;120:167–171.
9. Leber KA, Bergloff J, Pendl G. Dose-response tolerance of the visual pathways and cranial nerves of the cavernous sinus to stereotactic radiosurgery. J Neurosurg 1998;88:43–50.
10. Tishler RB, Loeffler JS, Lunsford D, et al. Tolerance of cranial nerves of the cavernous sinus to radiosurgery. Int J Radiat Oncol Biol Phys 1993;27:215–221.
11. Mitsumori M, Shrieve D, Alexander E, et al. Initial clinical results of LINAC-based stereotactic radiosurgery and stereotactic radiotherapy for pituitary adenomas. Int J Radiat Oncol Biol Phys 1998;42:573–580.
12. Perks JR, Jalali R, Cosgrove VP, et al. Optimization of stereotactically-guided conformal treatment planning of sellar and parasellar tumors, based on normal brain dose volume histograms. Int J Radiat Oncol Biol Phys 1999;45:507–513.
13. Jalali R, Brada M, Perks JR, et al. Stereotactic conformal radiotherapy for pituitary adenomas: technique and preliminary experience. Clin Endocrinol (Oxf) 2000;52: 695–702.
14. Khoo VS, Oldham M, Adams EJ, et al. Comparison of intensity-modulated tomotherapy with stereotactically guided conformal radiotherapy for brain tumors. Int J Radiat Oncol Biol Phys 1999;45:415–425.

15. Gittoes NJ, Bates AS, Tse W, et al. Radiotherapy for non-functioning pituitary tumours. Clin Endocrinol (Oxf) 1998;48:331–337.
16. Bradley KM, Adams CB, Potter CP, et al. An audit of selected patients with non-functioning pituitary adenoma treated by transsphenoidal surgery without irradiation. Clin Endocrinol (Oxf) 1994;41:655–659.
17. Lillehei KO, Kirschman DL, Kleinschmidt-DeMasters BK, et al. Reassessment of the role of radiation therapy in the treatment of endocrine-inactive pituitary macroadenomas. Neurosurgery 1998;43:432–438; discussion 438–439.
18. Brada M, Rajan B, Traish D, et al. The long-term efficacy of conservative surgery and radiotherapy in the control of pituitary adenomas. Clin Endocrinol (Oxf) 1993;38:571–578.
19. Grigsby PW, Simpson JR, Emami BN, et al. Prognostic factors and results of surgery and postoperative irradiation in the management of pituitary adenomas. Int J Radiat Oncol Biol Phys 1989;16:1411–1417.
20. McCollough W, Marcus RJ, Rhoton A, et al. Long-term follow up of radiotherapy for pituitary adenoma: the absence of late recurrence after 4500cGy. Int J Radiat Oncol Biol Phys 1991;21:607–614.
21. Davis DH, Laws ER, Jr, Ilstrup DM, et al. Results of surgical treatment for growth hormone-secreting pituitary adenomas. J Neurosurg 1993;79:70–75.
22. Freda PU, Wardlaw SL, Post KD. Long-term endocrinological follow-up evaluation in 115 patients who underwent transsphenoidal surgery for acromegaly. J Neurosurg 1998;89:353–358.
23. Fahlbusch R, Honegger J, Buchfelder M. Surgical management of acromegaly. Endocrinol Metab Clin North Am 1992;21:669–692.
24. Biermasz NR, Dulken HV, Roelfsema F. Postoperative radiotherapy in acromegaly is effective in reducing GH concentration to safe levels. Clin Endocrinol (Oxf) 2000;53:321–327.
25. Ciccarelli E, Corsello SM, Plowman PN, et al. Prolonged lowering of growth hormone after radiotherapy in acromegalic patients followed for over 15 years. In: Landolt AAM, Heitz PU, Zapf J, et al., eds. *Advances in Pituitary Adenoma Research.* Pergamon Press; 1988:269–272.
26. Littley MD, Shalet SM, Swindell R, et al. Low-dose pituitary irradiation for acromegaly. Clin Endocrinol (Oxf) 1990;32:261–270.
27. Lawrence AM, Pinsky SM, Goldfine ID. Conventional radiation therapy in acromegaly. A review and reassessment. Arch Intern Med 1971;128:369–377.
28. Feek CM, McLelland J, Seth J, et al. How effective is external pituitary irradiation for growth hormone- secreting pituitary tumors? Clin Endocrinol (Oxf) 1984;20:401–408.
29. Howlett TA, Plowman PN, Wass JA, et al. Megavoltage pituitary irradiation in the management of Cushing's disease and Nelson's syndrome: long-term follow-up. Clin Endocrinol (Oxf) 1989;31:309–323.
30. Estrada J, Boronat M, Mielgo M, et al. The long-term outcome of pituitary irradiation after unsuccessful transsphenoidal surgery in Cushing's disease. N Engl J Med 1997;336:172–177.
31. Jenkins PJ, Trainer PJ, Plowman PN, et al. The long-term outcome after adrenalectomy and prophylactic pituitary radiotherapy in adrenocorticotropin-dependent Cushing's syndrome. J Clin Endocrinol Metab 1995;80:165–171.
32. Mehta AE, Reyes FI, Faiman C. Primary radiotherapy of prolactinomas. Eight- to 15-year follow-up. Am J Med 1987;83:49–58.
33. Littley MD, Shalet SM, Reid H, et al. The effect of external pituitary irradiation on elevated serum prolactin levels in patients with pituitary macroadenomas. Q J Med 1991;81:985–998.
34. Bengtsson BA, Eden S, Ernest I, et al. Epidemiology and long-term survival in acromegaly. A study of 166 cases diagnosed between 1955 and 1984. Acta Med Scand 1988;223:327–335.
35. Bates AS, Van't Hoff W, Jones JM, et al. An audit of outcome of treatment in acromegaly. Q J Med 1993;86:293–299.

36. Orme SM, McNally RJ, Cartwright RA, et al. Mortality and cancer incidence in acromegaly: a retrospective cohort study. United Kingdom Acromegaly Study Group. J Clin Endocrinol Metab 1998;83:2730–2734.
37. Rosen T, Bengtsson BA. Premature mortality due to cardiovascular disease in hypopituitarism. Lancet 1990;336:285–288.
38. Bulow B, Hagmar L, Mikoczy Z, et al. Increased cerebrovascular mortality in patients with hypopituitarism. Clin Endocrinol 1997;46:75–81.
39. Bates AS, Van't Hoff W, Jones PJ, et al. The effect of hypopituitarism on life expectancy. J Clin Endocrinol Metab 1996;81:1169–1172.
40. Bates AS, Bullivant B, Sheppard MC, et al. Life expectancy following surgery for pituitary tumors. Clin Endocrinol (Oxf) 1999;50:315–319.
41. Nilsson B, Gustavasson-Kadaka E, Bengtsson BA, et al. Pituitary adenomas in Sweden between 1958 and 1991: incidence, survival, and mortality. J Clin Endocrinol Metab 2000;85:1420–1425.
42. Tomlinson JW, Holden N, Hills RK, et al. Association between premature mortality and hypopituitarism. West Midlands Prospective Hypopituitary Study Group. Lancet 2001;357:425–431.
43. Brada M, Ford D, Ashley S, et al. Risk of second brain tumor after conservative surgery and radiotherapy for pituitary adenoma. Br Med J 1992;304:1343–1346.
44. Jones AE: Complications of radiotherapy for acromegaly. In: Wass JAH, ed. *Treating Acromegaly*. Bristol: 1996:115–125.
45. Beaney RP, Gibbs JSR, Brooks DJ, et al. Absence of irradiation induced ischaemic temporal lobe damage in patients with pituitary tumors. J Neuro-oncol 1987;5:129–137.
46. Grattan-Smith PJ, Morris JG, Langlands AO. Delayed radiation necrosis of the central nervous system in patients irradiated for pituitary tumors. J Neurol Neurosurg Psychiatry 1992;55:949–955.
47. Guinan EM, Lowy C, Stanhope N, et al. Cognitive effects of pituitary tumors and their treatments: two case studies and an investigation of 90 patients. J Neurol Neurosurg Psychiatry 1998;65:870–876.
48. Peace KA, Orme SM, Thompson AR, et al. Cognitive dysfunction in patients treated for pituitary tumors. J Clin Exp Neuropsychol 1997;19:1–6.
49. Littley MD, Shalet SM, Beardwell CG, et al. Hypopituitarism following external radiotherapy for pituitary tumors in adults. Q J Med 1989;70:145–160.
50. Littley MD, Shalet SM, Beardwell CG, et al. Radiation-induced hypopituitarism is dose-dependent. Clin Endocrinol (Oxf) 1989;31:363–373.
51. Tsang RW, Brierley JD, Panzarella T, et al. Role of radiation therapy in clinical hormonally-active pituitary adenomas. Radiother Oncol 1996;41:45–53.
52. Shalet SM. Cancer treatment and hypopituitarism. In: Sheaves R, Jenkins JS, Wass JAH, eds. *Clinical Endocrine Oncology*. Oxford: Blackwell Science; 1997:502–509.
53. Ron E, Modan B, Boice JD, Jr, et al. Tumors of the brain and nervous system after radiotherapy in childhood. N Engl J Med 1988;319:1033–1039.
54. Neglia JP, Meadows AT, Robinson LL, et al. Second neoplasms after acute lymphatic leukemia in childhood. N Engl J Med 1991;325:1330–1336.
55. Walter AW, Hancock ML, Pui CH, et al. Secondary brain tumors in children treated for acute lymphoblastic leukaemia at St Jude Children's Research Hospital. J Clin Oncol 1998;16:3761–3767.
56. Tsang RW, Laperriere NJ, Simpson WJ, et al. Glioma arising after radiation therapy for pituitary adenoma. A report of four patients and estimation of risk. Cancer 1993;72:2227–2233.
57. Jones A. Radiation oncogenesis in relation to the treatment of pituitary tumors. Clin Endocrinol (Oxf) 1991;35:379–397.

58. Brada M, Burchell L, Ashley S, et al. The incidence of cerebrovascular accidents in patients with pituitary adenoma. Int J Radiat Oncol Biol Phys 1999;45:693–698.
59. Milker-Zabel S, Debus J, Thilmann C, et al. Fractionated stereotactically guided radiotherapy and radiosurgery in the treatment of functional and nonfunctional adenomas of the pituitary gland. Int J Radiat Oncol Biol Phys 2001;50:1279–1286.
60. Thapar K, Kovacs K, Scheithauer BW, et al. Proliferative activity and invasiveness among pituitary adenomas and carcinomas: an analysis using the MIB-1 antibody. Neurosurgery 1996;38:99–106; discussion 106–107.
61. Brada M, Ford D, Traish D, et al. Cerebrovascular mortality in patients with pituitary adenoma. Clin Endocrinol 2002;57:713–717.

14 Gamma Knife Radiosurgery for Secretory Pituitary Adenomas

Mary Lee Vance, MD, *and Edward R. Laws, Jr.,* MD, FACS

CONTENTS

INTRODUCTION

Radiation therapy for a secretory pituitary adenoma is most commonly used as adjunctive treatment for residual disease after pituitary surgery or unresponsiveness to medical therapy as may occur with a prolactin (PRL) secreting adenoma. Advances in the techniques of transsphenoidal removal of a pituitary adenoma have resulted in improved surgical results and safety for the patient. Despite these advances, in patients with a large invasive lesion, particularly with invasion of the cavernous sinus, it must be anticipated that additional treatment(s) will be necessary to control the disease. Thus, patients with an adenoma that is large or unresponsive to medical therapy should be informed of the need for multimodal therapy.

From: *Management of Pituitary Tumors: The Clinician's Practical Guide, Second Edition*
Edited by: M. P. Powell, S. L. Lightman, and E. R. Laws, Jr.

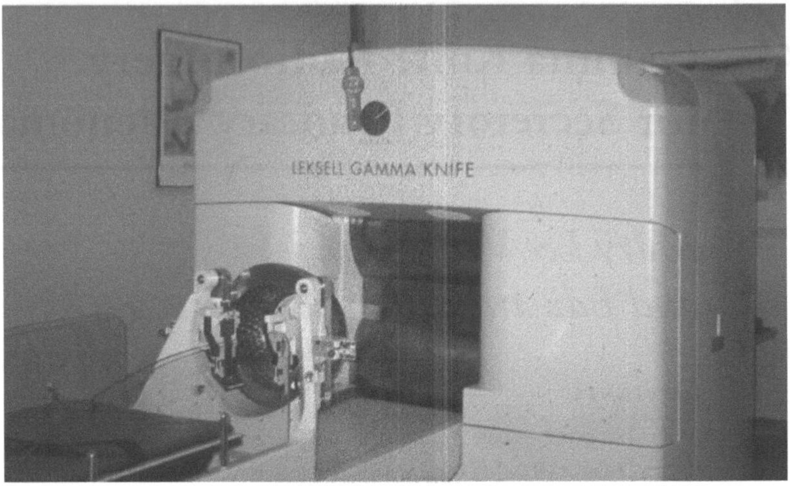

Fig. 1. The Gamma Knife machine.

Conventional fractionated radiation to a pituitary tumor has been used for more than 90 yr. The initial approaches used horizontally opposed temporal ports that resulted in effective control of some tumors but also caused radiation-induced damage to the carotid arteries and temporal lobes in some patients. The technique was modified by the introduction of multiport methodology followed by rotational and conformal techniques that are currently employed. Today, conventional radiotherapy is administered using a linear accelerator. Conventional radiotherapy to pituitary adenomas was usually beneficial in reducing the risk of continued growth and, in some cases, control of hormone hypersecretion. However, immediate or prompt control of hormone hypersecretion does not usually occur, and for several years, the patient experiences persistent active disease with its resultant complications.

In the 1960s, Dr. Lars Leksell developed the Gamma Knife as a method of delivering focused radiotherapy (radiosurgery), which consists of a large number of cobalt sources collimated to focus on a target area small enough to include a lesion in the sella turcica. Gamma Knife radiosurgery has achieved widespread use throughout the world and is theoretically ideal to treat a small pituitary lesion and reduce radiation exposure to the temporal and frontal lobes of the brain *(1–4)*. *See* Figs 1 and 2.

This discussion includes indications for Gamma Knife treatment of patients with a secretory pituitary adenoma, the need for adjunctive medical therapy to control hormone hypersecretion, the need for regular monitoring for development of new pituitary hormone deficiency, and the outcomes of Gamma Knife therapy.

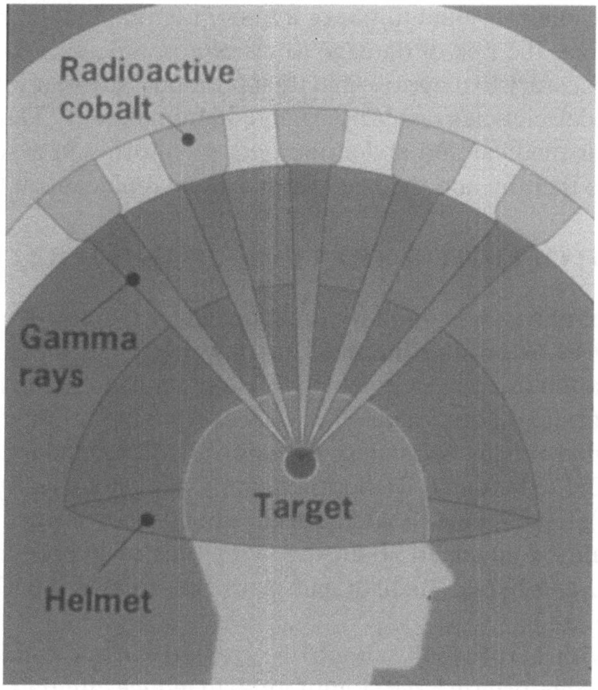

Fig. 2. The principals of focused targeting of gamma rays using Gamma Knife.

INDICATIONS FOR GAMMA KNIFE RADIOSURGERY

Patients with acromegaly, Cushing's disease (CD), Nelson's syndrome, or a prolactinoma unresponsive to dopamine agonist therapy are candidates for pituitary radiation therapy. Although medications may control excessive growth hormone (GH) secretion in patients with acromegaly and excessive cortisol production in patients with CD, no current medical therapy cures the disease. Thus, definitive therapy is necessary, and pituitary radiation offers the possibility of remission or cure. In patients with acromegaly, CD and Nelson's syndrome, the first treatment is usually surgery to remove as much of the tumor as possible. If there is residual disease, then medical therapy is given to control hormone hypersecretion (acromegaly, CD). In patients with a prolactinoma who do not respond to dopamine agonist therapy (approx 8% of patients), additional treatment, which may include surgery and radiation therapy, is indicated. Even though a large invasive tumor cannot be cured with surgery, the resulting reduction in the size of the lesion helps to decompress the optic chiasm, relieve the mass effect (e.g., headache, visual loss), and provide a small "target" for stereotactic radiotherapy. Because a limitation of Gamma Knife radiosurgery is the distance between the tumor margin and optic chiasm, the appropriate candidate for this treatment is a patient with a small residual tumor or a tumor confined to the cavernous sinus, which minimizes the risk of damage to vision.

It is also necessary to diagnose and treat promptly any new pituitary hormone deficiency or deficiencies resulting from radiation therapy. Thus, these patients require regular medical and endocrinologic monitoring to assess the effect of Gamma Knife therapy and the need for hormone replacement therapy.

PROTOCOL FOR TREATMENT AND FOLLOW-UP

Assessment of baseline pituitary function before Gamma Knife radiosurgery is mandatory to determine the need for any hormone replacement therapy. Because radiation therapy is expected to cause damage to the normal pituitary gland, patients should be evaluated at least every 6 mo for development of secondary hypothyroidism, secondary hypogonadism, secondary adrenal insufficiency, and GH deficiency. Radiation therapy does not usually cause diabetes insipidus (DI), but patients should be asked about excessive urination and thirst. Patients should be educated about the symptoms of hypothyroidism, adrenal insufficiency, and hypogonadism and instructed to return earlier should such symptoms develop.

Patients with acromegaly should be treated with a somatostatin analog (Sandostatin, Sandostatin LAR, Lanreotide) to reduce circulating GH- and insulin-like growth factor (IGF)-1 concentrations after treatment with the Gamma Knife. A report of a decrease in the efficacy of the Gamma Knife therapy in patients receiving a somatostatin analog at the time of radiosurgery compared with untreated patients resulted in the recommendation that medical therapy be given after Gamma Knife therapy *(5,6)*. Although these findings have not been confirmed, it is reasonable to withhold medical treatment until at least 6 wk after radiosurgery because medical treatment may delay the effectiveness of Gamma Knife treatment. Similarly, patients with a prolactinoma may have less favorable results from Gamma Knife treatment if they are receiving a dopamine agonist at the time of radiosurgery *(7)*. Although this observation has not been confirmed, it is prudent to delay adjunctive dopamine agonist therapy until 6 wk after Gamma Knife treatment if this observation is validated in studies of other patients. Patients with CD are treated with a drug to reduce adrenal cortisol production (e.g., ketoconazole, metopirone). Because these medications do not act on the pituitary gland and control of excessive cortisol production is important, these patients may be given medical therapy at the time of Gamma Knife treatment. Patients treated with ketoconazole must be followed closely for liver toxicity; regular measurement of liver enzymes is also indicated.

After Gamma Knife treatment patients are evaluated every 6 mo to determine if the therapy has reduced the excessive hormone level to normal and to identify new hormone deficiency or deficiencies. Because the patient with acromegaly or

CD will be taking medication to control hormone hypersecretion, the medication(s) should be discontinued for 1 mo before evaluation. In the case of patients with acromegaly receiving a long-acting somatostatin analog (Sandostatin LAR, Lanreotide), the suppressive effect may last longer than 1 mo. In this situation, if the serum IGF-1 level is normal, medication should be withheld and the serum IGF-1 level should be repeated 2 to 3 mo after stopping the medication. In patients with CD treated with ketoconazole to reduce adrenal cortisol secretion, a 24-h urine-free cortisol (UFC) should be measured 1 mo after discontinuation of the drug. Patients with a prolactinoma may have a partial response to a dopamine agonist drug (bromocriptine, norprolac, pergolide, cabergoline), and this medication should be administered if there is any evidence of a positive response. As with other medical therapies, the dopamine agonist should be discontinued every 6 mo for 4 to 6 wk, at which time a serum PRL is measured to evaluate the response to Gamma Knife treatment.

New hormone deficiency or deficiencies are identified by obtaining a thorough clinical history and physical examination and measurement of appropriate hormone concentrations. Fatigue, weight gain, decreased mental alertness, and constipation suggest hypothyroidism. Fatigue, orthostatic symptoms, diminished appetite, and weight loss suggest adrenal insufficiency. A decrease in libido or erectile dysfunction suggests hypogonadism in men and a change in menses (irregular menses, amenorrhea), diminished libido, or hot flashes suggest gonadal failure in women. The symptoms of GH deficiency overlap with other hormone deficiencies and include fatigue, decreased exercise tolerance, increase in abdominal adiposity, and diminished sense of well-being. Appropriate hormone studies include measurement of serum thyroxine (or free thyroxine, free T4), early morning cortisol, testosterone (men), and estradiol (women). Measurement of serum thyroid-stimulating hormone (TSH) is not helpful and may be misleading in a patient with secondary hypothyroidism. Assessment of GH production usually requires a stimulation test, because the serum IGF-1 (overall indicator of GH production) may be normal because IGF-1 production is influenced by nutrition and probably by other factors. The most rigorous test of GH secretion is the insulin-induced hypoglycemia test that also allows for assessment of adenocorticotropin hormone (ACTH)-cortisol reserve. Other acceptable stimulation tests for GH deficiency include iv arginine or arginine plus GH-releasing hormone (GHRH).

ASSESSMENT OF RESPONSE TO GAMMA KNIFE TREATMENT

A patient treated with Gamma Knife radiosurgery is considered to be in remission if the excessive hormone secretion becomes normal. In the case of patients with acromegaly, the definition of remission is a normal age- and gender-adjusted serum IGF-1 concentration. IGF-1 is the best indicator of overall GH secretion. Because GH production is influenced by age and gender (GH secretion declines with increasing age), it is necessary to have the IGF-1 level measured in a laboratory that provides normal values in relation to age and gender. In patients with CD, the 24-h UFC concentration is the best measure of integrated cortisol production. A normal 24-h UFC is an excellent measure of excessive cortisol production but is not helpful to assess adrenal insufficiency. A single serum PRL measurement in a patient with a prolactinoma is sufficient to assess the response to Gamma Knife therapy. Gonadal function is assessed by a history of normal libido and erectile function and a normal serum testosterone in men. In premenopausal women, regular menses indicate normal ovarian function. Men should have serum testosterone measured regularly, and menstrual history and serum estradiol levels should be measured in premenopausal women. In patients with Nelson's syndrome (increased serum ACTH after bilateral adrenalectomy), measurement of the serum ACTH level indicates the response to Gamma Knife treatment. Regular magnetic resonance imaging (MRI) examinations, usually once a year, are necessary to assess the effect of treatment on tumor volume. Both endocrine and imaging studies are necessary to properly evaluate the response to treatment and should be considered complementary. In the situation of patients with a secretory tumor, however, the definitive assessment of the response to treatment resides in the hormone measurements.

RESULTS OF GAMMA KNIFE TREATMENT

At the University of Virginia, 342 patients with pituitary lesions were treated with the Gamma Knife radiosurgery. Patients with a secretory adenoma included 85 patients with acromegaly, 65 patients with CD, 28 patients with a prolactinoma, and 23 patients with Nelson's syndrome. Because Gamma Knife treatment is not expected to be effective immediately, analysis of the effect of treatment was confined to patients with acromegaly followed 18 mo or more after treatment (conventional radiation is rarely effective before 3–5 yr after treatment). In patients with CD, a prolactinoma, or Nelson's syndrome, patients were considered evaluable 12 mo after treatment or if remission occurred within 12 mo of treatment. These times for evaluation are arbitrary but are based on comparison with the results of conventional fractionated pituitary radiation to provide a reasonable comparison of the results of both techniques. Because most of the patients do not reside in the immediate area, obtaining follow-up information is sometimes problematic. Thus, necessary information on some patients is lacking. If there was no follow-up information on these patients, they were excluded from analysis. When possible, follow-up information was obtained from visits to the Pituitary Clinic at the University of Virginia, contact with the referring physician, or contact with the patient.

Acromegaly

Eighty-five patients were treated and 58 were considered evaluable (followed >18 mo or remission before 18 mo). Serum IGF-1 became normal in 17 of 58 patients (29%) between 5 and 98 mo after treatment; the mean time to remission was 27 mo. A new hormone deficiency developed in 17 of 58 patients (29%). No patient who achieved remission had a subsequent serum IGF-1 increase; one patient was given a second Gamma Knife treatment 5 yr after the first treatment. There was no difference in the radiation dose between patients who achieved remission and those who did not achieved a normal serum IGF-1 concentration. One patient died of unknown cause during the follow-up period.

Cushing's Disease

Sixty-five patients were treated and 42 were evaluable (followed >12 mo or remission before 12 mo). A normal 24-h UFC measurement was achieved in 31 of 43 patients (74%); this occurred within 2 to 62 mo after treatment. The mean time to remission was 16 mo. A new hormone deficiency developed in 10 of 42 patients (24%). Two patients in remission subsequently developed elevated 24-h UFC levels and underwent a second Gamma Knife treatment. One patient had deterioration of vision; this patient had not received prior conventional radiation therapy. Three patients in this group died, one of progressive CD, one from a myocardial infarction, and one from sepsis. There was no difference in the total radiation dose administered to patients who achieved remission and those who did not achieve remission.

Prolactinoma

Twenty-eight patients with a PRL secreting adenoma received Gamma Knife therapy. These were patients who did not respond to medical therapy with a dopamine agonist and who underwent pituitary surgery to reduce tumor mass. Fifteen patients were considered evaluable (followed >12 mo). A normal serum PRL occurred in 4 of 15 patients (26%). Remission occurred at 18 to 51 mo after treatment; the mean time to remission was 30 mo. A new hormone deficiency occurred in 5 patients (33%). Three patients died, two from progressive disease and one from a myocardial infarction. No patient who achieved remission had a relapse.

Nelson's Syndrome

There were 23 patients with Nelson's syndrome treated. Sixteen were evaluable (followed >12 mo). A normal serum ACTH concentration occurred in one patient (6%). A new hormone deficiency developed in 3 of 16 patients (19%). Three patients in this group of 23 died, two of progressive disease and the one of unknown cause.

Pituitary radiation, regardless of delivery method, does not produce an immediate cure or reduction in tumor volume. Thus, it should be used as adjunctive therapy with the goal of controling tumor growth and excessive hormone production to prevent the complications and risk of premature mortality associated with hypersecretory states. Most of these patients have not been successfully treated with other modalities, including surgery and medical therapies, and radiation treatment is employed in the most difficult of circumstances.

COMPARISON OF GAMMA KNIFE RADIOSURGERY WITH CONVENTIONAL RADIATION

Precise comparison of many of the studies of conventional pituitary radiation and Gamma Knife radiosurgery is not truly possible because of limited information and because some of the conventional radiation studies are older and do not use modern criteria for cure or remission. Despite these limitations, some assessment is warranted. The most widely referenced study of conventional radiation for acromegaly is that of Eastman and colleagues. This study was published in 1979 and considered "remission" as a serum GH of <5 μg/L (10 mU/L) It is now known that this does not reflect remission or cure. In this study of 47 patients, 69% achieved a serum GH of ≤5 μg/L within 10 yr of treatment *(8)*. Another study of conventional radiation in 46 patients with acromegaly found that 26% of patients achieved a mean serum GH of <2.5 μg/L (5 mU/L) (an acceptable criterion for remission), seven within 5 yr, four within 10 yr, and one more than 10 yr after treatment *(9)*. A more recent study by Barkan and colleagues reported the effects of conventional radiation in 38 patients with acromegaly. Achievement of a normal serum IGF-1 occurred in two patients followed for an average of 6.8 yr *(10)*. In patients with CD, a study of 30 patients found that 25 patients (83%) treated with conventional radiation achieved remission at a median of 42 mo (range 18–114 mo) after treatment *(11)*. In 26 patients with a PRL-secreting adenoma treated with conventional radiation, 3 achieved a normal serum PRL within 4 yr of treatment *(12)*.

As noted, development of new pituitary hormone deficiency should be anticipated and treated promptly. Additional reported complications of Gamma Knife radiosurgery include development of a radiation-induced neoplasm. Two patients developed a glioblastoma multiforme 7.5 and 20 yr, respectively, after Gamma Knife treatment. One patient was treated for a vestibular schwannoma and the other for a cerebral arteriovenous malformation *(13,14)*. As in one patient in our series, damage to vision may occur, requiring regular ophthalmologic evalution.

Although it is difficult to compare precisely the results of conventional radiotherapy with Gamma Knife radiosurgery because of differences in criteria for remission, Gamma Knife radiosurgery is effective earlier than conventional radiotherapy in reducing excessive hormone secretion to normal. It is also evident that both conventional radiation and Gamma Knife treatment cause new pituitary hormone deficiencies requiring regular monitoring and hormone replacement as indicated.

SUMMARY AND CONCLUSIONS

Gamma knife radiosurgery is an effective method of delivering radiation to patients with a hypersecretory pituitary tumor when administered appropriately. This treatment should be administered only to patients who have not responded to other treatments, surgery, and/or medical treatment, with the goals of achieving restoration of normal secretion of the excessively produced pituitary hormone and of preventing tumor growth. The definitive results of Gamma Knife radiosurgery for pituitary adenomas remain to be determined. Improved outcomes for patients with a secretory tumor have occurred with more experience and a larger number of patients treated, as shown by our current results compared with an earlier report *(15)*. Gamma Knife radiosurgery is an evolving area of treatment that requires continued careful assessment.

REFERENCES

1. Backlund EO. The history and development of radiosurgery. In: Lunsford LS, ed. Stereotactic Radiosurgery Update. Proc Int Stereotactic Radiosurg Symp, Phildelphia: Elsevier Science; 1991: 463–465.
2. Lunsford LD, Flickinger JC, Linder G, et al. Stereotactic radiosurgery of the brain using the first United States 201 cobalt-60 source gamma knife. Neurosurgery 1989;24:151–159.
3. Rahn T, Thoren M, Hall K, et al. Stereotactic radiosurgery in Cushing's syndrome: acute radiation effects. Surg Neurol 1980;14:85–92.
4. Rocher FP, Sentenac I, Berger C, et al. Stereotactic radiosurgery: the Lyon experience. Acta Neurochir (Wein) 1995;63(suppl):109–114.
5. Landolt AM, Haller D, Lomax N, et al. Octreotide may act as a radioprotective agent in acromegaly. J Clin Endocrinol Metab 2000;85:1287–1289.
6. Landolt AM, Haller D, Lomax N, et al. Stereotactic radiosurgery for recurrent surgically treated acromegaly: comparison with fractionated radiotherapy. J Neurosurg 1998;88:1002–1008.
7. Landolt AM, Lomax N. Gamma knife radiosurgery for prolactinomas. J Neurosurg 2000;3(suppl):14–18.
8. Eastman RC, Gorden P, Roth, J. Conventional supervoltage irradiation is an effective treatment for acromegaly. J Clin Endocrinol Metab 1979;48:931–940.
9. Thalassinos NC, Tsagarakis S, Ioannides G, Tzavara I, Papavasiliou C. Megavoltage pituitary irradiation lowers but seldom leads to safe GH levels in acromegaly: a long-term follow-up study. Eur J Endocrinol 1998;138:160–163.
10. Barkan AL, Halasz I, Dornfeld KH, et al. Pituitary irradiation is ineffective in normalizing plasma insulin-like growth factor I in patients with acromegaly. J Clin Endocrinol Metab 1997;82:3187–3191.
11. Estrada J, Boronat M, Mielgo, M, et al. The long-term successful outcome of pituitary irradiation after unsuccessful transsphenoidal surgery in Cushing's disease. N Engl J Med 1997;336:172–177.

12. Frantz AG, Cogen PH, Chang CH, Holub DA, Jousepain EM. Long-term evaluation of the results of transsphenoidal surgery and radiotherapy in patients with a prolactinoma. In: Corsigani PG, Ruben BL, eds. *Endocrinology of Human Infertility: New Aspects*. New York: Grune and Strattton, 1981, pp. 161–170.
13. Shamisa A, Bance M, Nag S, et al. Glioblastoma multiforme occurring in a patient treated with gamma knife surgery. J Neurosurg 2001;94:816–821.
14. Kaido T, Hoshida T, Uranishi R, et al. Radiosurgery-induced brain tumor. J Neurosurg 2001;95:710–713.
15. Laws ER, Vance ML. Radiotherapy for pituitary tumors. Neurosurg Clin North Am 2000;11:1–9.

15 Parasellar Lesions Other Than Pituitary Adenomas

Kamal Thapar, MD, PhD, FRCS (C),
Tomohiko Kohata, MD,
and Edward R. Laws, Jr., MD, FACS

CONTENTS

INTRODUCTION

Pituitary adenomas are numerically the most significant of the sellar/parasellar lesions, but they represent only one of a multitude of pathologic processes occurring in the area *(1)*. Around the modest confines of the sella turcica are several intricate anatomical structures of neural, endocrine, vascular, osseous, and meningeal origins. It is remarkable that such morphologic and functional diversity can be so intimately represented in such a discrete area of the neuroaxis, and

From: *Management of Pituitary Tumors: The Clinician's Practical Guide, Second Edition*
Edited by: M. P. Powell, S. L. Lightman, and E. R. Laws, Jr. © Humana Press Inc., Totowa, NJ

that accompanying each anatomic component is a correspondingly diverse set of pathologic processes. A sprinkling of embryonic "rests" sequestrated in the vicinity provide the substrate for various sequelae of disordered embryogenesis. Surrounding neural, meningeal, and mesenchymal tissues further contribute an assortment of tumor types, so that few forms of intracranial neoplasia escape representation in the sellar and parasellar regions.

The spectrum of pathologic possibilities is supplemented further by a collection of nonneoplastic "tumor-like" afflictions, which can involve any of a variety of sellar region structures. Many of these are inflammatory in nature, ranging from acute suppuration to chronic granulomatous conditions to autoimmune processes. Others are structural abnormalities, such as the empty sella syndrome and aneurysms of the internal carotid artery. Although pituitary adenomas are the most common mass lesions encountered in the sellar region, several other pathologic processes do periodically involve the area. Because many of these conditions may mimic, clinically and radiologically, seemingly ordinary pituitary adenomas, both the clinician and the pathologist must always be prepared for unusual and, at times, unexpected pathology when approaching lesions of the sellar and parasellar regions.

In this chapter, we review the diagnosis and management of sellar and parasellar lesions, exclusive of pituitary adenomas. It is important to recognize that despite the etiologic, pathologic, and biologic diversity of the various tumor and tumor-like conditions represented in the sellar region, most are unified by a fairly generic pattern of clinical presentation—one dominated by the predictable ophthalmologic, endocrinologic, and neurologic sequelae of a sellar region mass. Furthermore, because many of these lesions share overlapping radiologic features—ones that frequently mimic seemingly typical pituitary adenomas—definitive preoperative diagnoses are often difficult to establish with certainty. Nonetheless, such distinctions should, if possible, be made because accompanying each of the different pathologic processes of the sellar region (Table 1) may be a different set of diagnostic and therapeutic imperatives that affect prognosis.

DIAGNOSIS OF SELLAR AND PARASELLAR LESIONS: *GENERAL PRINCIPLES*

The clinical features of sellar region pathology primarily represent the functional consequences of mass lesions, which, independently of histology, compress, distort, or otherwise compromise any of the parasellar structures. The optic apparatus, cranial nerves of the cavernous sinus, pituitary gland, hypothalamus, ventricular system, and brain are all vulnerable. Neurologic, neuro-ophthalmologic, endocrinologic, and neuroradiologic evaluations are all essential components of treatment. Each of these is fully discussed in the context of individual lesions throughout this and previous chapters.

Table 1
Differential Diagnoses of Neoplasms and Tumor-Like Lesions of the Sellar Region

Type	*Example*
Tumors of adenohypophyseal origin	Pituitary adenoma Pituitary carcinoma
Tumors of neurohypophyseal origin	Granular cell tumor Astrocytoma of posterior lobe and/or stalk (rare)
Tumors of nonpituitary origin	Craniopharyngioma Germ cell tumors Glioma (hypothalamic, optic nerve/chiasm, infundibulum) Meningioma Haemangiopericytoma Chordoma Haemangioblastoma Lipoma Giant cell tumor of bone Chondroma Fibrous dysplasia Sarcoma (chondrosarcoma, osteosarcoma, fibrosarcoma) Postirradiation sarcomas Paraganglioma Schwannoma Glomangioma Esthesioneuroblastoma Primary lymphoma Melanoma
Cysts, hamartomas, and malformations	Rathke's cleft cyst Arachnoid cyst Epidermoid cyst Dermoid cyst Gangliocytoma Empty sella syndrome
Metastatic tumors	Carcinoma Plasmacytoma Lymphoma Leukemia
Inflammatory conditions	Infection/abscess Mucocele Lymphocytic hypophysitis Sarcoidosis Langerhans' cell histiocytosis Giant cell granuloma
Vascular lesions	Internal carotid artery aneurysms Cavernous angioma

Sellar/parasellar lesions have specific endocrinologic effects that require special consideration. Moderate degrees of hyperprolactinemia (<6000 mU/L, <300 ng/mL) can occur with any of the mass lesions involving the sellar region. This phenomenon, frequently referred to as the "stalk effect" (*see* Chapter 2), is the result of compressive or destructive lesions involving the hypothalamus or pituitary stalk, particularly any structural, inflammatory, or neoplastic process occurring in the sella, and is fairly common.

It is, therefore, a nonspecific finding whose presence should not be routinely interpreted as being the result of a prolactin-secreting pituitary adenoma. Posterior pituitary failure in the form of diabetes insipidus (DI) is an occasional feature of sellar region pathology and is especially prominent among destructive lesions such as inflammatory processes, metastatic tumors, and primary tumors having an extra-adenohypophyseal origin. Unexplained, but of practical interest, is the fact that DI is rarely, if ever, a presenting feature of pituitary adenomas, and its preoperative presence strongly suggests an alternative diagnosis.

In all patients suspected of having sellar region pathology, a thorough laboratory evaluation of endocrine status is mandatory, being directed at identifying deficient hormone axes.

PRIMARY TUMORS OF THE SELLAR REGION

Craniopharyngiomas

Representing only 3% of all intracranial tumors overall, the craniopharyngioma is nonetheless one of the more common destructive lesions of the sellar region. Virtually every aspect of craniopharyngioma biology is the subject of ongoing debate. Nagging uncertainties regarding its cellular origins, opposing surgical philosophies concerning the need for a radical approach to resection, and the relative controversy over its natural history all provide immediate stimulus for intellectual discussion.

Craniopharyngiomas are generally believed to be developmental lesions that arise from remnants of Rathke's pouch. Such embryonic remnants assume the form of epithelial "rests," deposited between the tuber cinereum and the pituitary gland, along the tract of an incompletely involuted hypophyseal-pharyngeal duct *(1,2)*. Correspondingly, craniopharyngiomas can arise anywhere along this path. Craniopharyngiomas could also arise from the squamous metaplasia of normal cells situated on the pituitary stalk, as was once an alternative explanation of their origin. However, evidence in favor of such a view has been conflicting *(1)*.

From the standpoints of size, location, contents, pathologic appearance, and overall clinical behavior, craniopharyngiomas encompass a broad biologic spectrum. At the one extreme are minute tumors of microscopic proportions situated wholly within a normal pituitary gland. At the other and more common extreme are larger tumors, whose progressive growth enables them to compress the pituitary gland and stalk, optic apparatus, and hypothalamic structures. Frequently, these larger lesions also extend into the third ventricle causing hydrocephalus or permeate cerebrospinal fluid (CSF) spaces to gain access to the middle and posterior cranial fossae.

Craniopharyngiomas can be solid or cystic, and the overwhelming majority exhibit both features. The cyst contents, though classically described as "engine oil" in appearance and consistency, can range from a shimmering cholesterol-laden fluid to a brown-black purulent sludge mixed with desquamated debris. Calcification is a common feature of craniopharyngiomas, ranging from microscopic specks to palpable, even bone-like, concretions. Pathologically, the epithelial elements comprising these tumors can range from cuboidal to columnar, or squamous in appearance. There has been an increasing tendency to distinguish craniopharyngiomas as either classically adamantinomatous or papillary *(1,3)*. Although the latter has been proposed as a distinct clinicopathologic entity featuring a predilection for adults, a less aggressive biology, and an overall favorable prognosis *(4)*, so rigid a distinction may not be entirely justifiable, because papillary variants may simply reflect one component of the biologic heterogeneity so characteristic of craniopharyngiomas in general. More recent studies indicate no prognostic differences between these two variants *(5,6)*

Topologically, approx 80% of craniopharyngiomas arise in and maintain a suprasellar location (Fig. 1).

These lesions are often tenaciously adherent to, and occasionally invasive of, the optic apparatus, hypothalamus, pituitary stalk, cranial nerves, vascular structures, and surrounding brain parenchyma. Emphasis has also been placed on the exuberant gliotic nature of the brain parenchyma at the tumor-brain interface and its suitability as a safe surgical plane facilitating tumor removal. Approx 20% to 30% of craniopharyngiomas originate within the sella, resulting in its enlargement in a fashion similar to that seen with pituitary adenomas. Rare examples of craniopharyngiomas wholly situated within the third ventricle, optic chiasm, or sphenoid bone have been reported *(1,3)*.

The clinical presentation of craniopharyngiomas is determined by the age of the patient and the size and location of the tumor *(2,7)*. In general, symptoms can be categorized as endocrine, visual, cognitive, and those deriving from increased intracerebral pressure (ICP).

Endocrine dysfunction is more obvious in the pediatric population, primarily as retardation of growth and sexual development *(8)*. In adults, endocrine symptoms are often subtle, particularly those related to partial hypopituitarism. The effects of combined hypogonadotrophinemia, together with moderate hyperprolactinemia from stalk or hypothalamic compression, are generally more obvious, presenting in young women especially as amenorrhea and occasionally galactorrhea. DI may coexist in all age groups.

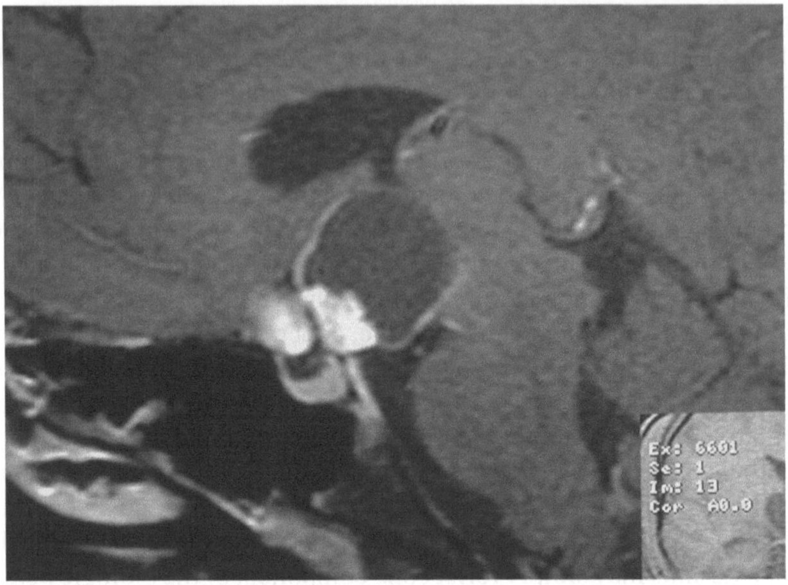

Fig. 1. A typical suprasellar craniopharyngioma with solid and cystic components. T1 sagittal MRI with gadolinium enhancement.

Visual dysfunction from chiasmatic or optic nerve compression occurs in patients of all ages, although children are more tolerant of, or more difficult to test for, visual field deficits. Cognitive symptoms in the form of memory loss, dementia, and psychiatric symptoms occur less frequently and are seen primarily in adults. Elevations in ICP, usually as the result of obstructive hydrocephalus, are common. Accordingly, headache, vomiting, papilledema, ataxia, and, rarely, cranial nerve palsies may all be additional presenting features.

All patients should have a comprehensive endocrine evaluation. Visual performance should be documented with fundoscopic examination, tangent screen, and perimetry. With computed tomography (CT) or magnetic resonance imaging (MRI), craniopharyngiomas typically appear as inhomogeneous lesions—ones in which cystic components can often be discerned from solid elements. Calcification is often present and can be a helpful diagnostic clue.

In newly diagnosed patients, maximum safe tumor resection is often a reasonable initial goal. In many instances, this can be achieved via craniotomy, although in selected cases transsphenoidal resection provides safer access. In others, complete excision requires a combination of both approaches. Tumors without sellar enlargement generally arise and remain suprasellar, and therefore are best managed by a transcranial (pterional, subfrontal, or anterior interhemispheric) route. When using any of these corridors of access, third ventricular components of the tumor can be exposed and resected by opening the lamina terminalis. When confronted with a wholly third ventricular tumor, particularly if solid and densely calcified, a transcallosal approach to the third ventricle may be necessary. During the course of tumor resection, it usually becomes evident whether complete removal is a safe and feasible strategy. Aggressive attempts to remove tumor fragments that are tenaciously adherent to neural and vascular structures are accompanied by a wholly unacceptable functional cost. Alternatively, other tumors are less adherent and complete excision can be safely achieved.

As a rule, craniopharyngiomas associated with sellar enlargement can be regarded as subdiaphragmatic. Even though such tumors may exhibit significant intracranial extension, they invariably maintain an "extra-pial" and "extra-arachnoid" disposition. Accordingly, they remain amenable to complete excision via a transsphenoidal route *(9,10)*. An interim analysis of experience with transsphenoidal management of craniopharyngiomas (1973–1996) included 138 patients *(7)*. Of these, 86 cases had involved primary operative attempts, with gross total removal the goal in virtually all. The remaining patients had been treated for palliation with goals of partial removal and decompression of cystic components. Collectively, the outcome for these patients has been satisfactory, with 82% of patients enjoying symptom-free survival at 5 or more years. Comparable results have been reported by others, particularly with regard to the primary use of transsphenoidal surgery for craniopharyngiomas *(11–14)*. Complete resection can be achieved in the majority of patients, and recurrence rates thereafter are less than 10%. Improvements in visual loss can be expected in the majority of affected patients. As mentioned, preservation of endocrine function is a major limitation of the transsphenoidal approach in this disease, with deterioration in anterior pituitary function reported in as many as 79% of treated patients and new onset DI occurring in up to half *(14)*. Still, when considered from the standpoints of survival, quality of life, recurrence rate after total removal, mortality, and morbidity, the results of transsphenoidal resection have been comparable to, and in most instances superior to, results reported in patients treated by craniotomy. This is especially true from the standpoint of recurrence, because several authors have commented on the significantly lower rate of recurrence of craniopharyngiomas amenable to transsphenoidal resection as compared with those patients who required transcranial procedures *(11–14)*. The difference is due to patient selection and reflects the fact that candidates suitable for transsphenoidal surgery are more likely to harbor tumors amenable to total removal than are the remaining population of craniopharyngiomas.

The prognosis of craniopharyngiomas depends, in large measure, on the completeness of tumor resection. For completely excised lesions, no adjuvant therapy is required. The outlook for these patients is favorable, although late recurrence occurs in as many as 25% of patients despite "total" removal. For incompletely resected tumors, symptomatic recurrence is virtually guaranteed; thus, radiation therapy is indicated to forestall recurrence. In one recent series, "radical subtotal resection" followed by radiotherapy provided progression-free survival in 91% of patients during a mean follow-up period of 4 yr (15). In attempting to isolate the efficacy of microsurgical management alone, Yasargil et al. reported a 90% rate of complete resection among 144 patients and a recurrence rate of 7%; the period of follow-up was not specified (16). In this series, 67% of patients experienced a "good" outcome; however, operative morbidity and overall mortality were 16% and 16.7%, respectively. Fahlbusch et al. reported their experience with 168 patients, followed for a mean period of almost 6 yr (12). In this report, gross total resection was achieved in approx half of all patients, leading to a cumulative recurrence-free survival of 87% and 81% at 5 and 10 yr, respectively. Of patients in whom only subtotal or partial resection could be achieved, the 5-yr recurrence-free survival dropped to 49% and 42%, respectively; approx 30% of patients received radiation therapy at some point in their course. The Mayo Clinic recently reported its long-term outcomes for 121 patients followed for a mean of 10 yr (6). In this report, gross total resection could be achieved in 69 of 121 (57%) patients. Radiologic recurrence/regrowth occurred in 24% of patients. Using a variety of outcome measures, "good outcomes" were achieved in approx 60% of patients. Among others, factors associated with poor outcomes included lethargy at presentation, visual loss, and hydrocephalus. Gross total resection favorably affected outcome and rate of recurrence, with the latter also being reduced by postoperative radiotherapy.

The management of the recurrent craniopharyngioma is more complex, because therapeutic goals must be especially well defined *(2,7,8,10,17)*. In some cases, and despite the technical demands of reoperation, total resection can still be achieved. However, for many recurrent tumors, palliative surgery is often the most realistic goal. Recurrent lesions with a significant cystic component can often be treated by repeat aspiration. This can be achieved by inserting a silastic tube attached to an Ommaya reservoir into the cyst cavity. Alternatively, the transsphenoidal insertion of a silastic tube from the tumor cavity into the posterior nasal space can provide prolonged drainage. In addition to conventional irradiation, there are several other radiotherapeutic options applicable for recurrent tumors *(18,19)*. For cystic lesions, intracavitary instillation of radioactive solutions containing colloidal phosphorus, yttrium, or gold has been of benefit. Solid recurrences have been treated with interstitial brachytherapy (the irradiation of lesions by insertion of an isotope within the tumor) and stereotactic radiosurgery.

Germ Cell Tumors

Although uncommon, germ cell tumors remain one of the principal diagnostic considerations in the evaluation of a sellar region mass, particularly in the pediatric population *(20)*. In North American and UK series, germ cell tumors account for only 1% of all intracranial tumors; however, approx 35% of these will involve the suprasellar regions. Why these tumors should be far more common in Japan, where they account for 10% of all intracranial tumors, remains an epidemiologic curiosity. Germ cell tumors typically occur during childhood and adolescence, having their peak incidence within the first two decades of life. Whereas those arising in the pineal region have a predilection for males, germ cell tumors of suprasellar origin appear notably more common in females.

It is important to recognize that germ cell tumors represent a collection of embryologically interrelated entities, each differing in germinal composition, degree of differentiation, and overall biological malignancy *(21,22)*. At the most benign extreme is the mature teratoma—a well-differentiated lesion composed of mature tissues derived from all three germ cell layers. The remaining germ cell tumors are fully malignant lesions, exhibiting both local invasiveness and metastatic capability. In order of increasing biologic aggression, germ cell tumors include germinoma, immature teratoma, embryonal carcinoma, endodermal sinus tumor, and choriocarcinoma *(196)*.

From practical and prognostic standpoints, malignant germ cell tumors are distinguished as being either germinomas or non-germinomatous germ cell tumors. The former account for 60% of all germ cell tumors and generally have a more favorable prognosis. By contrast, nongerminomatous germ cell tumors, being neoplastic counterparts of the most primitive of primordial tissues, can be considered among the most extreme examples of human malignancy—ones that usually prove fatal despite multimodality therapy. Mixed germ cell tumors composed of both germinomatous and nongerminomatous elements have also been increasingly recognized.

Germ cell tumors involving the sellar region are usually situated in the suprasellar cistern, tenaciously adherent to, if not frankly invasive of, the basal brain surface, hypothalamus, optic nerves, and pituitary stalk *(23–25)*. Larger lesions may extend upward into the anterior third ventricle and, less frequently, downward into the sella. Germ cell tumors of primary intrasellar origin are rare, although they have been known to cause sellar expansion, chiasmal compression, and cavernous sinus invasion in a fashion similar to pituitary adenomas *(26–28)*. Synchronous lesions occurring in both suprasellar and pineal locations are present in fewer than 10% of cases *(196)*.

The well-known clinical triad of DI, visual disturbance, and panhypopituitarism frequently characterizes the presentation of suprasellar germ cell tumors. DI is an important diagnostic feature—one that may occasionally antedate other clinical or radiological evidence of the tumor by years *(29)*. Panhypopituitarism is generally the result of hypothalamic or stalk compression and is usually manifested as delay or regression of sexual development or growth failure. Occasionally, a prepubertal child may present with precocious puberty, a phenomenon related to either hypothalamic compression/damage or the liberation of β-human chorionic gonadotropin (β-hCG) by the tumor *(30)*. Hydrocephalus, the result of third ventricular obstruction, is generally a late finding. MRI is the radiological investigation of choice; however, germ cell tumors lack any specific radiologic features that unequivocally distinguish them from other lesions (craniopharyngioma, chiasmatic glioma, hypothalamic hamartoma/glioma) occurring in the region.

Acknowledging the limitations of imaging to reliably predict tumor histology, practitioners have made use increasingly of various tumor markers as more accurate predictors of tumor histology *(20,22–25,31,32)*. α-Fetoprotein (AFP), β-hCG, and placental alkaline phosphatase (PLAP), as measured in both the blood and CSF, are most commonly measured. AFP elevations suggest an endodermal sinus tumor or a mixed tumor containing endodermal sinus elements. β-hCG elevations suggest a choriocarcinoma or a mixed tumor containing choriocarcinoma elements. When neither AFP nor β-hCG is elevated, a diagnosis of pure germinoma or teratoma is suspected. However, germinomas may also show variable elevations of β-hCG. High levels of PLAP suggest a diagnosis of germinoma; however, lesser elevations are compatible with any of the various germ cell entities. Despite their theoretic use, these tumor markers lack sufficient sensitivity and specificity to be routinely informative, and although they are frequently suggestive of tumor histology, only occasionally are they diagnostic. When elevated, however, these tumor markers are helpful in ongoing patient follow-up.

Although there is ongoing controversy over the optimal management of intracranial germ cell tumors in general, opinion appears less divided concerning suprasellar germ cell tumors *(23,25)*. The inability of MRI or tumor markers to distinguish reliably the radiosensitive germinomas from the aggressive nongerminomatous germ cell tumors (or, for that matter, other more common lesions occurring in the region, such as craniopharyngiomas) has placed increasing importance on obtaining a precise tissue diagnosis before instituting therapy. Accordingly, and after correction of any endocrine deficits, surgery plays both a diagnostic and a therapeutic role. Except for the rare germ cell tumors of intrasellar origin that have been successfully approached transsphenoidally *(26,28,33)*, most suprasellar germ cell tumors require craniotomy, usually through a subfrontal or subfrontal-pterional approach. Generous tissue sampling is obtained, the optic apparatus is decompressed, and a nonradical debulking procedure is undertaken. Except in the benign mature teratoma, where attempts at gross total excision may effect cure, there is little evidence that radical resection of malignant germ cell tumors supports any survival advantage.

Postoperatively, all malignant germ cell tumors require some form of adjuvant therapy, the nature of which is based on the histologic diagnosis and the degree of disseminated disease. The frequency of metastatic dissemination among these tumors has been variably reported between 10% and 57% *(22)*.

The majority of metastatic deposits occur within the neuroaxis; only 3% of all metastases occur systemically. The most important objective of staging is to exclude clinically occult subarachnoid deposits, the presence of which can be determined by studies of CSF cytology and spinal MRI. Germinomas, given their exquisite radiosensitivity, are treated with 1500 cGy to the tumor field, with additional craniospinal boosts should multifocal disease or positive CSF cytology be demonstrated. The prognosis of suprasellar germinomas is favorable, and contemporary series show that patient survival approaches 90% at 5 yr and longer *(34,35)*. On the other hand, nongerminomatous germ cell tumors continue to fare far worse despite surgery and radiation therapy; only exceptional cases are alive at 5 yr, as most patients succumb to local recurrence within 18 mo of diagnosis *(23,25)*. The effectiveness of chemotherapy for nongerminomatous germ cell tumors of the gonads has rejuvenated interest in applying the same to their intracranial counterparts. Postoperative neoadjuvant chemotherapy (cisplatin and VP-16), followed by craniospinal radiation, and followed again with chemotherapy (vinblastine, bleomycin, carboplatin, and VP-16), resulted in an encouraging tumor responses *(20,23–25)*. The evolution of aggressive chemotherapeutic regimens holds much promise in the management of nongerminomatous germ cell tumors—lesions that otherwise portend a uniformly terrible prognosis *(36)*.

Meningiomas of the Sellar Region

Approximately 10% of all intracranial meningiomas involve parasellar structures, and approx 10% of all parasellar tumors are meningiomas. The majority are situated in the suprasellar region, taking their dural origin from the tuberculum sellae, planum sphenoidale, olfactory groove, diaphragma sellae, medial sphenoid wing, optic nerve sheath, and anterior fossa floor/orbital roof. Although intrasellar extension may be an occasional, and typically late, feature of meningiomas arising at any of these sites, purely intrasellar meningiomas are exceptionally rare *(1,7,37–40)*. The majority of meningiomas involving the sellar region tend to be large circumscribed lesions that are compressive of adjacent structures. Less often, and notably in the case of sphenoid wing meningiomas, they grow in an *en plaque* configuration, so insinuating themselves around cranial nerves and blood vessels that surgical removal becomes a formidable and frequently pointless challenge. Erosion, hyperostosis, or frank invasion of bone may be features of any meningioma of the skull base, although they are especially prominent in the *en plaque* variety. All histopathologic variants of meningioma occur in and around the sella. Meningiomas in the parasellar region have also occurred after radiation therapy for a pituitary adenoma.

Although meningiomas situated at different parasellar sites will have, to some degree, certain unique site-specific presentation patterns, some clinical features are common to all meningiomas occurring in the region. Insidiously progressive visual loss is a common presenting symptom (*see* Chapter 6). Alterations in mental status may accompany those massive lesions compressing the basal frontal lobes or those large enough to cause elevated ICP. Hypopituitarism is uncommon and generally late in occurrence. Hyperprolactinemia on the basis of hypothalamic or pituitary stalk compression may occur and has, in some instances, been associated with the amenorrhea-galactorrhea syndrome. Lesions involving the cavernous sinus may present varying components of a cavernous sinus syndrome.

The CT, MRI, and angiographic characteristics of meningiomas are sufficiently well known that their preoperative diagnosis can usually be made with some degree of certainty (Fig. 2).

Rarely meningiomas of intrasellar origin and occasional suprasellar meningiomas descend into the sella, causing considerable diagnostic difficulties and may be mistaken for pituitary adenomas or other intrasellar pathologies.

In the past, parasellar meningiomas, whether primarily arising within the sella or secondarily extending into it from the cavernous sinus or a more superior site, were considered to fall exclusively within the domain of transcranial surgery. Indeed, when such meningiomas have been mistaken for pituitary adenomas, the transsphenoidal approach has proven disappointing. The inability to secure their vascular supply, together with their fibrous nature, which prevents their descent into the operative field, was believed to effectively contraindicate transsphenoidal removal. Accordingly, in such circumstances, after a frozen section has confirmed the diagnosis of meningioma, traditional teaching advises abandoning the procedure in favor of a transcranial approach at a later date. Whereas this traditional wisdom still holds true for many sellar region meningiomas, the development of the extended transsphenoidal approach now places selected meningiomas within the domain of transsphenoidal respectability *(41,42)*. This is usually so for small or medium tumors that are centered on or above the sella without significant parasellar extension. Using the same operative strategy employed for craniopharyngiomas, with resection of the sellar diaphragma, one can now completely resect such tumors transsphenoidally.

Chordomas

Chordomas are uncommon tumors of bone, presumed to arise as neoplastic derivatives of embryonal notochord remnants *(43–46)*. Accordingly, they can arise at any site along the axial skeleton, with 35% of all cases involving the clivus. Men are usually affected twice as often as women and curiously, despite their presumed embryonal origins, chordomas rarely affect individuals younger than 20 yr old. Although chordomas appear histologically benign, this aspect of their biology has been overemphasized because their locally destructive nature, unrelentingly progressive course, and variable metastatic potential collectively legitimize their inclusion as truly malignant tumors.

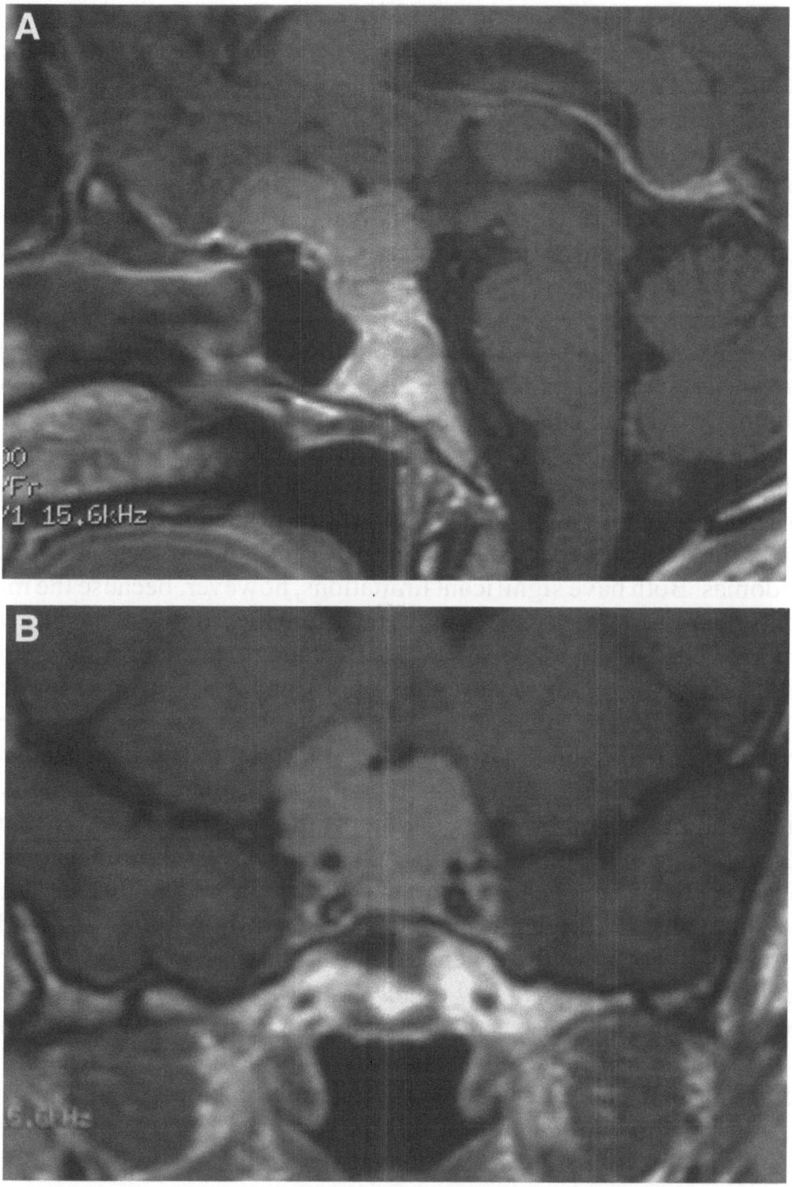

Fig. 2. Sagittal (A) and coronal (B) T1-weighted MRI of a sellar meningioma.

Usually, cranial chordomas are midline lesions and virtually all are, in some way, related to the clivus. Their precise site of origin determines their clinical presentation. Some arise in the mid and lower clival regions, producing multiple cranial nerve palsies and brain stem compression, whereas others originate from the ventral aspect of the clivus, producing symptoms of a nasopharyngeal mass. This discussion, however, concerns those chordomas whose origin in the most rostral extreme of the clivus and dorsum sellae warrants their inclusion as a sellar region mass (basis-sphenoidale chordomas) *(47)*. Such lesions may extend into the sella, producing hypopituitarism or, with suprasellar extension, a chiasmal syndrome. Lateral penetration into the cavernous sinus may compromise cranial nerves transiting therein. Headache, usually the result of bony destruction, is a common accompaniment. All chordomas are locally invasive extra-axial lesions that begin with expansile bony destruction at their site of origin, followed later by infiltration and transgression of the dura, with eventual and widespread intracranial extension and encasement of cranial nerves, brain stem, and vascular structures. Metastatic dissemination is usually a late occurrence—one encountered clinically in 10%–20% of cases and at autopsy in up to 40% of cases.

The radiographic appearance of chordoma, as determined by CT and MRI, is fairly characteristic, consisting of a destructive and expansile process of the skull base in association with a coarsely calcified soft tissue mass (Fig. 3).

The combination of surgery and radiation therapy constitutes standard therapy for chordomas. Both have significant limitations, however, because the majority of patients treated eventually succumb to recurrent local disease. Surgical access to chordomas can be provided by a variety of standard intradural and extradural approaches. Selection of the most suitable approach for any given lesion depends primarily on whether the tumor is midline or lateral, and whether it is intradural or extradural. For intradural rostrally placed lesions of the parasellar region, particularly those having significant lateral, suprasellar, or cavernous sinus extension, a pterional or subfrontal craniotomy provides good access to the intracranial component of the tumor. When such tumors have a significant extradural component or for basis-sphenoidal chordomas, which are wholly extradural and midline, an anterior extradural approach is generally required. Accordingly, extradural involvement of the sphenoid sinus, sella, or upper clivus can best be approached by the transsphenoidal route. When the area or disease is below the anterior fossa floor, the transbasal/subcranial approach provides ideal exposure. Given the anatomic limits of all standard approaches, certain chordomas, depending on their particular geometry, require combined or multiple procedures. Although gross "total" removal is the surgical objective in most cases, it is difficult to achieve, even with the benefit of elaborate skull-base operation strategies currently employed.

Radiation therapy offers some measure of temporary tumor control, but because tumoricidal doses generally exceed levels of central nervous system (CNS) tolerance, tumor recurrence has proven to be inevitable. Stereotactic radiosurgical approaches continue to be evaluated.

As determined by various series, the mean survival of patients with chordoma ranged from 4.2 to 5.2 yr *(43)*. The average time to first recurrence is approx 3 yr.

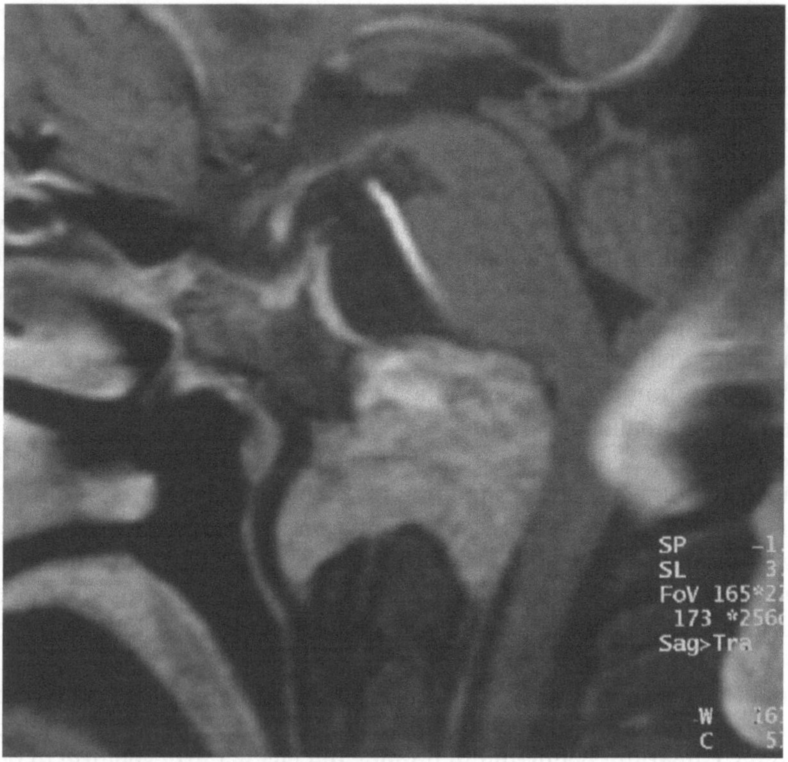

Fig. 3. Sagittal T1-weighted MRI of a caudally extending chordoma of the clivus. Note the extensive bony destruction of the clivus.

A variant of chordoma, containing conspicuous foci of cartilaginous material intertwined between tumor cells, is the chondroid chordoma. The variant accounts for approx one third of all cranial chordomas. Although its clinical presentation is indistinguishable from the standard chordoma, its prognosis is more favorable. The mean survival of patients with chondroid chordoma is almost 16 yr.

Parasellar Gliomas

Mass lesions involving parasellar structures occasionally arise from glial tissues *(1)*. This is especially true in the pediatric population wherein the possibility of a glial tumor is commonly considered in the differential diagnosis of a suprasellar mass. The majority of these are astrocytomas, whose anatomic origins include the optic nerve/chiasm, hypothalamus, and third ventricular walls. In many instances, however, assignment of a precise anatomic origin is difficult, if not impossible, given the infiltrative nature of most astrocytic tumors and the sleek anatomic continuity of the third ventricular floor, hypothalamus, and optic chiasm. Rarely, astrocytomas may arise from the infundibular stalk and even more rarely from the posterior pituitary *(48–52)*. Finally, occasional glial tumors, such as ependymomas or choroid plexus papillomas, arise within the anterior third ventricle, secondarily descending into the suprasellar space.

Collectively, visual pathway and hypothalamic gliomas account for approx 5% of all pediatric intracranial tumors, with most occurring during the first decade of life. Most of these lesions are low-grade astrocytomas of pilocytic type; low-grade fibrillary variants also occur, but less frequently. Rarely, and notably in the adult patient, gliomas located here tend to be higher grade lesions—ones assuming the histology and behavior of glioblastoma multiforme. Between 15% and 35% of patients with visual pathway gliomas will also have neurofibromatosis (NF-1) *(53)*. Whether tumors occurring in the presence of NF-1 behave differently from sporadic ones remains uncertain.

The clinical presentation of these lesions depends primarily on their location. Diagnostic features of intraorbital tumors and intracranial tumors confined to the optic nerve include decreased visual acuity, optic atrophy, proptosis, and, in the young child, strabismus and/or nystagmus. Chiasmatic-hypothalamic lesions also present with visual loss, often with bilateral field deficits. In addition, these lesions may also be accompanied by hydrocephalus and elevated ICP as the result of ventricular obstruction.

Endocrine dysfunction is frequently reported with these lesions, assuming the form of growth failure, precocious puberty, and occasionally the diencephalic syndrome. Generally occurring in infants, the last is fairly specific to processes involving the anterior hypothalamus and is characterized by failure to thrive, emaciation, hyperkinesis, nystagmus, and inappropriate euphoria. The anatomic diagnosis is best provided by MRI. The presence of a suprasellar lesion with contiguous optic nerve and/or optic tract thickening is characteristic.

The optimal management of these lesions remains a subject of ongoing debate. The necessity of tissue diagnosis, the indications for treatment, and the timing and form of intervention are all issues steeped in controversy. Much of the uncertainty stems from the seemingly erratic natural history of these tumors. In many instances, their natural history is one of quiescence and negligible growth over long periods of time *(53)*. In a significant yet uncertain proportion of cases, however, their behavior is unpredictable, with periods of quiescence abruptly giving way to progressive growth, visual and neurologic compromise, and eventually death *(32,54–58)*. In nonprogressive lesions—ones in which the radiologic diagnosis of glioma is near certain and the patient remains neurologicly stable—careful observation is often prescribed as the wisest course. In progressive lesions, such as those associated with increasing neuroendocrine deficits and ICP elevations, some form of intervention is required. Therapeutic options include surgery, irradiation, or chemotherapy. The main indication for surgical resection is in the circumstance of disfiguring proptosis or severe visual loss occurring with a tumor confined to the optic nerve. In this situation, en bloc excision of the involved optic nerve-associated tumor is generally curative. This is achieved by either a transcranial approach through the orbital roof or a lateral orbitotomy, depending on the precise location and extent of the tumor.

For chiasmatic-hypothalamic gliomas, surgery, irradiation, and chemotherapy have all been applied as either primary or adjuvant therapy. A surgical debulking procedure carried out through a variety of transcranial approaches has proven beneficial in some circumstances; visual improvement, ICP reduction, and amelioration of hydrocephalus have all been observed, sometimes with involution of the residual tumor *(32,54–58)*. By delaying the time to disease progression, surgical intervention may also postpone the need for immediate radiation therapy—an issue important in the young child *(59)*. Furthermore, surgical therapy has a definite beneficial role in the management of recurrent postirradiation tumors. The devastating neuroendocrine and developmental consequences of cranial radiation in young children notwithstanding, radiation therapy does have a beneficial antitumor effect for these lesions. In one report, radiation therapy increased the median time to tumor progression by 40 mo and led to clinical and radiologic improvement in 45% of patients *(58)*. Chemotherapy is emerging as an increasingly used option in young children in whom there is a desire to defer the deleterious effects of radiation. In one report, actinomycin D and vincristine induced remission in 63% of patients during a median follow-up of 4.3 yr *(57)*. In several of these, tumor shrinkage was also demonstrated. Petronio and colleagues, using several nitrosurea-based cytotoxic regimens, induced clinical remission, stabilization/improvement in visual and neurologic deficits, and tumor shrinkage in up to 88% of patients during a median follow-up period of 18 mo *(60)*. Chemotherapy may also have a role in the management of recurrent postirradiation tumors. The overall 5-yr survival rate of patients with chiasmatic-hypothalamic gliomas has been variably reported between 40% and 88% *(32)*.

Hamartomas (Gangliocytomas) of the Sellar Region

Tumor-like lesions composed of neurons can, on rare occasions, present as symptomatic masses in the sellar region *(1)*. Although the nomenclature of these lesions has been confusing, including designations such as hamartoma, gangliocytoma, and choristoma, the basic lesions in all cases are the same: mature neurons of varying size clustered among axons and astroglial elements. Because of their benign nature, uniformly slow growth, and histologic resemblance to fully differentiated hypothalamic tissue, they are generally considered hamartomatous. In some instances, the neuronal elements of these lesions secrete hypophysiotropic factors, producing a clinically manifest hypersecretory state. Hamartomas of the sellar region are distinguished according to their state of origin. Those arising in the hypothalamus are referred to as hypothalamic neuronal hamartomas, whereas those arising in the sella are designated as adenohypophyseal neuronal choristomas.

Hypothalamic Neuronal Hamartomas

When carefully sought, ectopic foci of hypothalamic tissue are not unusual as autopsy findings, appearing as minute macroscopic masses attached to the ventral hypothalamus, the adjacent pia, or on the surface of the proximal posterior cerebral arteries. Although such hamartomatous nodules are clinically insignificant, on occasion they may be several centimeters, extend into the third ventricle, descend into the sella, or hang in the interpeduncular cistern, producing a variety of compressive and endocrinologic effects. Most symptomatic examples occur in young males, in whom precocious puberty is the best known manifestation *(61)*. The latter features may simply be the result of hypothalamic compression; however, in some instances, these lesions contain gonadotropin-releasing hormone (GnRH), thus providing an endocrine basis for accelerated sexual maturation. Other hypothalamic neuronal hamartomas liberate growth hormone-releasing hormone (GHRH), which may induce GH cell hyperplasia and GH adenomas in the pituitary, with acromegaly being the clinical result *(62–68)*. Aside from other features, hypothalamic hamartomas are associated with a peculiar form of epilepsy—one characterized by laughing fits (gelastic seizures).

As a rule, hypothalamic hamartomas are generally quiescent lesions; however, others may be slowly progressive, causing visual and neurologic deficits and death. Given their eloquent hypothalamic origins, the management of these lesions is often difficult. Establishing a histologic diagnosis is an important initial objective, thus excluding inflammatory conditions and other tumors that may be radiosensitive (germinomas, possibly gliomas). Large masses are often amenable to significant surgical debulking—a procedure generally reserved for those lesions having documented radiologic or clinical progression and one that occasionally provides marked symptomatic benefit.

Adenohypophyseal Neuronal Choristoma

This lesion is histologically similar to the hypothalamic variant but has a primary intrasellar origin, lacks anatomic continuity with the hypothalamus, and is almost invariably associated with a hypersecretory pituitary adenoma. The basic lesion consists of neurons and associated neuropil interspersed within the substance of a pituitary adenoma. It has been proposed that by way of paracrine mechanisms, choristomas release hypothalamic trophic hormones, which may induce a change in adjacent adenohypophyseal cells. Of reported cases, most have occurred in the context of acromegaly, wherein the neuronal choristoma contains GHRH and is associated with a GH-producing pituitary adenoma *(62,63,66,67)*. Similar lesions producing corticotroph-releasing hormone (CRH) have also been associated with corticotroph adenomas in the context of Cushing's disease (CD) *(1)*.

Because of their near-uniform association with a hypersecretory state, adenohypophyseal neuronal choristomas are always preoperatively mistaken for functioning pituitary macroadenomas, both clinically and radiographically. Their diagnosis is revealed only after pathologic examination of the surgical specimen. Given the limited number of cases reported, the long-term outcome of these lesions is uncertain but is likely to be comparable to that of the hypersecretory tumors with which they are associated.

Parasellar Granular Cell Tumors

Although symptomatic parasellar granular cell tumors are rare, they are nonetheless the most common primary tumor of the neurohypophysis *(1)*. Historically, these lesions have been subject to a confusing terminology, one in which "choristoma," "granular cell myoblastoma," and "pituicytoma" have been so variably and inconsistently applied that such nomenclature has lost any specific meaning. As incidental autopsy findings, minute granular cell tumors or "tumorlets" are seen with surprising regularity, being present in up to 17% of carefully studied adult autopsy pituitary glands *(69)*. Barely visible macroscopically, these tumorlets assume the form of cryptic aggregates, often multiple, and are equally distributed between the infundibulum and posterior lobe. That such incidental granular cell tumors are rarely present postmortem in individuals younger than 20 yr of age suggests that they are acquired lesions. The most likely progenitor of these tumors is the pituicyte—a glial element that is the dominant cell type of the neurohypophysis.

Symptomatic granular cell tumors are rare. Of reported cases, the majority have occurred during the fourth and fifth decades of life *(70–79)* . Most symptomatic granular cell tumors arise from the infundibulum and present as suprasellar masses. Less frequently, others originate from the posterior pituitary, causing sellar enlargement and eventual extension to the suprasellar region. Although globular growth in an upward direction is the rule, parasellar and retrosellar extensions are occasionally encountered. Rarely, granular cell tumors wholly situated within the third ventricle have been reported. The clinical presentation is nonspecific; visual loss, hypopituitarism, increased ICP, and DI are all features attributable to the tumor's compressive effects *(73)*. Aside from a single instance, wherein a granular cell tumor occurred in association with acromegaly and the liberation of a GH-secreting peptide was invoked, all other clinically significant examples presented as clinically nonfunctioning sellar/suprasellar masses. With CT and MR imaging, these lesions appear as large globular well-demarcated homogeneously enhancing suprasellar masses *(80)*. Sellar enlargement may be a feature of those tumors originating below the diaphragma. In those studied by angiography, a vascular blush is characteristically present. Given their globular well-demarcated nature and vascularity a granular cell tumor may mimic a suprasellar meningioma.

Large suprasellar granular cell tumors unaccompanied by sellar enlargement are approached transcranially, usually by a subfrontal or pterional approach. Intraoperatively, they appear as firm pale masses, often with a rubbery texture. As a rule, granular cell tumors are not invasive of surrounding brain, although they are occasionally strongly adherent to it. Given their marked vascularity, bleeding can usually be anticipated during the course of tumor removal. The surgical objective is chiasmal and hypothalamic decompression, although gross total resection may be attempted if it can be easily and safely accomplished. The presence of a ballooned sella in association with a granular cell tumor indicates a tumor of subdiaphragmatic origin. Accordingly, these lesions are best approached transsphenoidally.

Because of their rarity, the natural history of either untreated lesions or those treated with surgery and/or radiotherapy has not been precisely defined. Schaller et al. in their review of 43 cases from the literature, noted that the natural history of symptomatic lesions is unfavorable with conservatively managed patients, most dying as the result of their tumor within 2 to 26 mo *(73)*. Of 19 patients treated with surgery alone, a 12% recurrence rate was recorded at mean time of 46 mo postsurgery. Of 17 patients treated with surgery and radiotherapy, a 7% recurrence rate was seen, occuring at a mean postoperative period of 70 mo. Accordingly, the prognosis for granular cell tumors is generally favorable, with total/subtotal resection generally providing long-term remission *(73)*. Symptomatic recurrences, although uncommon, are managed with repeat resection. In the past, radiation therapy was generally considered unnecessary *(79)*; however, the literature review of Schaller et al. does suggest that radiation therapy delays symptomatic recurrence.

Miscellaneous Tumors of the Sellar Region

In addition to the major forms of sellar and parasellar neoplasia reviewed, a variety of other rare and occasionally exotic tumors periodically involve the sellar region *(1)* (Table 1). Despite the diversity of tumor types represented, most have a fairly nonspecific clinical profile, characterized by a radiologically evident sellar/parasellar mass in association with visual dysfunction, low-grade hyperprolactinemia, and/or varying hypopituitarism. Given their rarity, these tumors are seldom considered in the preoperative differential diagnosis, because most are managed as if they were seemingly ordinary endocrinologically inactive pituitary adenomas. With their true identity being revealed only after pathologic examination of the surgical specimen, their diagnosis often arrives as something of a surprise.

Schwannomas

Nerve sheath tumors, although accounting for almost 10% of all intracranial tumors, rarely occur in the sellar and parasellar regions. In fact, only six such cases have been reported to date, with four arising from within the sella proper showing suprasellar extension, one arising from the tuberculum sellae with suprasellar extension, and one originating from the extracavernous trigeminal nerve, which also extended into the suprasellar space *(81–84)*. Schwannomas that do not arise from a cranial nerve, such as those of intrasellar origin, are presumed to arise from ectopic Schwann cell rests or from autonomic vasomotor fibers. With the evolution of cavernous sinus surgery, schwannomas arising from cranial nerves within the cavernous sinus are increasingly recognized and surgically managed. In a recent review by Sekhar et al. 12% of 103 benign cavernous sinus tumors were schwannomas *(85)*.

Paragangliomas

Paragangliomas are tumors of neural crest origin, the majority of which arise in the adrenal medulla and paraganglia. More than 80% of extra-adrenal cases involve the head and neck, with the carotid body, temporal bone, and vagal body being the classic and most common sites. Though rare, there have been periodic reports of paragangliomas arising in the parasellar region *(86–92)*. Some have a primary intrasellar origin, whereas others have arisen in the cavernous sinus and secondarily involving the sella. Headache, hypopituitarism, and diplopia were variably present, with a sizeable sellar region mass being a uniform finding. Some are amenable to transsphenoidal removal, whereas others have been treated transcranially. Three of these cases were treated with postoperative radiation therapy. Given that neither the pituitary gland nor adjacent parasellar structures contain paraganglionic tissue, the cellular origins of these tumors is obscure. Persistent embryonic "rests" of paraganglionic tissue and/or abnormal migration of neural crest cells into the parasellar region have been invoked as possible mechanisms accounting for their origin in or around the sella.

Hemangioblastomas

Isolated accounts of sellar region hemangioblastomas, both sporadic and in association with the von Hippel-Lindau (VHL) syndrome, have appeared in the literature *(93)*. Of reported examples in the sellar region, most originated from the anterior pituitary, pituitary stalk, optic nerves, and upper clivus *(94–96)*. The treatment is surgical resection with a goal of gross total resection. In all seemingly sporadic cases, one must undertake investigations to exclude an underlying VHL syndrome.

Lipomas

Rarely, incidental lipomas of the hypothalamus are seen at autopsy, appearing as discrete pedunculated masses hanging down from the tuber cinereum. Genuine symptomatic examples are exceptional and are not only more adherent to but also have parenchymal involvement with the hypothalamus, tuber cinereum, and mammillary bodies *(97,98)*. Depending on their size, hypothalamic dysfunction, hyperprolactinemia, and varying degrees of hypopituitarism may all be presenting features. Although benign and slow growing, symptomatic lipomas are often so intimately related to surrounding nervous tissue that complete resection is seldom possible.

Other Tumors

An additional spectrum of rare and peculiar tumors of the parasellar region are the subjects of isolated case reports. These include fibrosarcoma *(99)*, glomangioma *(100)*, cavernous hemangioma *(93,101–103)*, primary lymphoma *(104)*, primary melanoma *(105,106)*, myxoma *(107)*, osteogenic sarcoma *(108)*, and pseudotumor *(109)*.

UNCOMMON OSSEOUS LESIONS OF THE SKULL BASE

In addition to chordomas, several variably aggressive osseous lesions involve the skull base. Their relevance to parasellar pathology derives from their occasional tendency to involve the sphenoid bone and bony sella, resulting in neurologic, ophthalmologic, and, occasionally, endocrine dysfunction.

Fibrous Dysplasia

Fibrous dysplasia is a non-neoplastic developmental abnormality of bone characterized by the gradual replacement of normal bone by an abnormal fibro-osseous proliferation. Generally presenting during childhood, fibrous dysplasia may progress slowly during the first three decades of life. Thereafter, the process spontaneously stops and active lesions can no longer be detected. The disorder has, by convention, been divided into three forms, depending on the extent of bony involvement: monostotic, polyostotic, and lesions occurring in the context of McCune-Albright's syndrome (polyostotic fibrous dysplasia, short stature, pigmented cutaneous lesions, and precocious puberty occurring most commonly in females). Craniofacial involvement may be a feature of any of these, although most skull-base lesions are of the monostotic variety.

McCune-Albright syndrome is associated with a mutation of the α gene of a G protein linked to a family of membrane-bound receptors. This mutation must be a somatic rather than germ-line mutation, resulting in chimeric distribution of affected cells and variable presentation.

It is found in the affected bone but not in adjacent normal tissue. The pathologic process begins with proliferation of fibrous tissue in which irregularly arranged bony spicules are embedded. The lack of osteoblastic activity prevents conversion to lamellar bone, even after many years. At the skull base, involved bones undergo exuberant thickening, leading to displacement of surrounding structures and foraminal encroachment. Intraosseous hemorrhage with cystic degeneration is commonly observed. Malignant transformation (osteosarcoma, chondrosarcoma, fibrosarcoma) is exceedingly rare; most reported cases have incurred in previously irradiated lesions *(108)*. Depending on the relative proportion of bone, soft fibrous tissue, and cystic areas, the process may manifest itself radiologically as sclerotic, cystic, or a mixture of the two. In the skull-base series of Derome, the relative proportion of each was 50%, 15%, and 35%, respectively *(110)*.

Cranial involvement most commonly affects the frontal, ethmoid, and sphenoid bones. The most common presenting feature is progressive orbitocranial swelling, which not infrequently assumes enormous proportions, producing significant craniofacial deformity. Proptosis and secondary exposure keratitis, restriction in globe mobility, and diplopia are common accompanying features. The most important concern with this condition is blindness—a process occurring as the result of compression of the optic nerve from a thickened optic canal or, less commonly, the ischemic result of ophthalmic artery compression. Depending on the extent of the disease, visual loss may be bilateral. In most instances, the visual deterioration is slowly progressive; however, the occasional and dramatic occurrence of sudden blindness is a well-known feature of the condition *(111)*. Encroachment upon other cranial nerve foramina may produce additional cranial palsies. Unexplained is the rare association of fibrous dysplasia with several endocrinologic conditions, including hyperthyroidism, acromegaly, and CD.

CT scanning, like skull X-rays, reveals obliteration of the medullary canal of involved bone by an expansile homogeneous matrix that is denser than that of normal bone, but occasionally contains focal sclerotic and lytic areas. Optic canal compromise is usually obvious. Basal and *en plaque* meningiomas occasionally show similar findings, although they can now be differentiated by MRI. Three-dimensional reconstructed images are indispensable when extensive craniofacial corrective procedures are anticipated. Because involved bone is typically vascular, preoperative angiography/embolization is often helpful.

Beyond cosmetic considerations, which are often of foremost concern to the patient, additional issues surrounding the management of fibrous dysplasia include: (1) the non-neoplastic nature of the condition; (2) the self-limiting nature of the process, which rarely progresses beyond age 30; and (3) the ominous concern of progressive or sudden visual loss. Visual loss from foraminal encroachment or threatened globe viability as the result of severe proptosis is generally considered an absolute indication for surgical management. In this situation, the optic canal and/or orbit are decompressed, with the removal of all involved bone. Depending on the degree of craniofacial abnormality, elaborate reconstructive procedures may also be necessary. In patients without neuro-ophthalmologic symptomatology, no treatment is generally required because virtually all cases eventually stabilize spontaneously. Derome, in addressing the unpredictable occurrence of sudden visual loss, has also advocated "prophylactic" decompressive surgery in visually asymptomatic patients younger than 25 yr old, in whom optic canal compression is demonstrated *(110)*. In patients for whom cosmetic complications are the only concern, particularly in those with extensive craniofacial deformity requiring complex craniofacial reconstruction, surgery is generally deferred until adolescence or early adulthood.

Giant Cell Tumors of Bone

Best known for their epiphyseal origin in long bones, giant cell tumors of bone only rarely involve the cranial vault. Of the exceptional cases that do, virtually all arise in the sphenoid or temporal bones. The predilection for giant cell tumors to arise here has been related to the unique embryology of the sphenoid and temporal bones. Unlike the remaining osseous components of the cranial vault, the sphenoid and temporal bones share with long bones of the skeleton an origin via endochondral bone formation. Fewer than 40 cases of giant cell tumor of the sphenoid bone have been reported, with most occurring in the third and fourth decades of life *(112,113)*. Beginning in the floor of the sella, these are destructive lesions that spread laterally and inferiorly as cohesive soft tissue masses. Destruction of the dorsum sellae is typically an early radiologic feature—one eventually followed by destruction of the sphenoid wings, petrous apex, and clivus. Headaches, visual loss, and cranial nerve palsies are the most frequent presenting symptoms; pituitary insufficiency is rarely a feature. In the past, most cases were treated with surgical resection followed by radiation therapy. More recently, particularly with the evolution of skull-base surgery, as well as the concern of radiation-induced sarcomatous degeneration, there has been increasing emphasis on radical resection as the sole form of therapy *(112)*.

Radiation therapy is reserved for incompletely excised and recurrent tumors, in addition to those with obvious malignant history. The prognosis is both variable and unpredictable. In some cases, long-term quality survival is achieved; however, in others, progressive or recurrent disease is accompanied by significant disability or death.

Chondrosarcomas

Cranial chondrosarcomas are rare tumors of adult life and are occasionally difficult to differentiate from chordoma. Their preferred site of origin is the sphenoid bone, particularly in or near the sella turcica. Additional favored sites include the petrous temporal bone and clivus. Most chondrosarcomas of the skull base are primary lesions, although a minority may arise from preexisting chondromas or enchondromas of Ollier's disease and the related Maffucci's syndrome. Because these tumors are slow growing, local pain of long duration is the most common and frequently the only presenting complaint. With time, additional symptoms of mass effects, including cranial nerve palsies and occasionally pituitary dysfunction, emerge. Metastases, typically to the lungs, occur primarily in high-grade tumors. Bony destruction is a uniform radiologic feature; fine stippled calcification is often characteristic. CT and MRI define the extent of the soft tissue mass. Radical surgical excision is the treatment of choice, whose curability diminishes as tumor size and grade increase. Periodic recurrence is frequent and often necessitates subsequent surgical procedures. Although most often used for incompletely resected, recurrent, and high-grade tumors, the effectiveness of radiation therapy has yet to be established. The prognosis for these tumors is variable, with 5-yr survival rates approaching 60% *(114)*.

EXTRACRANIAL TUMORS OF THE HEAD SECONDARILY INVOLVING THE PARASELLAR REGION

Although primarily of interest to the head and neck surgeon, there are several extracranial skull base tumors whose tendency for intracranial extension is an occasional source of neurosurgical concern. These include the juvenile angiofibroma, esthesio-neuroblastomas, and nasopharyngeal carcinomas.

Juvenile Angiofibroma

The juvenile angiofibroma is an uncommon tumor that primarily affects adolescent males. Although a histologically benign tumor, and one whose growth characteristics are often expansive rather than invasive, the destruction potential of juvenile angiofibromas should not be overlooked; their capacity for aggressive local growth remains an ongoing and significant source of morbidity. Most of these tumors arise extracranially, with the medial pterygoid region being their most common site of origin. With progressive growth, they involve the nose, nasopharynx, infratemporal fossa, sphenoid bone, cavernous sinus, inferior and superior orbital fissures, and middle cranial fossae. Because one of their routes of intracranial access involves superior extension through the roof of the sphenoid sinus into the sella, sellar and/or parasellar involvement is occasionally a feature of juvenile angiofibromas. Their most common presenting symptoms include recurrent nasal obstruction and epistaxis, the latter occasionally being quite dramatic. Additional symptoms include facial swelling, proptosis attendant to orbital extension, and cranial nerve palsies owing to optic nerve compression and cavernous sinus involvement. Evidence of pituitary dysfunction is unusual. In addition to demonstrating an enhancing soft tissue mass involving the nasopharynx and the skull base, the classic CT finding is widening of the pterygopalatine fossa. MRI clearly identifies the extent of both intracranial and extracranial disease and provides some indication of the vascularity of the tumor mass. Angiography is useful not only because of its classic appearance (early arterial blush with external carotid artery feeders) but also because of its therapeutic value, serving as a prelude to embolization.

Therapeutic options for angiofibromas, depending on their extent, include surgical resection, radiotherapy, and chemotherapy, either alone or in combination. Surgery and radiotherapy are each sufficiently effective as primary treatment modalities so that the relative role of each is controversial *(115,116)*. Nevertheless, surgical resection remains the most widely used form of therapy, particularly in the case of smaller tumors, where complete surgical resection alone is often curative. Larger and incompletely removed tumors are often treated with adjuvant radiotherapy. Because these tumors arise extracranially and the bulk of the tumor resides there, most tumors are approached extracranially. Tumors with significant intracranial extension require combined craniofacial (extracranial-intracranial) approaches. Harrison, in a personal series of 44 patients, found that curative resections were achieved in 77% of patients. Recurrent tumors were often successfully treated by repeat resections *(116)*.

Esthesio-Neuroblastomas

Esthesio-neuroblastoma, or olfactory neuroblastoma, is a rare tumor of neural crest origin that arises from olfactory epithelium *(117)*. Having a peak incidence in the third decade of life and occurring most commonly in males, esthesioblastomas usually begin high in the nasal cavity, extend into the paranasal sinuses, and eventually erode intracranially via the cribriform plate. Transgression of dura, brain invasion, intraorbital extension, and cavernous sinus infiltration are potential sequelae of intracranial disease. Metastatic dissemination, usually to regional lymph nodes, lungs, or bones, occurs in up to 30% of patients at some time during their lifetime. Nasal obstruction, epistaxis, ocular symptoms, and headache are the most common presenting features. More than half of all tumors are of advanced stage at the time of diagnosis. The optimal treatment for this tumor is unsettled *(117–119)*. When intracranial extension is demonstrated, a common, but not universally endorsed treatment protocol includes preoperative radiation, preoperative and postoperative chemotherapy, and craniofacial resection. At the University of Virginia, this strategy provided 5- and 10-yr survival rates of 81% and 55%, respectively *(120)*. Local recurrence is common, which, in some instances, may occur a decade or more after initial therapy.

Nasopharyngeal Carcinoma

Nasopharyngeal carcinoma is an aggressive tumor with a propensity for skull-base invasion. Although rare in North America, its dramatically increased incidence in China remains an epidemiologic curiosity. The incidence peak of nasopharyngeal carcinomas approaches 50 yr of age, with males being most commonly affected. Most nasopharyngeal carcinomas arise in the superior aspect of the nasopharynx and promptly invade the skull base, often extending intracranially through bony foramina. Secondary involvement of the sphenoid sinus occurs commonly, with occasional extension into the sella, cavernous sinus, and parasellar region. The clinical presentation is usually one of pain, epistaxis, nasal obstruction, and eventual cranial neuropathies (especially the trigeminal nerve). Radiation therapy is the primary mode of treatment, surgery being reserved for recurrent tumors, often in the context of salvage surgery. Depending on the radiosensitivity and degree of differentiation, 10-yr survival rates are approx 30% *(121)*.

CYSTIC LESIONS OF THE PARASELLAR REGION

Rathke's Cleft Cyst

Rathke's cleft cyst is an epithelial cyst apparently derived from remnants of Rathke's pouch, the embryologic anlage of the anterior pituitary *(1)*. At approx wk 4 of gestation, Rathke's pouch arises as a stomadeal evagination that extends cranially to form the craniopharyngeal duct and later the anterior lobe of the pituitary gland. The eventual obliteration of the craniopharyngeal duct is normally accompanied by involution of Rathke's pouch. In some pituitary glands, however, discontinuous cystic remnants of the pouch may persist within the pars intermedia—the interface between the anterior and posterior lobes of the gland. Such cystic remnants, usually only of microscopic dimensions, are readily identified in up to 25% of autopsy pituitaries as incidental clinically insignificant findings *(122)*. Occasionally, such cysts, presumably by way of progressive accumulation of colloidal material, attain sufficient size to be clinically relevant. When symptomatic, such a cyst usually manifests itself between the third and fifth decades, and a slight female preponderance has consistently been noted.

Most symptomatic Rathke's cleft cysts arise within and remain confined to the sella turcica, causing sellar enlargement and compression of the pituitary gland and stalk *(123)* (Fig. 4).

An additional third of cases exhibit significant suprasellar extension, causing visual loss, hypothalamic dysfunction, and, if sufficiently large, hydrocephalus. On rare occasions, pure suprasellar Rathke's cleft cysts have also been documented *(124–126)*. Local compressive effects are the usual basis for presentation in symptomatic cases, with headache, partial hypopituitarism, low-grade hyperprolactinaemia, visual disturbance, and, rarely, DI being the principal clinical features. Unusual complications include chemical meningitis arising from the leakage of irritative cyst contents into the CSF and infection with abscess formation. The characteristic radiologic appearance of Rathke's cleft cysts is not particular. Sellar enlargement is a common feature, except in those wholly suprasellar in location. On CT scanning, most, but not all, appear as homogeneous noncalcified low-density nonenhancing lesions. Their MR signal characteristics are variable, depending on the composition and consistency of their fluid contents. Nonetheless, in many instances a presumptive diagnosis of Rathke's cleft cyst can be made on radiologic grounds. The difficulty arises in the occasional

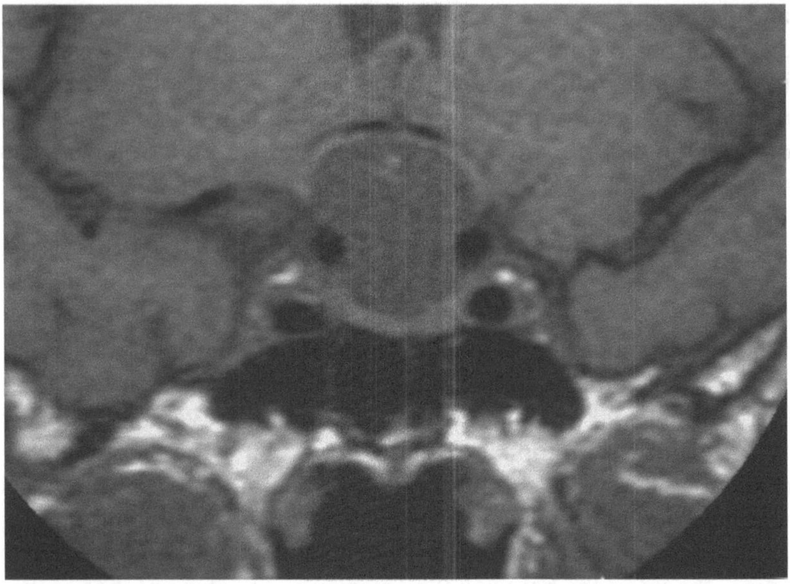

Fig. 4. Coronal T1 MRI with downward compression of the pituitary and stretching and thinning of the chiasm from a Rathke's cleft cyst presenting with visual symptoms alone.

case having a heterogeneous fluid content, particularly one in which cellular debris is abundant. In such cases the imaging characteristics may resemble craniopharyngioma, cystic pituitary adenoma, or other suprasellar tumors. It is of great practical importance to distinguish Rathke's cleft cysts from other tumors, particularly craniopharyngiomas, because the therapeutic strategies are quite different. Such distinctions can sometimes by made only by gross inspection at the time of surgery or by biopsy.

Symptomatic Rathke's cleft cysts are treated by surgical decompression *(7,14,123,127–130)*. Once a diagnosis of craniopharyngioma or other tumor has been excluded with an intraoperative biopsy of the cyst wall, simple transsphenoidal drainage with conservative partial resection of the cyst wall usually effects a cure. Because most patients have dramatic resolution of symptoms and because few will recur, more aggressive surgical approaches are unjustified. The outcome for this lesion is generally favorable. In their recent review, El-Mahdy and Powell restored visual deficits in almost 70% of cases, normalized prolactin (PRL) levels in 63%, and restored one or more axes of preoperative hormone deficiency in 15–20% of cases *(128)*. No patient experienced recurrence over the period of this study. The issue of recurrence was, however, highlighted by Mukherjee et al. who noted recurrence in fully one third of patients *(127)*. However, we have not encountered so high rate of symptomatic reexpansion. This may, in part, result from our strategy of marsupializing such cysts and maintaining a communication between the cyst and the sphenoid sinus without reconstruction of the sellar floor. We believe this to be important in preventing symptomatic intracranial reexpansion of such cysts.

Epidermoid Tumor (Cyst)

Epidermoid cysts account for fewer than 1% of all intracranial tumors. Presumed to be products of disordered embryogenesis, epidermoid cysts arise from the aberrant inclusion of epithelial tissue or "rests" at the time of neural tube closure or cerebral vesicle formation. Their predilection for basal brain areas and their ability to permeate along cisternal pathways accounts for approx one third of all intracranial epidermoids involving the suprasellar and parasellar regions. Despite their embryonic origins, few epidermoids are symptomatic before middle age.

Grossly, epidermoid cysts appear as glistening "pearly" white encapsulated lesions having a waxy texture and a friable flaky consistency. Their growth is slow—a process involving progressive desquamation of capsular elements and the accumulation of keratin and cholesterol debris. Displacing rather than invading anatomic structures, parasellar epidermoid cysts are frequently seen to encase chiasmatic, cranial nerve, and basal arterial structures and are often tenaciously adherent to the same. Although pure intrasellar epidermoid cysts have been reported *(131)*, most epidermoids have a sellar component as the result of secondary extension from a contiguous suprasellar or parasellar lesion (Fig. 5A,B).

When symptomatic, headaches and visual dysfunction are their most common symptoms; endocrine abnormalities occur much less frequently, and hydrocephalus is rare. Because parasellar epidermoids embed themselves in the mesial temporal lobe, partial complex seizures are an occasional accompaniment. The major complications of epidermoid cysts are chemical meningitis as the result of leakage of irritative cyst contents into the CSF and the rare phenomenon of malignant transformation into squamous cell carcinoma *(132)*.

The treatment of symptomatic parasellar epidermoid cysts is operative. The surgical objective is to decompress the optic apparatus and other compromised structures, removing as much tumor as is safely possible. Although a substantial portion of these cysts is easily removed, fragments densely adherent to neural and vascular structures should be left. Regrowth of residual fragments is so slow that symptomatic recurrence is infrequent. Although pure intrasellar epidermoid cysts, including those having a suprasellar component, can be approached transsphenoidally, the majority of epidermoids in this location, because of their frequent and often extensive lateral extensions, are approached transcranially.

Dermoid Tumor (Cyst)

Occurring with one tenth the frequency of epidermoid cysts, dermoid cysts are rare. Given their affinity for midline intracranial sites, their occasional occurrence in the sellar and parasellar regions is well recognized, although published

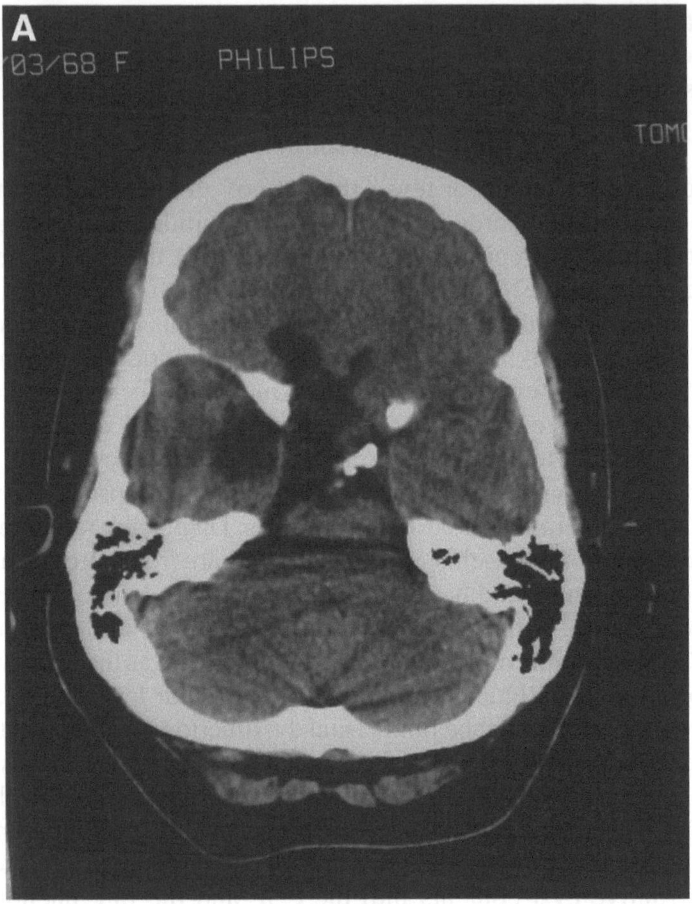

Fig. 5. Massive suprasellar and sellar epidermoid presenting with epilepsy and irregular menses. Axial CT (A) and sagittal unenhanced T1 MRI (B, *facing*).

reports of such cases have been few *(133)*. In addition to the epidermal elements present in epidermoid cysts, dermoid cysts have the additional features of hair follicles, sweat glands, and sebaceous glands. These lesions typically have a firm fibrous capsule that is often densely adherent to surrounding structures.

Dermoid cysts occur in younger patients, with most cases occurring within the first two decades of life. Their clinical presentation in the sellar region is variable, and DI, visual dysfunction, precocious puberty, and mild hyperprolactinemia have all been associated with dermoid cysts in this area. Some are confined exclusively to the sella, others are exclusively suprasellar, and some involve both sites. Radiologically, dermoid cysts appear as inhomogeneously enhancing masses, sometimes calcified, and often containing fat.

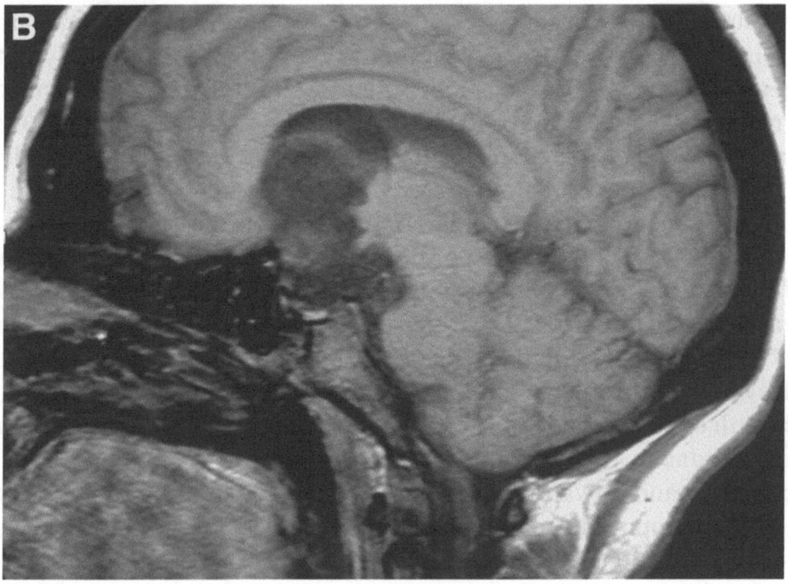

Fig. 5B.

Like epidermoid cysts, dermoid cysts are also prone to spontaneous bouts of chemical meningitis caused by seepage of their irritative cyst contents into the CSF, and they too may, rarely, undergo malignant transformation to squamous cell carcinoma *(134)*. As a rule, dermoid cysts grow more quickly than epidermoid cysts and recur more frequently.

Therapy for parasellar dermoid cysts is surgical removal. Although complete surgical excision of these lesions is always desirable, their frequent adherence to cranial nerves and blood vessels often necessitates a safer subtotal resection. Postoperative radiotherapy has not shown any benefit in either shrinking residual tumor or forestalling recurrence, and as such is not recommended. Fortunately, subtotal resection alone usually provides long-term symptom-free survival.

Arachnoid Cysts

Although uncommon, arachnoid cysts periodically arise in the region of the sella turcica, serving as an occasional source of neurologic and endocrinologic dysfunction in both pediatric and adult age groups *(123,135–141)*. With 15% of all arachnoid cysts occurring in the sellar region, this site represents the second most common intracranial location for such lesions. Arachnoid cysts are presumed to be developmental in origin, arising as the consequence of splitting or duplication of the arachnoid membrane, forming an arachnoid-lined sac in which CSF is entrapped.

The natural history of these lesions remains uncertain, with some arachnoid cysts remaining quiescent for years and others demonstrating symptomatic enlargement. The basis for such enlargement is similarly uncertain, with osmotic gradients, endogenous CSF production, and progressive accumulation of CSF through a "ball-valve" mechanism all being invoked as potential growth mechanisms. Although most arachnoid cysts are topologically related to a normal subarachnoid cistern, macroscopic continuity with the subarachnoid space is rarely apparent. Arachnoid cysts of the sellar region are distinguished as being one of two types, intrasellar and suprasellar—each is discussed separately.

Intrasellar arachnoid cysts are the least common of the two, arising from arachnoid remnants within the sella *(135)*. In contrast to arachnoid cysts occurring elsewhere, intrasellar arachnoid cysts tend to occur in older patients, usually in the fourth or fifth decade of life. They behave as expansile intrasellar masses, causing headache, sellar enlargement, hypopituitarism, moderate hyperprolactinemia, and upward displacement of the diaphragma sellae, resulting in visual loss. An important anatomic feature of these lesions is that, even with large suprasellar extensions, the diaphragma is always intact and the cysts remain entirely subdiaphragmatic. In rare instances, a pinhole communication with the suprasellar subarachnoid space is noted; however, as evidenced by their failure to admit contrast agents delivered cisternally, most intrasellar arachnoid cysts lack free communication with the subarachnoid space. Radiologically, these lesions are associated with sellar enlargement, appearing as homogeneous cysts whose fluid contents exhibit density and signal characteristics identical to CSF. Intrasellar arachnoid cysts are distinguished from the intrasellar herniation of the chiasmatic cistern that occurs with the empty sella syndrome and other cystic pathologies that occur in the region (craniopharyngioma, Rathke's cleft cyst, cystic pituitary adenoma, epidermoids, dermoids). Symptomatic intrasellar arachnoid cysts, as well as those in which imaging studies fail to exclude a cystic neoplasm, are best managed by transsphenoidal exploration, excision of the cyst wall for diagnosis, and marsupialization of the cyst cavity. Symptomatic improvement is the rule, headache, visual function, and hyperprolactinemia improving virtually always; however, anterior pituitary deficits, particularly if long-standing, are generally less responsive to surgical decompression.

Suprasellar arachnoid cysts are predominantly lesions of the pediatric population, with the majority of patients presenting within the first two decades of life *(32,136)*. Arising within the chiasmatic cistern, suprasellar arachnoid cysts may become sizeable, causing compression of the hypothalamus and third ventricle, stretching of the optic nerve, and distortion of the pituitary stalk. Lateral and posterior extensions into the medial temporal lobe and interpeduncular cistern, respectively, may also occur. Hydrocephalus, on the basis of third ventricular compression or aqueductal distortion, is often the dominant presenting feature, resulting in headache, macrocephaly, and retardation; precocious puberty or hypopituitarism reflects hypothalamic and/or stalk compression. Visual field deficits and loss of acuity are often present. A peculiar and intermittent pattern of head movements dubbed the "bobble-head doll" syndrome is a rare but classic presentation of arachnoid cysts in this location.

The management of suprasellar arachnoid cysts is surgical; however, the optimal form of intervention remains a matter of debate. Marsupialization of the cyst wall, with or without some form of shunting procedure, is the principal therapeutic option; ventriculoperitoneal shunting alone rarely produces a satisfactory or durable response *(32,136)*. Access to the cyst wall for purposes of marsupialization can be accomplished by a variety of approaches, including subfrontal, transcortical-transventricular, transsylvian, or transcallosal routes. Once a wide excision of the cyst wall has been achieved, some authors advocate the routine placement of a cystoperitoneal or ventriculoperitoneal shunt, because marsupialization alone may fail to improve hydrocephalus, despite seemingly adequate decompression of the cyst.

Empty Sella Syndrome

The term "empty sella" refers to the anatomic state occurring as the result of intrasellar herniation of the subarachnoid space through an incompetent and enlarged diaphragma sellae. The result is a compressed and posteriorly displaced pituitary gland housed within an enlarged and demineralized sella. These features lend a seemingly "empty" appearance to the sella, both grossly and radiographically. It is of clinical, pathophysiologic, and occasionally therapeutic importance to distinguish those cases occurring without an identifiable cause ("primary" empty sella) from those arising as the result of loss of intrasellar volume, which may accompany infarction, surgical resection, or radionecrosis of an intrasellar tumor ("secondary" empty sella).

Primary Empty Sella Syndrome

Though frequently considered the simple consequence of a developmentally enlarged diaphragmatic aperture, the primary empty sella syndrome is a far more complex condition, in which diaphragmatic defects represent only one of several incompletely understood pathophysiologic components. Autopsy studies have repeatedly shown that anatomic defects of the diaphragma sellae of 5 mm or more are present in almost 40% of consecutive autopsies, with more than 20% exhibiting intrasellar extension of the subarachnoid space and 5% showing a fully developed empty sella *(142)*. Insofar as the majority of these findings are incidental autopsy findings in persons without neurological or endocrine symptoms, it is likely that additional factors contribute to the development of the clinical syndrome. One potentially important contributing factor is elevated intracranial pressure. ICP elevations have been documented in patients with the empty sella syndrome, and at least 10% of patients with benign intracranial hypertension also have a coexisting empty sella *(143)*. The latter relationship is especially intriguing in that both syndromes share overlapping clinical profiles.

The overwhelming majority of patients with primary empty sella syndrome are asymptomatic, with their empty sellae being an incidental radiographic finding typically discovered during the investigation of an unrelated complaint. Of the minority of patients who are symptomatic, their clinical profile is often characteristic. More than 80% of symptomatic patients are middle-aged women, many of whom are obese, multiparous, and hypertensive *(144)*. Long-standing headache is the most common and frequently the only presenting complaint. Only rarely are visual field deficits attributable to this syndrome, because symptomatic compression or intrasellar prolapse of the optic chiasm rarely occurs. Complaints of blurred vision or ophthalmologic findings such as papilledema, decreased acuity, enlarged blind spot, and optic atrophy are likely to be the result of coexisting intracranial hypertension. Isolated accounts of atypical facial pain and sensory loss in the distribution of the trigeminal nerve have been noted. Clinically apparent pituitary dysfunction is unusual, although instances of pituitary deficiency, ranging from subtle abnormalities on dynamic endocrine testing (blunted GH response to insulin-induced hypoglycemia) to rare cases of panhypopituitarism, have periodically been reported *(144,145)*. Moderate hyperprolactinemia, as the result of stalk compression, has been variably reported in approx 5% of patients *(146)*. Hypersecretion of other anterior pituitary hormones suggests a coexisting pituitary adenoma. Finally, CSF rhinorrhea is a complication of empty sella syndrome in approx 10% of patients *(147,148)*. As the result of CSF pulsations, the sella floor becomes progressively thinned, eventually providing communication between the intrasellar subarachnoid space and the sphenoid sinus.

The radiologic diagnosis of this entity is usually straightforward. Lateral skull X-rays reveal a symmetrically enlarged and thin-walled sella, one that retains its normal configuration. Both CT and MRI scanning show clearly the CSF space extending from the hypothalamus down to a flattened pituitary gland, a finding that virtually excludes the possibility of other cystic lesions. If the diagnosis is still in doubt, CT cisternography demonstrates filling of the sella and conclusively secures a diagnosis of empty sella syndrome.

Secondary Empty Sella Syndrome

This entity is the occasional consequence of prior surgical therapy or radionecrosis of an intrasellar tumor. Occasionally, the condition may occur long after auto-infarction of a pituitary adenoma or a nontumorous pituitary gland, as may occur with apoplexy and Sheehan's syndrome, respectively. The diaphragma may be either developmentally deficient, eroded by the tumor, or disrupted by therapeutic intervention, thus permitting the descent of the chiasmatic cistern into the sella. Intrasellar prolapse of the optic chiasm is a frequent accompaniment, wherein it becomes entrapped and kinked by adhesions and scar tissue.

Clinically, the secondary empty sella syndrome is distinct from the primary form. Both sexes are equally affected, and there is no predilection for any particular body habitus. Visual dysfunction is the most common presenting symptom and may occur weeks or even years after surgery or radiotherapy. Bitemporal and binasal hemianopic defects, as well as asymmetrical deficits in the form of constrictions, segmental defects, or scotomas, may occur. The visual loss is often progressive; however, abrupt deterioration has also been known to occur. Endocrine dysfunction is not unusual and is likely to be the residual effect of prior surgery and/or radiation for an intrasellar tumor and not the result of secondary empty sella. Elevated ICP, headache, and CSF rhinorrhea are occasional features of this condition.

Treatment

Relatively few patients with primary or secondary empty sella syndrome require surgical intervention. After establishing the diagnosis and excluding other intrasellar cystic pathologies, the management of these conditions rests primarily on the recognition and treatment of potential complications (endocrine, ophthalmologic, and CSF rhinorrhea). The endocrine status of the patient requires careful laboratory evaluation, both at the time of diagnosis and periodically thereafter. Hypopituitarism, if present, requires appropriate hormone replacement therapy. Except for the case of low-grade hyperprolactinemia, hormonal hypersecretion warrants the exclusion of a coexisting hypersecreting microadenoma with MRI. When radiologically occult GH, adrenocorticotrophic hormone (ACTH), or prolactin-secreting microadenomas are suspected, transsphenoidal exploration may be necessary. Low-grade hyperprolactinemia (of stalk compression origin), because of its long-term adverse effects, should be treated if associated with symptoms of hypogonadism, such as amenorrhea, and is often exquisitely responsive to low-dose dopamine agonist therapy.

Deteriorating visual function necessitates careful evaluation. In primary empty sella syndrome, this is usually the result of benign intracranial hypertension. Accordingly, appropriate therapy for the latter should be initiated. Documented progressive visual loss in the case of the secondary empty sella syndrome is usually the result of chiasmal prolapse, the extent of which can be assessed with MRI. In such cases, transsphenoidal exploration and elevation of the chiasm with fat or muscle ("chiasmopexy") may halt progression of visual loss, and in some instances may actually improve vision *(149)*, although this is controversial.

CSF rhinorrhea, because it seldom stops spontaneously, virtually always requires definitive operative repair. The usual cause is a transsellar fistula into the sphenoid sinus; however, occasionally the site of leak may be along the anterior fossa floor. Accordingly, preoperative radiologic visualization of the precise site of leak is always desirable. This is best achieved by high-resolution coronal CT cisternography. For transsellar leaks, transsphenoidal exploration, sealing the leak with fibrin glue, and packing the sella and sphenoid sinus with fat or fascia constitute the treatment of choice. Leaks from the anterior fossa floor require repair by frontal craniotomy. Transnasal endoscopic methods are sometimes useful for the repair of such leaks.

METASTATIC TUMORS TO THE SELLAR REGION

Metastatic deposits from any systemic and hemopoietic malignancies occasionally involve the sellar region *(1)*. A favored anatomic target for such deposits is the posterior lobe of the pituitary. The predilection of metastatic tumors for the posterior lobe of the pituitary relates to its blood supply. In contrast to the anterior pituitary, which has a somewhat tenuous and indirect supply from the portal circulation, the posterior lobe derives its circulation directly from the carotid arterial system. Although the majority of metastatic tumors in this region occur in the context of advanced malignancy, occasional posterior lobe metastases may be the first sign of an unrecognized neoplastic process *(150,151)*. Of the metastatic cancers, breast is the most common primary, followed by lung and prostate *(150,151)*. Hemopoietic malignancies that may present with a posterior lobe deposit include the solitary plasmacytomas (which usually evolve into multiple myelomas) as well as various lymphomas and leukemias *(150,152)*. DI is often an accompanying feature, and its presence in association with a sellar mass should raise the possibility of a metastatic tumor. Additional symptoms include headache, visual field defects, hypopituitarism, and cranial nerve palsies related to cavernous sinus infiltration. With the exception of DI, which is rarely a feature of pituitary adenoma, it is often impossible in the absence of a known history of malignancy to distinguish a metastatic tumor to the sella from a pituitary adenoma. Transsphenoidal sellar exploration and decompression provide the tissue diagnosis and often effect symptomatic improvement and are, therefore, the treatment of choice in appropriate patients. Adjuvant radiation therapy is usually required postoperatively. Depending on the responsiveness of the primary tumor and the clinical status of the patient, chemotherapy may also be considered.

INFLAMMATORY DISEASES OF THE SELLAR REGION

The sellar region is host to a diverse collection of inflammatory disorders, the pathogenesis of which can range from acute suppuration through chronic granulomatous infiltration to autoimmune processes. Only in a minority of cases is the presenting clinical or radiologic appearance suggestive of the pathologic diagnosis; in many cases, the inflammatory basis is revealed only after careful pathologic examination of the surgical specimen.

Infections

Pituitary Abscess

Acute bacterial infection of the sella turcica is a rare event *(153–161)*. Whereas in many instances the pathogenesis of pituitary infection is not apparent, those instances in which an etiology has been established suggest that pituitary abscess arises in two clinical settings. The first is the result of secondary extension from a preexisting anatomically contiguous purulent focus. Acute sphenoid sinusitis, osteomyelitis of the sphenoid bone, mastoiditis, cavernous sinus thrombophlebitis, peritonsillar abscess, purulent otitis media, and bacterial meningitis have all been implicated as the primary infectious source. The other principal pathogenetic mechanism relates to generalized sepsis and hematogenous dissemination from a variety of distant septic foci (pneumonia, osteomyelitis, endocarditis, retroperitoneal abscess, tooth abscess). Isolated pituitary abscesses are extremely rare. More commonly (although still extremely unusual) abscesses have been reported in association with pre-existing sellar lesions (pituitary adenoma, craniopharyngioma, Rathke's cyst) *(154,160)*. Why such lesions should be especially vulnerable to abscess formation is unclear but may be related to the impaired vascularity and/or areas of necrosis within such lesions.

The symptoms of pituitary abscess are nonspecific and frequently indistinguishable from those of other sellar mass lesions (headache, visual field deficits, hypopituitarism). When these symptoms are accompanied by fever, leukocytosis, and meningismus, the possibility of a pituitary abscess should be strongly considered. Admittedly, so florid an infectious presentation tends to occur in only a minority of patients, being present in only a third of the 24 examples of Vates et al. *(160)*. In only 20% of their patients could the correct diagnosis be made preoperatively. Most patients will have some radiologic evidence of sellar pathology, the result of either a preexisting lesion or of the abscess itself. The bacteriology of pituitary abscess is variable. When organisms have been isolated, *Staphylococcus aureus*, *Diplococcus pneumoniae*, group A *Streptococcus*, *Klebsiella* species, *Escherichia coli*, and *Citrobacter divercusis* are most frequently reported *(160)*. In this series, definitive organisms were isolated in fewer than 60% of cases, whereas in the remainder, it was either intraoperative appearance or histopathologic evidence of necrosis and inflammation that prompted a diagnosis of pituitary abscess. One must recognize, however, that both intraoperative appearance and inflammatory histopathology can be misleading, particularly when dealing with certain cystic pathologies in the sella (notably Rathke's cleft cysts and craniopharyngiomas) whose cyst contents may fully mimic the appearance, consistency, and texture of suppuration. Accordingly, one must exercise caution in labeling a sellar process as being infectious when neither the clinical presentation nor the microbiologic diagnosis are confirmatory.

The management of a suspected pituitary abscess includes transsphenoidal exploration of the sella, drainage of the inflammatory mass, and antibiotic therapy. Selection of antimicrobial agents is based ideally on culture reports; however, empiric broad-spectrum therapy should include a combination of a third-generation cephalosporin, a synthetic penicillin, and metronidazole for their Gram-negative, staphylococcal, and anaerobic sensitivities, respectively. The optimal duration of antibiotic therapy has not been established.

Because pituitary abscesses are rare, recent data concerning long-term outcome are not available. Based on their review of 29 cases, Domingue and Wilson identified an overall mortality rate of 28% for pituitary abscess, which further increased to 45% if meningitis was also present *(154)*. In a more contemporary series of Vates et al., which also included seven patients reported by Domingue and Wilson, the overall mortality rate was 8.3% *(160)*.

Miscellaneous Infections

A variety of other rare nonbacterial or atypical bacterial infective agents may also be responsible for pituitary and sellar region infection. Tuberculosis, still endemic in certain areas, has historically been an important etiology for destructive granulomatous inflammatory lesions involving the hypothalamus and sellar region *(162–164)*. In most instances, parasellar involvement has been a complication of its dense plaque-like basilar meningitis. Such "tuberculomas" are often associated with near-total anterior and posterior pituitary failure, are frequently calcified, and often, but not invariably, associated with evidence of active tuberculosis elsewhere (Fig. 6).

Brucellosis, a common zoonosis in many parts of the world, has in rare instances presented as a sellar mass *(165,166)*.

Syphilis, now extremely uncommon in its consummate forms, represents another granulomatous infection involving the hypothalamus and sellar region *(153)*. Historical accounts suggest that the clinical features of syphilitic gumma in the sellar region were typical of other destructive processes of the sella and were usually associated with syphilitic lesions elsewhere in the neuroaxis.

Mycotic infection, notably aspergillosis, has also been reported to involve the sellar, parasellar, and orbital regions, often presenting as a discrete inflammatory mass *(167,168)*. Rare examples of candidal abscess in the pituitary are also known to occur *(169)*. Parasitic infiltration of the sellar and parapituitary regions by cystercosis *(170)* and echinococcus *(171)* have both produced a mass in this region. Finally, in the context of AIDS and other immunosuppressed states, an additional spectrum of pituitary infection has emerged, including agents such as *Pneumocystis carinii*, *Toxoplasma gondii*, and cytomegalovirus *(172)*.

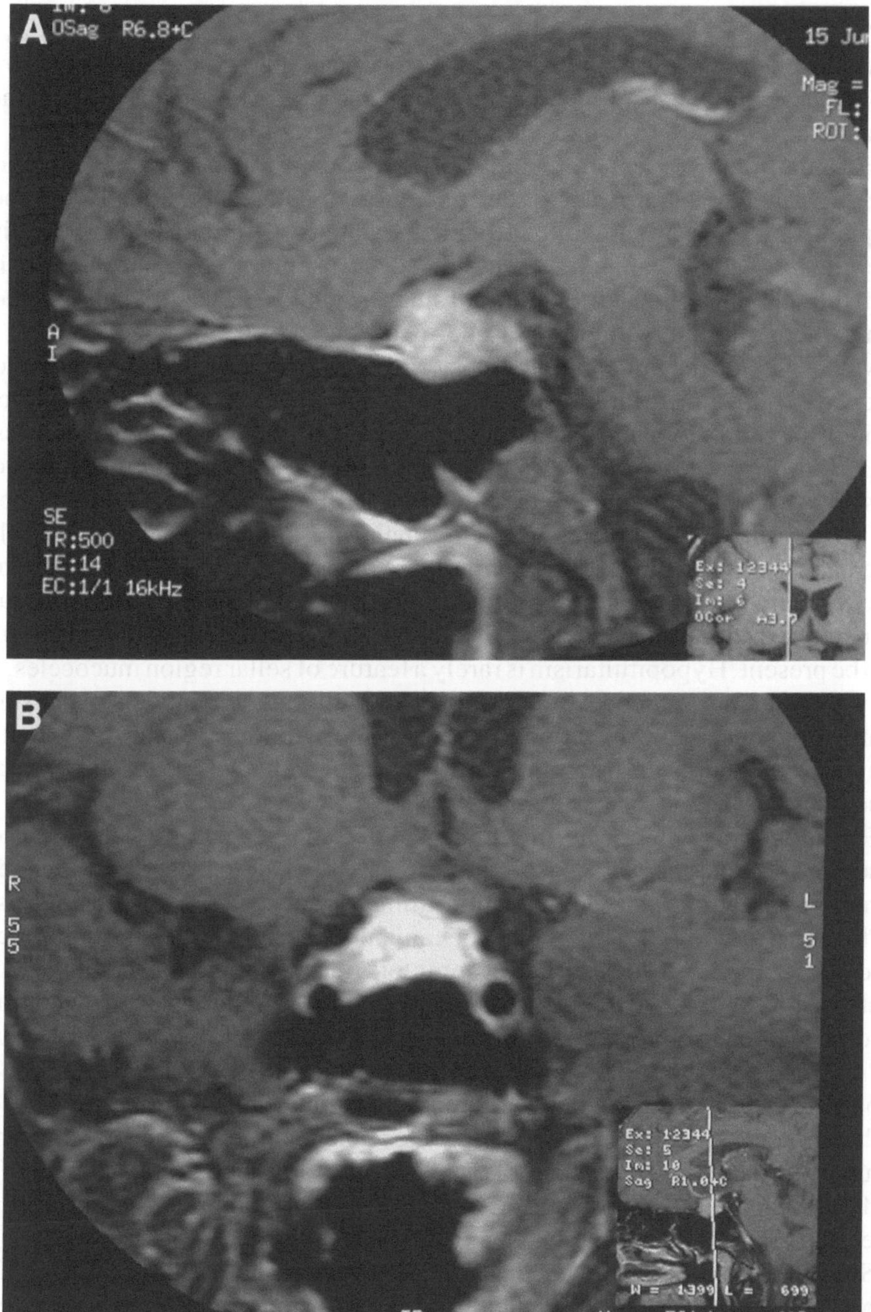

Fig. 6. Tuberculous granuloma of the sella. T1-weighted MRI with gadolinium sagittal (A) and coronal (B).

Mucoceles

Mucoceles are benign slowly expansile mucous-filled cystic lesions that arise in paranasal sinuses. Their neurosurgical relevance derives primarily from their occasional tendency to erode intracranially, wherein they may present as an intracranial mass or, less frequently, offer a source for intracranial infection. Although mucoceles arising in the maxillary sinus are numerically the most frequent, and those arising in the frontal and anterior ethmoid sinuses are clinically the most significant, this discussion concerns those rare mucoceles arising from the sphenoid or posterior ethmoid sinuses, whose intracranial involvement brings them into the realm of parasellar pathology.

Mucoceles of the sphenoid and posterior ethmoid sinuses (spheno-ethmoid mucoceles) are rare. Rarer still is the occasion when these mucoceles erode through the sellar floor and present as intrasellar, parasellar, or suprasellar masses *(173–176)*. In some instances their clinical features are indistinguishable from those of a nonfunctioning pituitary adenoma (NFPA); the sella is eroded, showing balloon-like enlargement, and a chiasmal syndrome attendant to suprasellar extension is documented. In other cases there may be morc extensive intracranial involvement, with extensions into the orbital apex and superior orbital fissure. In such cases additional symptoms of exophthalmos and oculomotor palsies may also be present. Hypopituitarism is rarely a feature of sellar region mucoceles. On CT scanning, most mucoceles appear isodense, although their walls may exhibit contrast enhancement of varying degree. Bone windows reveal the extent of bony erosion and/or destruction. Their MRI signal characteristics are variable, depending on the viscosity of contents.

Pathologically, mucoceles are encapsulated masses whose walls are composed of the mucoperiosteal lining of the involved sinus. Their pathogenesis remains conjectural. Although postinflammatory obstruction of the sinus ostia is the most commonly invoked mechanism underlying their development, mucoceles appear to be neither a common nor an inevitable result of such obstruction. Whatever the basis for their initiation, mucoceles are generally chronic lesions, frequently exhibiting years of subclinical growth before causing symptoms. Ongoing accumulation of mucoid material gives rise to expansile growth, causing bony erosion of the sinus walls, and eventual access to the intracranial compartment. Mucoceles that become infected are known as "mucopyoceles" and, unexpectedly, have an abruptly accelerated course, often with rapid bony destruction and an increased risk of intracranial or intraorbital infection (Fig. 7).

Sphenoido-ethmoidal mucoceles are effectively treated by transsphenoidal or transethmoidal exploration, depending on their sinus of origin. Drainage of mucocele contents and mucosal exenteration of the involved sinus is generally curative. Radical removal of the intracranial portion of the mucocele wall is neither necessary nor advisable.

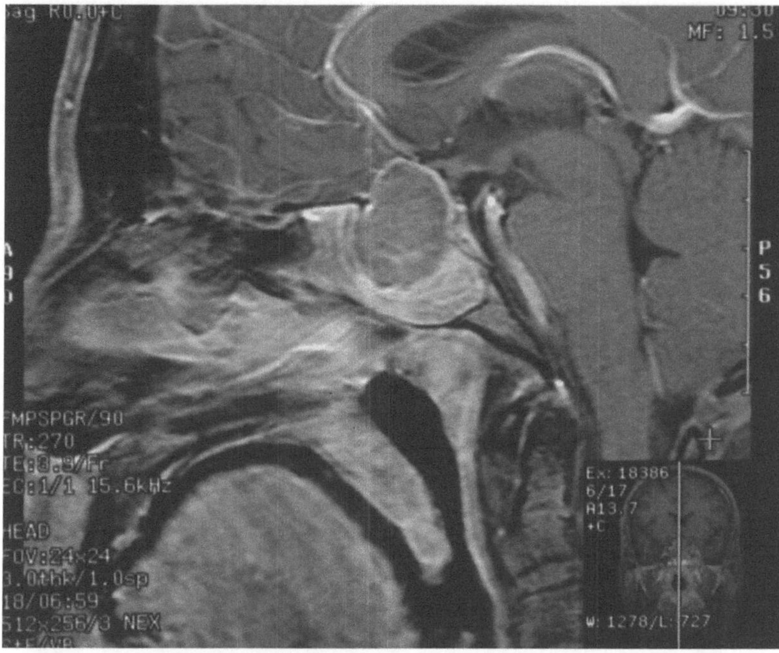

Fig. 7. Sagittal T1-weighted gadolinium-enhanced MRI of a mucopyocele of the sphenoid sinus with an associated pituitary adenoma.

Rarely, mucoceles are a complication of previous transsphenoidal or more particularly trans-ethmoidal surgery.

Noninfectious Inflammatory Lesions of the Sellar Region

Lymphocytic Hypophysitis

Lymphocytic hypophysitis is a destructive inflammatory disorder of the anterior pituitary, presumed to be autoimmune in origin. Although the earliest descriptions of this condition stemmed from necropsy studies wherein the potentially lethal nature of the disorder was emphasized, improved recognition of the condition, coupled with hormone replacement therapy, has since rendered lymphocytic hypophysitis an entirely treatable condition.

The basic lesion consists of a destructive inflammatory infiltrate of lymphocytes, plasma cells, and macrophages that is restricted exclusively to the anterior lobe of the gland. The result is a firm and enlarged gland that often extends into the suprasellar space and microscopically exhibits effacement of the normal glandular architecture and disruption of the structural and immunohistochemical integrity of all anterior lobe secretory elements *(177)*. Lymphoid follicles and loosely organized germinal centers may be present, as are varying degrees of

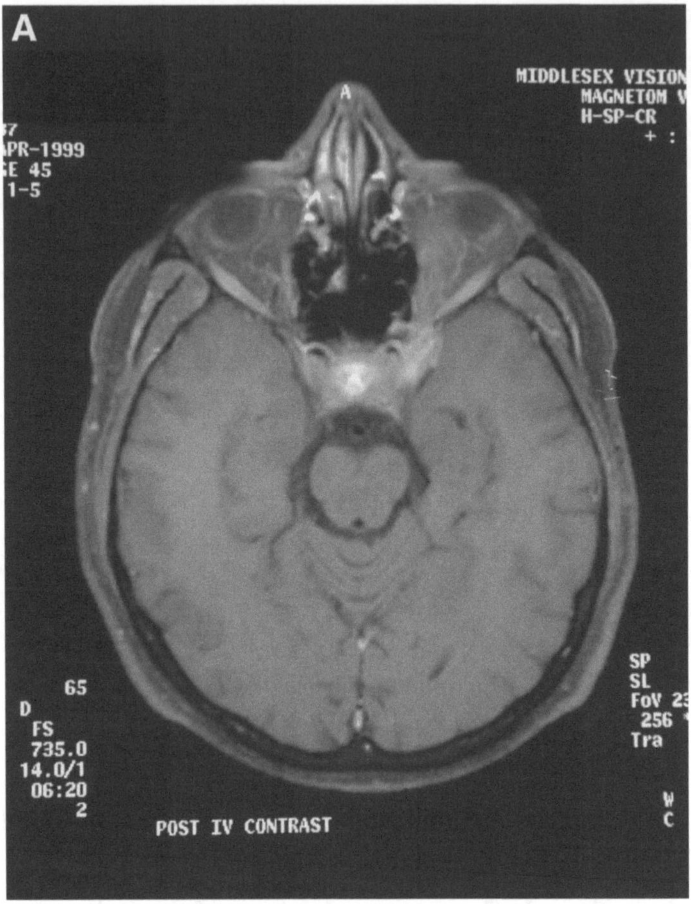

Fig. 8. Lymphocytic hypophysitis with cavernous sinus extension presenting in a male. Enhanced T1 MRI axial (A) and coronal (B, *facing*).

fibrosis, depending on the chronicity of the condition. Several lines of evidence suggest that this process has an autoimmune basis *(177–180)*. First, the cellular infiltrate present in affected glands is similar to other autoimmune reactions occurring in other organs. Antipituitary antibodies have been identified in the serum of some patients with the condition. Finally, patients with lymphocytic hypophysitis frequently have a concurrent or prior history of other autoimmune diseases (Hashimoto's thyroiditis, idiopathic adrenalitis, pancreatitis, and others), thus suggesting that lymphocytic hypophysitis is but one component of a generalized polyglandular autoimmune disorder.

The clinical profile of lymphocytic hypophysitis is fairly characteristic. Although the condition was once believed to affect women exclusively, ever-

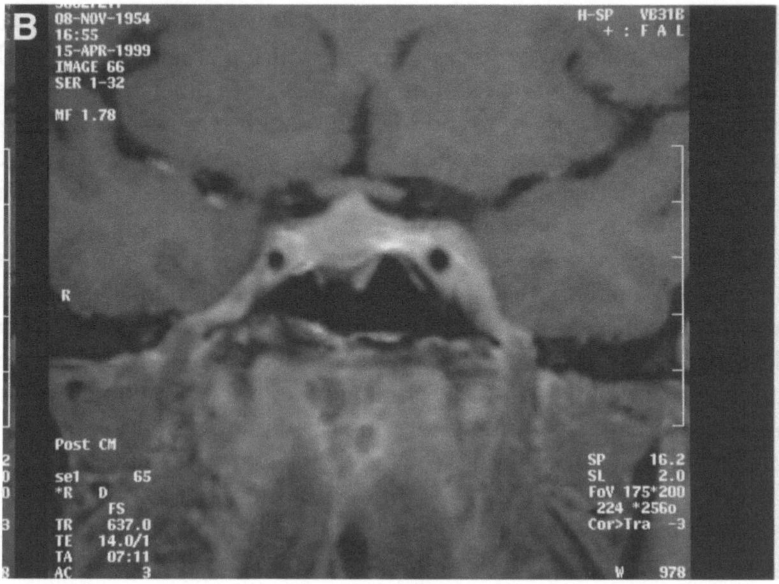

Fig. 8B.

increasing reports of its occurrence in men have established that males, too, may be affected, although considerably less often *(181,182)* (Fig. 8). One of the most typical features of the condition concerns its temporal association with pregnancy; almost 70% of reported cases occur during pregnancy or more commonly during the first postpartum year. Indeed the condition is sometimes called postpartum hypophysitis. Clinically, the picture is one of progressive anterior pituitary failure in association with an expansile sellar mass. The pituitary insufficiency may involve any or all anterior pituitary hormones; manifestations of hypocortisolism have been especially prominent among reported cases.

Amenorrhea or failure of appropriate resumption of menses following parturition is a common presenting complaint; galactorrhoea occurs less frequently. The amenorrhoea is at least in part related to the compression, a common accompaniment to the condition. Because the posterior lobe escapes injury, DI is not ordinarily a feature of the condition. Because there is often considerable enlargement of the gland, the majority of patients also have symptoms of mass effect, including headache and visual loss. The radiologic appearance of lymphocytic hypohysitis is nonspecific. Plain films may demonstrate sellar enlargement and suprasellar extension, and MRI scanning shows a sellar/suprasellar mass that is homogeneously isointense to brain parenchyma.

In its most typical clinical context, such as that involving the pregnant or postpartum female presenting with a sellar region mass, lymphocytic hypophysitis should be an obvious diagnostic consideration. Prolactin-producing pituitary adenomas, given their known tendency to enlarge during pregnancy, are probably the most commonly considered differential diagnosis. In other clinical situations not related to pregnancy, or those involving male patients, a prospective diagnosis of a lymphocytic hypophysitis cannot be made with any certainty. In all cases, however, the definitive diagnosis requires histologic confirmation. Accordingly, the management of this condition involves establishing a tissue diagnosis and chiasmal decompression—objectives best served by the transsphenoidal route. The gland typically appears firm and diffusely enlarged and has a pale-yellow appearance. The surgical goal is to remove sufficient tissue for histologic diagnosis and chiasmal decompression while preserving as much of the viable gland as possible, thus maximizing prospects for residual pituitary function.

Given the presumed autoimmune origins of lymphocytic hypophysitis, the therapeutic use of immunosuppressive agents has met with some success as an adjuvant form of therapy for this condition. In some patients, corticosteroid therapy has resulted in reduction in the size of the sellar mass and improvement in visual function, prompting some authors to recommend such therapy from the start, thus avoiding the immediate need for surgical decompression or tissue diagnosis *(179)*. It is acknowledged, however, that experience with this approach has been limited and that steroids have not proven uniformly successful in ameliorating the inflammatory process *(183)*.

Endocrine replacement therapy is an essential component of the management of this disorder. Pituitary insufficiency should be carefully assessed and appropriately treated both at presentation and during long-term follow-up. Because the degree of anterior pituitary destruction is typically quite severe, most patients with lymphocytic hypophysitis require chronic long-term replacement therapy.

Sarcoidosis

Known as one of the "great imitators," sarcoidosis is well recognized for its periodic affinity for parasellar structures, serving as an occasional diagnosis of exclusion for masses and other inflammatory processes affecting this region *(178,184,185)*. As a chronic multisystem granulomatous disease of unknown origin, sarcoidosis can affect any organ or tissue, with uveoparotitis, pulmonary, and lymph node involvement being its classical manifestations.

Five percent of all cases exhibit nervous system involvement, most commonly in the form of dense adhesive granulomatous arachnoiditis involving the base of the brain *(185)*. Cranial nerves, the pituitary gland stalk, hypothalamic, and anterior third ventricular structures may all be engulfed in the inflammatory process. Less frequently, neurosarcoidosis can assume the form of discrete masses, both in the parasellar region and elsewhere in the neuroaxis.

The clinical features of neurosarcoidosis are variable and reflect the degree of anatomic involvement. The hypothalamus and pituitary stalk are favored targets, and accordingly features of hypothalamic dysfunction often predominate *(186)*. The single most common feature of CNS involvement—one occasionally serving as the presenting feature of the disease in general—is DI. This usually reflects hypothalamic involvement and, less often, damage to the stalk. Additional evidence of hypothalamic disease in the form of somnolence and alterations of eating, emotion, and thermoregulation often coexist. Damage to hypophysiotropic areas of the hypothalamus or the stalk can result in hypopituitarism and low-grade hyperprolactinemia. Primary involvement of the anterior pituitary may also be the source of hypopituitarism, but less commonly. Visual dysfunction secondary to optic nerve and chiasmal involvement also occurs. Depending on the extent of basilar meningeal involvement, other cranial nerve palsies may also occur. Hydrocephalus, reflecting basilar meningeal or third ventricular obstruction, may be present.

Imaging studies, when positive, generally reveal an enhancing meningeal process, or evidence of a discrete mass of the sellar region. A search for active disease in the lungs or elsewhere is often informative in providing corroborative evidence of sarcoidosis; however, definite diagnosis requires biopsy. Because the histopathology of sarcoidosis is often characteristic but falls short of being diagnostic, this is a diagnosis of exclusion. A compatible clinical profile, histologic evidence of noncaseating granulomas, and negative bacterial and fungal cultures of biopsy specimens are the practical diagnostic criteria used for this entity. CSF studies, though frequently abnormal (lymphocytic pleocytosis, elevations of protein and immunoglobins, decreased glucose concentrations), are nonspecific.

From the surgical perspective most cases of sarcoidosis involving the sellar region present as undiagnosed mass lesions, occurring in the absence of recognized systemic sarcoidosis. Therefore, the surgical objectives primarily include establishing a tissue diagnosis and decompression of the visual apparatus. Once the diagnosis is established, corticosteroids are often effective therapy. In cases unresponsive to steroids, chloroquine, azathioprine, and methotrexate have all been used with varying degrees of success. The prognosis is variable, being most favorable in patients with limited disease, where spontaneous remission is also occasionally seen. In other patients, particularly those with pulmonary involvement and disease in more than three organ systems, the prognosis is poor.

Langerhans Cell Histiocytosis (Histiocytosis X)

Langerhans cell histiocytosis is an umbrella term encompassing a collection of poorly understood clinically heterogeneous but pathologically interrelated entities. Unified pathologically and pathognomonically by a destructive infiltrate of foamy histiocytes in affected organs, the clinical expression of Langerhans cell histiocytes is variable, depending on the extent and nature of organ involvement. Ranging from the fulminant, disseminated, and frequently fatal Letterer-Siwe disease seen in childhood, through the multifocal eosinophilic

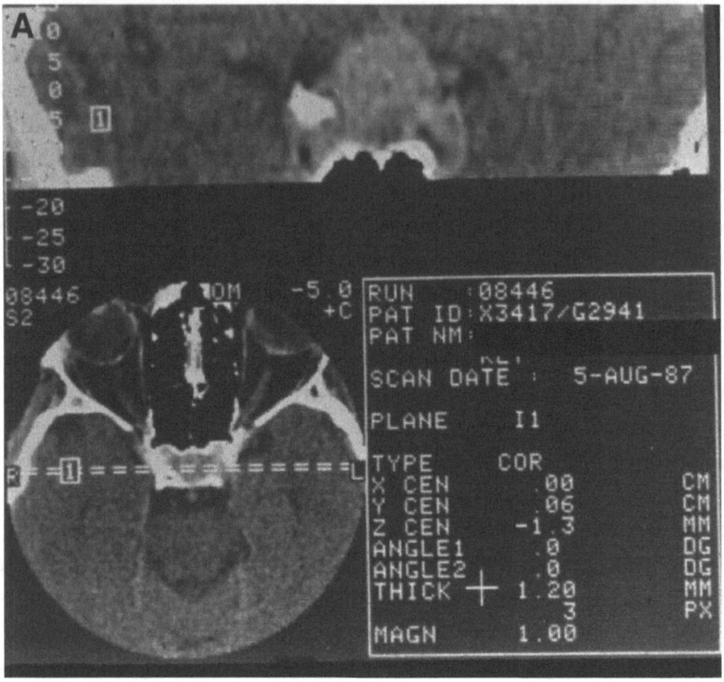

Fig. 9 . Sellar aneurysm presenting with bitemporal hemianopia axial CT scan (A) AP carotid angiogram (B, *facing*).

granulomas of Hand-Schuller-Christian disease, and to the relatively innocent solitary eosinophilic granulomas of bone, involvement of parasellar structures may be a feature of each.

CNS involvement, usually in association with multifocal bony lesions, occurs in almost one quarter of all patients with systemic Langerhans cell histiocytosis; isolated CNS involvement is, however, rare *(187)*. There is an apparent predilection for involvement of the hypothalamus, infundibulum, and posterior pituitary, with adenohypophyseal involvement occurring less frequently *(188–194)*. In some cases, the disease is discretely localized in the hypothalamus or posterior pituitary. In other cases the process is less restricted, with bony disease of the skull base and secondary infiltrates both compressing and permeating meningeal and multiple parasellar structures. DI is the most common presenting feature of CNS disease and commonly is the first sign of unrecognized systemic disease. Hyperprolactinemia on the basis of stalk or hypothalamic involvement may also present. Involvement of the optic apparatus occurs less frequently, and anterior pituitary function is often spared. Imaging studies are nonspecific, typically revealing obvious bony disease, with a contiguous soft tissue component.

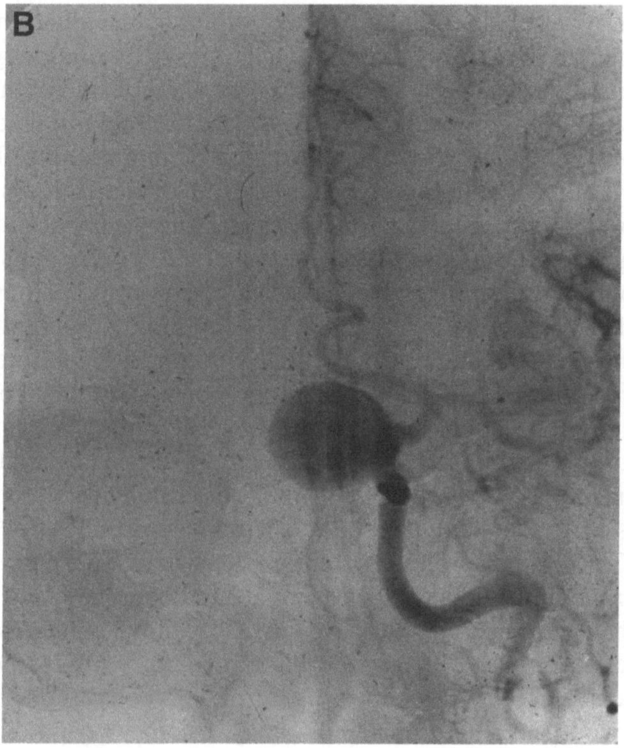

Fig. 9B.

If the diagnosis is already known, owing to the multisystem nature of the disease, there is no role for surgical intervention. In the rare situation of an isolated parasellar granuloma, the surgical objective in this condition is directed primarily at establishing a histologic diagnosis, and possibly decompression of compromised sellar structures. A definitive diagnosis rests on the identification of the intracytoplasmic organelles known as Birbeck granules, the demonstration that cells of the histiocytic infiltrate bear the CD1 antigenic determinant, and the confirmation that bacterial and fungal cultures of the surgical specimen are negative.

ANEURYSMS OF THE SELLAR REGION

Although uncommon, the possibility of a cerebral aneurysm masquerading as a pituitary adenoma has always been an important, if not a nagging, diagnostic consideration in the evaluation of an endocrine-inactive sellar mass (Fig. 9).

Indeed, the inadvertent rupture of an unsuspected intrasellar aneurysm during the course of transsphenoidal exploration for a presumed pituitary adenoma represents one of the classic neurosurgic disasters. That cerebral angiography was, until recently, a regular practice in the radiological evaluation of pituitary adenomas further emphasizes the fact that aneurysms do periodically involve the sellar region, and their exclusion is essential. Fortunately, one of the many benefits of MRI is its ability to exclude an aneurysm as a potential aetiology of a sellar region mass, thus obviating the routine use of angiography. The majority of aneurysms involving the sellar region derive from the intracavernous segment of the carotid artery, and less often from the supraclinoid carotid and the anterior communicating artery complex. The clinical picture may be indistinguishable from a NFPA or other sellar mass; headache and retro-orbital pain, visual symptoms, low-grade hyperprolactinemia, and, less commonly, hypopituitarism and DI may all be presenting features. Should such aneurysms erode into and occupy the sella, the resulting sellar enlargement can be indistinguishable from that occurring with pituitary adenomas or other intrasellar mass lesions.

In addition to mimicking pituitary adenomas, aneurysms have also coexisted with pituitary adenomas. As reviewed by Weir, the incidence of coexisting pituitary adenomas and incidental cerebral aneurysms approaches 7.4% in various reports *(195)*. GH-producing pituitary tumors in particular have been repeatedly reported to coexist with incidental aneurysms at a frequency above what would be expected by chance alone. The basis of this association is uncertain. Because generalized arterial ectasia is a recognized feature of acromegaly, some have speculated that the local effects of GH or, more likely, of IGF-1 on cerebral blood vessels (which are known to have IGF-1 receptors) may in some way predispose or contribute to aneurysm formation.

REFERENCES

1. Thapar K, Kovacs K. Tumors of the sellar region. In: Bruner JM, ed. *Russel and Rubinstein's Pathology of Tumors of the Nervous System.* 6th ed. Baltimore: Williams & Wilkins; 1998:561–677.
2. Laws ER. Craniopharyngiomas: diagnosis and treatment. In: Schramm V, ed. *Tumors of the Cranial Base: Diagnosis and Treatment.* Mount Kisco, NY: Futura; 1987:347–371.
3. Burger P, Scheithauer B. *Tumors of the Central Nervous System.* Third Series, Fascicle 10. Washington, DC: Armed Forces Institute of Pathology; 1994.
4. Adamson TE, Wiestler OD, Kleihues P, Yasargil MG. Correlation of clinical and pathological features in surgically treated craniopharyngiomas. J. Neurosurg. 1990;73(1):12–17.
5. Weiner HL, Wisoff JH, Rosenberg ME, et al. Craniopharyngiomas: a clinicopathological analysis of factors predictive of recurrence and functional outcome. Neurosurgery 1994;35(6):1001–1010.
6. Duff JM, Meyer FB, Ilstrup DM, Laws ER, Schleck CD, Scheithauer BW. Long-term outcomes for surgically resected craniopharyngiomas. Neurosurgery 2000;46(2):291–302; discussion 302–305.
7. Thapar K, Laws ER. Unusual lesions of the sella turcica: craniopharyngiomas, benign cysts, and meningiomas. In: Black M, ed. *Operative Neurosurgery.* London: Harcourt Publishers; 2000:723–740.
8. Laws ER, Thapar K. The diagnosis and management of craniopharyngioma. Growth Gen Horm 1994;10(3):6–11.

9. Laws ER. Transsphenoidal microsurgery in the management of craniopharyngioma. J Neurosurg1980;52:661–666.
10. Laws ER Jr. Transsphenoidal removal of craniopharyngioma. Pediatr Neurosurg 1994;21(Suppl 1):57–63.
11. Honegger J, Buchfelder M, Fahlbusch R, Däubler B, Dörr HG. Transsphenoidal microsurgery for craniopharyngiomas. Surg Neurol 1992;37:189–196.
12. Fahlbusch R, Honegger J, Paulus W, Huk W, Buchfelder M. Surgical treatment of craniopharyngiomas: experience with 168 patients. J Neurosurg 1999;90(2):237–250.
13. Maira G, Anile C, Rossi GF, Colosimo C. Surgical treatment of craniopharyngiomas: an evaluation of the transsphenoidal and pterional approaches. Neurosurgery 1995;36(4):715–724.
14. Landolt AM, M. Z. Results of transsphenoidal extirpation of craniopharyngiomas and Rathke's cysts. Neurosurgery 1991;28:410–415.
15. Baskin DS, Wilson CB. Surgical management of craniopharyngiomas. A review of 74 cases. J Neurosurg 1986;65(1):22–27.
16. Yasargil MG, Curcic M, Kis M, Siegenthaler G, Teddy PJ, Roth P. Total removal of craniopharyngiomas. Approaches and long-term results in 144 patients. J Neurosurg 1990;73(1):3–11.
17. Laws ER, Jr. Craniopharyngioma: transsphenoidal surgery. Curr Ther Endocrinol Metab 1997;6:35–38.
18. Voges J, Sturm V, Lehrke R, Treuer H, Gauss C, Berthold F. Cystic craniopharyngioma: long-term results after intracavitary irradiation with stereotactically applied colloidal beta-emitting radioactive sources. Neurosurgery 1997;40(2):263–269; discussion 269–270.
19. Vitaz TW, Hushek S, Shields CB, Moriarty T. Changes in cyst volume following intraoperative MRI-guided Ommaya reservoir placement for cystic craniopharyngioma. Pediatr Neurosurg 2001;35(5):230–234.
20. Hooda BS, Finlay JL. Recent advances in the diagnosis and treatment of central nervous system germ-cell tumors. Curr Opin Neurol 1999;12(6):693–696.
21. Sano K. Intracranial dysembryogenetic tumors: pathogenesis and their order of malignancy. Neurosurg Rev 2001;24(4):162–167; discussion 168–170.
22. Jennings MT, Gelman R, Hochberg F. Intracranial germ-cell tumors: natural history and pathogenesis. J Neurosurg 1985;63(2):155–167.
23. Packer RJ, Cohen BH, Cooney K. Intracranial germ cell tumors. Oncologist 2000;5(4):312–320.
24. Brandes AA, Pasetto LM, Monfardini S. The treatment of cranial germ cell tumors. Cancer Treat Rev 2000;26(4):233–242.
25. Allen JC. Controversies in the management of intracranial germ cell tumors. Neurol Clin 1991;9(2):441–452.
26. Baskin D, Wilson C. Transsphenoidal management of intrasellar germinomas. J Neurosurg 1983;59:1063–1066.
27. Muzumdar D, Goel A, Desai K, Shenoy A. Mature teratoma arising from the sella—case report. Neurol Med Chir (Tokyo) 2001;41(7):356–359.
28. Nishioka H, Ito H, Haraoka J, Akada K. Immature teratoma originating from the pituitary gland: case report. Neurosurgery 1999;44(3):644–647; discussion 647–648.
29. Saeki N, Uchida D, Tatsuno I, Saito Y, Yamaura A. MRI detection of suprasellar germinoma causing central diabetes insipidus. Endocr J 1999;46(2):263–267.
30. Starzyk J, Starzyk B, Bartnik-Mikuta A, Urbanowicz W, Dziatkowiak H. Gonadotropin releasing hormone-independent precocious puberty in a 5 year-old girl with suprasellar germ cell tumor secreting beta-hCG and alpha-fetoprotein. J Pediatr Endocrinol Metab 2001;14(6):789–796.
31. Baumgartner JE, Edwards MS. Pineal tumors. Neurosurg Clin North Am 1992;3(4):853–862.
32. Rutka JT, Hoffman HJ, Drake JM, Humphreys RP. Suprasellar and sellar tumors in childhood and adolescence. Neurosurg Clin North Am 1992;3(4):803–820.

33. Page R, Ploude R, Coldwell D, Heald J, Weinstein J. Intrasellar mixed germ-cell tumor. Case report. J Neurosurg 1983;58:766–770.
34. Horowitz M, Hall W. Central nervous system germinomas. Arch Neurol 1991;48:652–657.
35. Legido A, Packer R, Sutton L, et al. Suprasellar germinomas of childhood: a reappraisal. Cancer 1989;63:340–344.
36. Robertson PL, DaRosso RC, Allen JC. Improved prognosis of intracranial non-germinoma germ cell tumors with multimodality therapy. J Neurooncol 1997;32(1):71–80.
37. Kumar PP, Good RR, Skultety FM, Masih AS, McComb RD. Spinal metastases from pituitary hemangiopericytic meningioma. Am J Clin Oncol 1987;10:422–428.
38. Kinjo T, Al-Mefty O, Ciric I. Diaphragma sellae meningiomas. Neurosurgery 1995;36:1082–1092.
39. Grisoli F, Vincentelli F, Raybaud C, et al. Intrasellar meningioma. Surg Neurol 1983;20:36–41.
40. Beems T, Grotenhuis JA, Wesseling P. Meningioma of the pituitary stalk without dural attachment: case report and review of the literature. Neurosurgery 1999;45(6): 1474–1477.
41. Kouri JG, Chen MY, Watson JC, Oldfield EH. Resection of suprasellar tumors by using a modified transsphenoidal approach. Report of four cases. J Neurosurg 2000;92(6): 1028–1035.
42. Kaptain GJ, Vincent DA, Sheehan JP, Laws ER, Jr. Transsphenoidal approaches for the extracapsular resection of midline suprasellar and anterior cranial base lesions. Neurosurgery 2001;49(1):94–100; discussion 100–101.
43. Black K. Chordomas of the clival region. Contemp Neurosurg 1990;12:1–7.
44. Mathews W, Wilson C. Ectopic intrasellar chordoma. J Neurosurg 1974;40:260–263.
45. Wold L, Laws ER. Cranial chordomas in children and young adults. J Neurosurg 1983;59:1043–1047.
46. Laws E. Clivus chordomas. In: Janecka I, ed. *Surgery of Cranial Base Tumors*. New York: Raven Press;1993:679–686.
47. Thodou E, Kontogeorgos G, Scheithauer BW, et al. Intrasellar chordomas mimicking pituitary adenoma. J Neurosurg 2000;92(6):976–982.
48. Uesaka T, Miyazono M, Nishio S, Iwaki T. Astrocytoma of the pituitary gland (pituicytoma): case report. Neuroradiology 2002;44(2):123–125.
49. Schultz AB, Brat DJ, Oyesiku NM, Hunter SB. Intrasellar pituicytoma in a patient with other endocrine neoplasms. Arch Pathol Lab Med 2001;125(4):527–530.
50. Brat DJ, Scheithauer BW, Staugaitis SM, Holtzman RN, Morgello S, Burger PC. Pituicytoma: a distinctive low-grade glioma of the neurohypophysis. Am J Surg Pathol 2000;24(3):362–368.
51. Hurley TR, D'Angelo CM, Clasen RA, Wilkinson SB, Passavoy RD. Magnetic resonance imaging and pathological analysis of a pituicytoma: case report. Neurosurgery 1994;35(2):314–317; discussion 317.
52. Rossi ML, Bevan JS, Esiri MM, Hughes JT, Adams CB. Pituicytoma (pilocytic astrocytoma). Case report. J Neurosurg 1987;67(5):768–772.
53. Cohen ME, Duffner PK. Optic pathway tumors. Neurol Clinics 1991;9(2):467–477.
54. Grill J, Laithier V, Rodriguez D, Raquin MA, Pierre-Kahn A, Kalifa C. When do children with optic pathway tumors need treatment? An oncological perspective in 106 patients treated in a single centre. Eur J Pediatr 2000;159(9):692–696.
55. Janss AJ, Grundy R, Cnaan A, et al. Optic pathway and hypothalamic/chiasmatic gliomas in children younger than age 5 years with a 6-year follow-up. Cancer 1995;75(4):1051–1059.
56. Elster AD. Modern imaging of the pituitary. Radiology 1993;187(1):1–14.
57. Packer RJ, Sutton LN, Bilaniuk LT, et al. Treatment of chiasmatic/hypothalamic gliomas of childhood with chemotherapy: an update. Ann Neurol 1988;23(1):79–85.

58. Rodriguez LA, Edwards MS, Levin VA. Management of hypothalamic gliomas in children: an analysis of 33 cases. Neurosurgery 1990;26(2):242–246.
59. Wisoff JH, Abbott R, Epstein F. Surgical management of exophytic chiasmatic-hypothalamic tumors of childhood. J Neurosurg 1990;73(5):661–667.
60. Petronio J, Edwards MS, Prados M, et al. Management of chiasmal and hypothalamic gliomas of infancy and childhood with chemotherapy. J Neurosurg 1991;74(5):701–708.
61. Albright L, Lee PA. Neurosurgical treatment of hypothalamic hamartomas causing precocious puberty. J Neurosurg 1993;78:77–82.
62. Asa S, Kovacs K, Tindall G, Barrow D, Horvath E, Vecsei P. Cushing's disease associated with an intrasellar gangliocytoma produing corticotropin-releasing factor. Ann Intern Med 1984;101:789–793.
63. Towfighi J, Salam M, McLendon R, Powers S, Page R. Ganglion cell-containing tumors of the pituitary gland. Arch Pathol Lab Med 1996;120:369–377.
64. Asa S, Bilbao J, Kovacs K, Linfoot J. Hypothalamic neuronal hamartoma associated with pituitary growth hormone cell adenoma and acromegaly. Acta Neuropathol (Berlin) 1980;52:231–234.
65. Saeger W, Puchner M, Lüdecke D. Combined sellar gangliocytoma and pituitary adenoma in acromegaly or Cushing's disease. Virchows Arch Pathol Anat 1994;425:93–99.
66. Horvath E, Kovacs K, Scheithauer BW, Lloyd RV, Smyth HS. Pituitary adenoma with neuronal choristoma (PANCH): composite lesion or lineage infidelity? Ultrastruct Pathol 1994;18:565–574.
67. Scheithauer BW, Kovacs K, Randall RV, Horvath E, Okazaki H, Laws ER Jr. Hypothalamic neuronal hamartoma and adenohypophyseal neuronal: Their association with growth hormone adenoma of the pituitary gland. J Neuropathol Exp Neurol 1983;42:633–648.
68. Asa SL, Scheithauer BW, Bilbao J, et al. A case for hypothalamic acromegaly: a clinicopathologic study of six patients with hypothalamic gangliocytomas producing growth hormone releasing factor. J Clin Endocrinol Metab 1984;59:796–803.
69. Luse S, Kernohan J. Granular cell tumors of the stalk and posterior lobe of the pituitary gland. Cancer 1955;8:616–622.
70. Bubl R, Hugo HH, Hempelmann RG, Barth H, Mehdorn HM. Granular-cell tumor: a rare suprasellar mass. Neuroradiology 2001;43(4):309–312.
71. Ogata S, Shimazaki H, Aida S, Miyazawa T, Tamai S. Giant intracranial granular-cell tumor arising from the abducens. Pathol Int 2001;51(6):481–486.
72. Iglesias A, Arias M, Brasa J, Paramo C, Conde C, Fernandez R. MR imaging findings in granular cell tumor of the neurohypophysis: a difficult preoperative diagnosis. Eur Radiol 2000;10(12):1871–1873.
73. Schaller B, Kirsch E, Tolnay M, Mindermann T. Symptomatic granular cell tumor of the pituitary gland: case report and review of the literature. Neurosurgery 1998;42(1):166–170; discussion 170–171.
74. Nishio S, Takeshita I, Yoshimoto K, Yamaguchi T. Granular cell tumor of the pituitary stalk. Clin Neurol Neurosurg 1998;100(2):144–147.
75. Ji CH, Teng MM, Chang T. Granular cell tumor of the neurohypophysis. Neuroradiology 1995;37(6):451–452.
76. Lafitte C, Aesch B, Henry-Lebras F, Fetissof F, Jan M. Granular cell tumor of the pituitary stalk. Case report. J Neurosurg 1994;80(6):1103–1107.
77. Boecher-Schwarz HG, Fries G, Bornemann A, Ludwig B, Perneczky A. Suprasellar granular cell tumor. Neurosurgery 1992;31(4):751–754; discussion 754.
78. Chimelli L, Symon L, Scaravilli F. Granular cell tumor of the fifth cranial nerve: further evidence for Schwann cell origin. J Neuropathol Exp Neurol 1984;43:634–642.
79. Becker DH, Wilson C. Symptomatic parasellar granular cell tumors. Neurosurgery 1981;8:173–180.

80. Losa M, Saeger W, Mortini P, Pandolfi C, Terreni MR, Taccagni G, Giovanelli M. Acromegaly associated with a granular cell tumor of the neurohypophysis: a clinical and histological study. Case report. J Neurosurg 2000;93(1):121–126.
81. Perone TP, Robinson B, Holmes SM. Intrasellar schwannoma: case report. Neurosurgery 1984;14(1):71–73.
82. Whee SM, Lee JI, Kim JH. Intrasellar schwannoma mimicking pituitary adenoma: a case report. J Korean Med Sci 2002;17(1):147–150.
83. Wilberger JE, Jr. Primary intrasellar schwannoma: case report. Surg Neurol 1989;32(2):156–158.
84. Civit T, Pinelli C, Klein M, Auque J, Baylac F, Hepner H. Intrasellar schwannoma. Acta Neurochir (Wien) 1997;139(2):160–161.
85. Sekhar L, Ross D, Sen C. Cavernous sinus and sphenocavernous neoplasms: anatomy and surgery. In: Janecka I, ed. *Surgery of Cranial Base Tumors*. New York: Raven Press;1993: 521–604.
86. Bilbao JM, Horvath E, Kovacs K, Singer W, Hudson AR. Intrasellar paraganglioma associated with hypopituitarism. Arch Pathol Lab Med 1978;102(2):95–98.
87. Del Basso De Caro ML, Siciliano A, Cappabianca P, Alfieri A, de Divitiis E. Intrasellar paraganglioma with suprasellar extension: case report. Tumori 1998;84(3):408–411.
88. Flint EW, Claassen D, Pang D, Hirsch WL. Intrasellar and suprasellar paraganglioma: CT and MR findings. AJNR Am J Neuroradiol 1993;14(5):1191–1193.
89. Mokry M, Kleinert R, Clarici G, Obermayer-Pietsch B. Primary paraganglioma simulating pituitary macroadenoma: a case report and review of the literature. Neuroradiology 1998;40(4):233–237.
90. Sambaziotis D, Kontogeorgos G, Kovacs K, Horvath E, Levedis A. Intrasellar paraganglioma presenting as nonfunctioning pituitary adenoma. Arch Pathol Lab Med 1999;123(5):429–432.
91. Scheithauer BW, Parameswaran A, Burdick B. Intrasellar paraganglioma: report of a case in a sibship of von Hippel-Lindau disease. Neurosurgery 1996;38(2):395–399.
92. Steel TR, Dailey AT, Born D, Berger MS, Mayberg MR. Paragangliomas of the sellar region: report of two cases. Neurosurgery 1993;32(5):844–847.
93. Thapar K, Laws ER. Vascular tumors: haemangioblastomas, haemangiopericytomas and cavernous haemangiomas. In: Wass J, ed. *Clinical Endocrine Oncology*. Oxford: Blackwell Science; 1996.
94. Dan NG, Smith DE. Pituitary hemangioblastoma in a patient with von Hippel-Lindau disease. Case report. J Neurosurg 1975;42(2):232–235.
95. Goto T, Nishi T, Kunitoku N, et al. Suprasellar hemangioblastoma in a patient with von Hippel-Lindau disease confirmed by germline mutation study: case report and review of the literature. Surg Neurol 2001;56(1):22–26.
96. Grisoli F, Gambarelli D, Raybaud C, Guibout M, Leclercq T. Suprasellar hemangioblastoma. Surg Neurol 1984;22(3):257–262.
97. Esposito S, Nardi P. Lipoma of the infundibulum: case report. J Neurosurg 1987;67:304–306.
98. Discepoli S. The lipoma of the tuber cinereum. Tumori 1980;66:123–130.
99. Lopes MB, Lanzino G, Cloft HJ, Winston DC, Vance ML, Laws ER, Jr. Primary fibrosarcoma of the sella unrelated to previous radiation therapy. Mod Pathol 1998;11(6):579–584.
100. Asa S, Kovacs K, Horvath E, Ezrin C, Weiss M. Sellar glomangioma. Ultrastruct Pathol 1984;7:49–54.
101. Mohr G, Hardy J, Gauvin P. Chiasmal apoplexy due to ruptured cavernous hemangioma of the optic chaism. Surg Neurol 1985;24:636–640.
102. Sansone M, Liwnicz B, Mandybur T. Giant pituitary cavernous hemangioma. J Neurosurg 1980;53:124–126.
103. Buonaguidi R, Canapicci R, Mimassi N, Ferdeghini M. Intrasellar cavernous hemangioma. Neurosurgery 1984;14:732–734.

104. Kaufmann TJ, Lopes MB, Laws ER, Jr., Lipper MH. Primary sellar lymphoma: radiologic and pathologic findings in two patients. AJNR Am J Neuroradiol 2002;23(3):364–367.
105. Scholtz C, Siu K. Melanoma of the pituitary. J Neurosurg 1976;45:101–103.
106. Copeland D, Sink J, Seigler H. Primary intracranial melanoma presenting as a suprasellar tumor. Neurosurgery 1980;6:542–545.
107. Nagatoni M, Mori M, Takomoto N, et a;. Primary myxoma in the pituitary fossa:case report. Neurosurgery 1987;20:329–331.
108. Amine A, Sugar O. Suprasellar osteogenic sarcoma following radiation for pituitary adenomas. Case report. J Neurosurg 1976;44:88–91.
109. Olmos P, Falko J, Rea G, Boesel C, Chakeres D, McGhee D. Fibrosing pseudotumor of the sellar and parasellar area producing hypopituitarism and multiple cranial nerve palsies. Neurosurgery 1993;32:1015–1021.
110. Derome P, Visot A. Bony lesions of the anterior and middle cranial fossae. In: Schramm VL, ed. *Tumors of the Cranial Base: Diagnosis and Treatment*. Mout Kisco, NY: Futura;1987:304–317.
111. Weisman JS, Hepler RS, Vinters HV. Reversible visual loss caused by fibrous dysplasia. Am J Ophthalmol 1990;110(3):244–249.
112. Watkins L, Uttley D, Archer D, Wilkins P, Plowman N. Giant cell tumors of the sphenoid bone. Neurosurgery 1992;30:576–581.
113. Wolfe J, Scheithauer B, Dahil D. Giant cell tumors of the sphenoid bone. Review of 10 cases. J Neurosurg 1983;59:322–327.
114. Stapleton SR, Wilkins PR, Archer DJ, Uttley D. Chondrosarcoma of the skull base: a series of eight cases. Neurosurgery 1993;32(3):348–355; discussion 355–356.
115. Cummings BJ, Blend R, Keane T, et al. Primary radiation therapy for juvenile nasopharyngeal angiofibroma. Laryngoscope 1984;94(12 Pt 1):1599–1605.
116. Harrison DF. The natural history, pathogenesis, and treatment of juvenile angiofibroma. Personal experience with 44 patients. Arch Otolaryngol Head Neck Surg 1987;113(9):936–942.
117. Dulguerov P, Allal AS, Calcaterra TC. Esthesioneuroblastoma: a meta-analysis and review. Lancet Oncol 2001;2(11):683–690.
118. Simon JH, Zhen W, McCulloch TM, et al. Esthesioneuroblastoma: the University of Iowa experience 1978–1998. Laryngoscope 2001;111(3):488–493.
119. Chao KS, Kaplan C, Simpson JR, et al. Esthesioneuroblastoma: the impact of treatment modality. Head Neck 2001;23(9):749–757.
120. Polin RS, Sheehan JP, Chenelle AG, et al. The role of preoperative adjuvant treatment in the management of esthesioneuroblastoma: the University of Virginia experience. Neurosurgery 1998;42(5):1029–1037.
121. Erkal HS, Serin M, Cakmak A. Nasopharyngeal carcinomas: analysis of patient, tumor and treatment characteristics determining outcome. Radiother Oncol 2001;61(3):247–256.
122. Kovacs K, Horvath E. *Tumors of the Pituitary Gland.* Washington, DC: Armed Forces Institute of Pathology;1986.
123. Baskin DS, Wilson CB. Transsphenoidal treatment of non-neoplastic intrasellar cysts. A report of 38 cases. J Neurosurg 1984;60(1):8–13.
124. Barrow DL, Spector RH, Takei Y, Tindall GT. Symptomatic Rathke's cleft cysts located entirely in the suprasellar region: review of diagnosis, management, and pathogenesis. Neurosurgery 1985;16(6):766–772.
125. Itoh J, Usui K. An entirely suprasellar symptomatic Rathke's cleft cyst: case report. Neurosurgery 1992;30:581–585.
126. Wenger M, Simko M, Markwalder R, Taub E. An entirely suprasellar Rathke's cleft cyst: case report and review of the literature. J Clin Neurosci 2001;8(6):564–567.
127. Mukherjee JJ, Islam N, Kaltsas G, et al. Clinical, radiological and pathological features of patients with Rathke's cleft cysts: tumors that may recur. J Clin Endocrinol Metab 1997;82(7):2357–2362.

128. el-Mahdy W, Powell M. Transsphenoidal management of 28 symptomatic Rathke's cleft cysts, with special reference to visual and hormonal recovery. Neurosurgery 1998;42(1):7–16; discussion 16–7.
129. Voelker JL, Campbell RL, Muller J. Clinical, radiographic, and pathological features of symptomatic Rathke's cleft cysts. J Neurosurg 1991;74(4):535–544.
130. Midha R, Jay V, Smyth HS. Transsphenoidal management of Rathke's cleft cysts. A clinicopathological review of 10 cases. Surg Neurol 1991;35(6):446–454.
131. Boggan J, Davis R, Zorman G, Wilson C. Intrasellar epidermoid cyst: case report. J Neurosurg 1983;58:411–415.
132. Lewis A, Cooper P, Kasel E, Schwartz M. Squamous cell carcinoma arising in a suprasellar epidermoid cyst: case report. J Neurosurg 1983;59:538–541.
133. Klonoff D, Kahn D, Rosenzweig W, Wilson C. Hyperprolactinemia in a patient with a pituitary and ovarian dermoid tumor: case report. Neurosurgery 1990;26:335–339.
134. Cohen JE, Abdallah JA, Garrote M. Massive rupture of suprasellar dermoid cyst into ventricles. Case illustration. J Neurosurg 1997;87(6):963.
135. Meyer F, Carpenter S, Laws EJ. Intrasellar arachnoid cysts. Surg Neurol 1987;28:105–110.
136. Jones R, Warnock T, Nayanar V, Gupta J. Suprasellar arachnoid cysts: management by cyst wall resection. Neurosurgery 1989;25:554–561.
137. Pierre-Kahn A, Capelle L, Brauner R, et al. Presentation and management of suprasellar arachnoid cysts. Review of 20 cases. J Neurosurg 1990;73(3):355–359.
138. Mohn A, Fahlbusch R, Dorr HG. Panhypopituitarism associated with diabetes insipidus in a girl with a suprasellar arachnoid cyst. Horm Res 1999;52(1):35–38.
139. Miyajima M, Arai H, Okuda O, Hishii M, Nakanishi H, Sato K. Possible origin of suprasellar arachnoid cysts: neuroimaging and neurosurgical observations in nine cases. J Neurosurg 2000;93(1):62–67.
140. Thompson TP, Lunsford LD, Kondziolka D. Successful management of sellar and suprasellar arachnoid cysts with stereotactic intracavitary irradiation: an expanded report of four cases. Neurosurgery 2000;46(6):1518–1522; discussion 1522–1523.
141. Weil RJ. Rapidly progressive visual loss caused by a sellar arachnoid cyst: reversal with transsphenoidal microsurgery. South Med J 2001;94(11):1118–1121.
142. Bergland RM, Ray BS, Torack RM. Anatomical variations in the pituitary gland and adjacent structures in 225 human autopsy cases. J Neurosurg 1968;28(2):93–99.
143. Weisberg LA, Housepian EM, Saur DP. Empty sella syndrome as complication of benign intracranial hypertension. J Neurosurg 1975;43(2):177–180.
144. Neelon FA, Goree JA, Lebovitz HE. The primary empty sella: clinical and radiographic characteristics and endocrine function. Medicine 1973;52(1):73–92.
145. Gharib H, Frey HM, Laws ER, Jr., Randall RV, Scheithauer BW. Coexistent primary empty sella syndrome and hyperprolactinemia. Report of 11 cases. Arch Intern Med 1983;143(7):1383–1386.
146. Weisberg LA, Zimmerman EA, Frantz AG. Diagnosis and evaluation of patients with an enlarged sella turcica. Am J Med 1976;61(5):590–596.
147. Applebaum EL, Desai NM. Primary empty sella syndrome with CSF rhinorrhea. JAMA 1980;244(14):1606–1608.
148. Garcia-Uria J, Ley L, Parajon A, Bravo G. Spontaneous cerebrospinal fluid fistulae associated with empty sellae: surgical treatment and long-term results. Neurosurgery 1999;45(4):766–773; discussion 773–774.
149. Welch K, Stears JC. Chiasmapexy for the correction of traction on the optic nerves and chiasm associated with their descent into an empty sella turcica. Case report. J Neurosurg 1971;35(6):760–764.
150. Branch CL, Laws ER Jr. Metastatic tumors of the sella turcica masquerading as primary pituitary tumors. J Clin Endocrinol Metab 1987;65:469–474.

151. Morita A, Meyer FB, Laws ER, Jr. Symptomatic pituitary metastases. J Neurosurg 1998;89(1):69–73.
152. Dhanani A-N, Bilbao J, Kovacs K. Multiple myeloma presenting as a sellar plasmacytoma and mimicking a pituitary tumor:report of a case and review of the literature. Endocr Pathol 1990;1:245–248.
153. Berger SA, Edberg SC, David G. Infectious disease of the sella turcica. Rev Infect Dis 1986;8:747–755.
154. Domingue JN, Wilson CB. Pituitary abscesses. Report of seven cases and review of the literature. J Neurosurg 1977;46(5):601–608.
155. Jain KC, Varma A, Mahapatra AK. Pituitary abscess: a series of six cases. Br J Neurosurg 1997;11(2):139–143.
156. Kroppenstedt SN, Liebig T, Mueller W, Graf KJ, Lanksch WR, Unterberg AW. Secondary abscess formation in pituitary adenoma after tooth extraction. Case report. J Neurosurg 2001;94(2):335–338.
157. Martines F, Scarano P, Chiappetta F, Gigli R. Pituitary abscess. A case report and review of the literature. J Neurosurg Sci 1996;40(2):135–138.
158. Scanarini M, Cervellini P, Rigobello L, Mingrino S. Pituitary abscesses: report of two cases and review of the literature. Acta Neurochir (Wien) 1980;51(3–4):209–217.
159. Somali MH, Anastasiou AL, Goulis DG, Polyzoides C, Avramides A. Pituitary abscess presenting with cranial nerve paresis. Case report and review of literature. J Endocrinol Invest 2001;24(1):45–50.
160. Vates GE, Berger MS, Wilson CB. Diagnosis and management of pituitary abscess: a review of twenty-four cases. J Neurosurg 2001;95(2):233–241.
161. Wolansky LJ, Gallagher JD, Heary RF, et al. MRI of pituitary abscess: two cases and review of the literature. Neuroradiology 1997;39(7):499–503.
162. Paramo C, de L, Nodar A, Miramontes S, Quintela JL, Garcia-Mayor RV. Intrasellar tuberculoma—a difficult diagnosis. Infection 2002;30:35–37.
163. Patankar T, Patkar D, Bunting T, Castillo M, Mukherji SK. Imaging in pituitary tuberculosis. Clin Imag 2000;24(2):89–92.
164. Sharma MC, Arora R, Mahapatra AK, Sarat-Chandra P, Gaikwad SB, Sarkar C. Intrasellar tuberculoma—an enigmatic pituitary infection: a series of 18 cases. Clin Neurol Neurosurg 2000;102(2):72–77.
165. Ciftci E, Erden I, Akyar S. Brucellosis of the pituitary region: MRI. Neuroradiology 1998;40(6):383–384.
166. Guven MB, Cirak B, Kutluhan A, Ugras S. Pituitary abscess secondary to neurobrucellosis. Case illustration. J Neurosurg 1999;90(6):1142.
167. Ramos-Gabatin A, Jordan RM. Primary pituitary aspergillosis responding to transsphenoidal surgery and combined therapy with amphotericin-B and 5-fluorocytosine: case report. J Neurosurg 1981;54(6):839–841.
168. Endo T, Numagami Y, Jokura H, Ikeda H, Shirane R, Yoshimoto T. Aspergillus parasellar abscess mimicking radiation-induced neuropathy. Case report. Surg Neurol 2001;56(3):195–200.
169. Heary RF, Maniker AH, Wolansky LJ. Candidal pituitary abscess: case report. Neurosurgery 1995;36(5):1009–1012; discussion 1012–1013.
170. Del Brutto O, Guevara J, Sotelo J. Intrasellar cysticercosis. J Neurosurg 1988;69:58–60.
171. Osgen T, Bertan V, Kansu T, Akalin S. Intrasellar hydatid cyst. Case report. J Neurosurg 1984;60:647–648.
172. Sano T, Kovacs K, Scheithauer BW, Rosenblum MK, Petito CK, Greco CM. Pituitary pathology in acquired immunodeficiency syndrome. Arch Pathol Lab Med 1989;113:1066–1070.
173. Delfini R, Missori P, Iannetti G, Ciappetta P, Cantore G. Mucoceles of the paranasal sinuses with intracranial and intraorbital extension: report of 28 cases. Neurosurgery 1993;32:901–906.

174. Abla A, Maroon J, Wilberger JJ, Kennerdell J, Deeb J. Intrasellar mucocele simulating pituitary adenoma: case report. Neurosurgery 1986;197–199.
175. Close N, O'Conner W. Sphenoethmoidal mucoceles with intracranial extension. Otolaryngol Head Neck Surg 1983;91:350–357.
176. Gore RM, Weinberg PE, Kim KS, Ramsey RG. Sphenoid sinus mucoceles presenting as intracranial masses on computed tomography. Surg Neurol 1980;13(5):375–379.
177. Asa SL, Bilbao JM, Kovacs K, Josse RG, Kreines K. Lymphocytic hypophysitis of pregnancy resulting in hypopituitarism: a distinct clinicopathologic entity. Ann Intern Med 1981;95(2):166–171.
178. Thorner MO, Vance ML, Horvath E, Kovacs K. The anterior pituitary. In: Foster DW, ed. *Williams Textbook of Endocrinology.* Philadelphia: WB Saunders;1992:221–310.
179. Cosman F, Post K, Holub DA, Wardkaw SL. Lymphocytic hypophysitis. Report of 3 new cases and review of the literature. Medicine 1989;68:24–56.
180. Feigenbaum S, Martin M, Wilson C, Jaffe R. Lymphocytic adenohypophysitis: a pituitary mass lesions occurring in pregnancy. Proposal for medical treatment. Am J Obstet Gynecol 1991;164:1549–1555.
181. Lee JH, Laws ER, Jr., Guthrie BL, Dina TS, Nochomovitz LE. Lymphocytic hypophysitis: occurrence in two men. Neurosurgery 1994;34(1):159–162; discussion 162–163.
182. Tubridy N, Saunders D, Thom M, et al. Infundibulohypophysitis in a man presenting with diabetes insipidus and cavernous sinus involvement. J Neurol Neurosurg Psychiatry 2001;71(6):798–801.
183. Reusch JE, Kleinschmidt-DeMasters BK, Lillehei KO, Rappe D, Gutierrez-Hartmann A. Preoperative diagnosis of lymphocytic hypophysitis (adenohypophysitis) unresponsive to short course dexamethasone: case report. Neurosurgery 1992;30(2):268–272.
184. Lara Capellan JI, Cuellar Olmedo L, Martinez Martin J, et al. Intrasellar mass with hypopituitarism as a manifestation of sarcoidosis. Case report. J Neurosurg 1990;73(2):283–286.
185. Stern BJ, Krumholz A, Johns C, Scott P, Nissim J. Sarcoidosis and its neurological manifestations. Arch Neurol 1985;42(9):909–917.
186. Scott IA, Stocks AE, Saines N. Hypothalamic/pituitary sarcoidosis. Aust N Z J Med 1987;17(2):243–245.
187. Grois NG, Favara BE, Mostbeck GH, Prayer D. Central nervous system disease in Langerhans cell histiocytosis. Hematol Oncol Clin North Am 1998;12(2):287–305.
188. Bakshi R, Fenstermaker RA, Bates VE, Ravichandran TP, Goodloe S, Jr., Kinkel WR. Neurosarcoidosis presenting as a large suprasellar mass. Magnetic resonance imaging findings. Clin Imaging 1998;22(5):323–326.
189. Loh KC, Green A, Dillon WP, Jr., Fitzgerald PA, Weidner N, Tyrrell JB. Diabetes insipidus from sarcoidosis confined to the posterior pituitary. Eur J Endocrinol 1997;137(5):514–519.
190. Guoth MS, Kim J, de Lotbiniere AC, Brines ML. Neurosarcoidosis presenting as hypopituitarism and a cystic pituitary mass. Am J Med Sci 1998;315(3):220–224.
191. Chevrette E, Morissette L, Gould P. Neurosarcoidosis presenting as an intrasellar pseudotumoral mass: case report. Can Assoc Radiol J 1999;50(6):407–412.
192. Christoforidis GA, Spickler EM, Recio MV, Mehta BM. MR of CNS sarcoidosis: correlation of imaging features to clinical symptoms and response to treatment. AJNR Am J Neuroradiol 1999;20(4):655–669.
193. Bullmann C, Faust M, Hoffmann A, et al. Five cases with central diabetes insipidus and hypogonadism as first presentation of neurosarcoidosis. Eur J Endocrinol 2000;142(4):365–372.
194. Konrad D, Gartenmann M, Martin E, Schoenle EJ. Central diabetes insipidus as the first manifestation of neurosarcoidosis in a 10-year-old girl. Horm Res 2000;54(2):98–100.
195. Weir B. Pituitary tumors and aneurysms: case report and review of the literature. Neurosurgery 1992;30(4):585–591.
196. Jennings MT, Gelman R, Hochberg F. Intracranial germ cell tumors: Natural history and pathogenesis. J. Neurosurg 1985;63:155–167.

16 A Patient's Perspective on Pituitary Tumors

Patsy Perrin

Contents

INTRODUCTION

My goal in writing has been to describe—primarily for medical readers—what it's like to be on the receiving end of diagnosis and treatment for pituitary disorders. I have described our responses to diagnosis and treatment, coping strategies and social and family concerns as a way to identify specific actions and steps that medical professionals can take to ease the patient's journey through what may appear to some of us as a strange world. What patients actually do experience is conveyed here by direct quotations gathered from many pitutiary patients, including myself. While based on experience in the UK, many of the points raised are adaptable to treatment worldwide. I want to note also that where I use the term "patient" I often mean "patients and their supporters."

From: *Management of Pituitary Tumors: The Clinician's Practical Guide, Second Edition*
Edited by: M. P. Powell, S. L. Lightman, and E. R. Laws, Jr.

About the Author

Diagnosed with acromegaly in my late 40s, I have since had transsphenoidal surgery and radiotherapy, and I am now balancing a drug regimen that gives me the optimum feeling of well-being. During the course of treatment it was discovered that I had enlarged parathyroid glands as well, so I am, perhaps, more "complicated" than other pituitary patients. However, I believe I share with others a feeling that a return to what I remember as being "fit and well" is elusive. I am lucky to have been treated in a medical center committed to excellence.

As a trustee of The Pituitary Foundation, a UK-based patient support organization, I have met many pituitary patients during the last four years and conversations with them have contributed to this chapter.

ACCESS TO INFORMATION

"I've got what? ....A tumor?... Do you mean cancer?

....At the base of my brain? ...Is it a brain tumor?"

Why Information Is Important for Patients and Their Supporters

In my experience gathering and digesting information is one of the best ways of handling the shock, bewilderment, stress, and the many other emotions that are experienced both at diagnosis and in subsequent years.

As a patient you have a need to understand what is happening to you for your own sake. It can help you handle the procedures and treatment that follow when you have an idea of what to expect, how you may feel afterward, and what the expected outcomes may be. You need to be able to explain the situation to family, friends, employers, and coworkers among others: they may be equally in the dark. In the longer term, all those whose lives are affected by your condition will benefit from understanding it. You have to come to grips, too, with the complexity of the illness and develop ways of explaining the progress of treatment without sounding freakish, or by treating it superficially. This is made harder by the fact that you may appear to others as you always did, possibly better than you did before your operation, and suspicions of malingering can and do arise.

You may have had no idea of why you were sent to see a specialist. You may not have even heard of the pituitary gland and have no idea where it is and what it does. In addition, "tumor" is not a friendly word and it is made even more frightening because the brain or head are also involved. Suddenly being faced with a medical problem you have never heard of before is a very stressful moment.

Can my medical readers imagine how they would feel in a comparable situation?

Sources

How can the patient and their supporters acquire this knowledge?

"Initially I didn't get any information. Neither my GP nor my endocrine consultant offered me information, nor was I given the names of organizations that would be able to offer information and support. Things changed when I was forced to give up work as a result of ill health and I found myself at home with a pile of my sister's medical textbooks. I read through every section that I could find on anything to do with the endocrine system to try and get an idea of what was going on in my body. It was around this time that I found the address for The Pituitary Foundation. Approximately six months later I set up my computer to access the Internet and now find most of my information from there."

- Medical sources include the doctors and nurses who work in endocrine and other hospital departments, the patient's local doctor (who may have no direct experience of the condition) and other medical professionals who will treat the patient (for radiotherapy, MRI scans, and so forth).
- Written material can be found in many ways. General medical encyclopedias are vague regarding pituitary disease. The local library or bookshop may have medical textbooks, parts of which will be intelligible to the layperson. The book I found, aimed at medical students, has been invaluable, but I didn't understand much of it in the early days.
- The Internet is a first port of call for many. It can be a vast minefield waiting to confuse and alarm. It can also be the source of wonderfully clear patient-oriented information (*see* Table 1).
- Occasionally articles appear in the media, but often they are rather sensationalized—gigantism is a common example of pituitary disease. A recent television program on that topic talked about "this fatal tumor."
- Patient support organizations are an invaluable source of patient-oriented information and are likely to provide leaflets on specific conditions as well as a help line service.

"I came across a leaflet the night before my operation. It was marvellous. I slept with it under my pillow."

- Patient support groups may be invaluable to some people, as will be personal contacts (face-to-face or by telephone). Their down side is that experiences may be out-of-date, frightening, or depressing.
- Government-provided telephone support services may have some information, but in my experience pituitary disease is too specialized for them.

The sources are many. You can influence some of the patient's searching by pointing them in the right directions. Tell them when you use the words "pituitary tumor."

"To me this was a key moment when a leaflet or phone number would have been of invaluable help."

"Initially I got quite detailed information from the Encyclopaedia Britannica, and medical books. In later years, both ACTH [a UK-based Cushing's support group] and The Pituitary Foundation have been helpful; also I have learned a lot from the Internet."

"I did not really start to understand my condition until the day I was admitted for surgery when the doctor spent a long time explaining things to me."

Sorting Out the Good, the Bad, and the Ugly

Table 1 gives some examples of the results I found with my favorite search engine. There are thousands of sites to choose from, so which would a newly diagnosed patient, desperate for information, read? How would you react when you saw references to cancer, even though your doctor said your tumor was benign? The text of these sites may confirm that your tumor is benign, but the thought can be distressing. Some sites are too technical for the layman, and in my view—reinforced by phone calls from distressed newly diagnosed patients—is that some are alarmist.

Patient's Comments

"So, somewhat amazed [at the diagnosis] I went home and looked up acromegaly in my Family Health *book with limited success. I also searched the Internet. This had too many medically oriented articles to choose from, and the couple I picked at random were not enlightening. The main thing was that they reinforced that wonderful word "benign." What did I tell my family and colleagues? I can't remember now, but it must have been a good mixture of half-understood confused facts."*

"With a lot more knowledge under my belt my opinion is that some Internet articles present a very pessimistic view of pituitary disease and its treatment, especially to a "new' patient."

"The impact of this leaflet on my morale cannot be overestimated. It explained in clear language about pituitary tumors and acromegaly. It was a contact with other people who had this mysterious condition and was a great help not only to me but also to family and friends who were struggling to understand what was happening to me."

Table 1
World Wide Web Search Results
for Pituitary Disease-Related Sites[a]

Search for	*ALL/ UK*	*Total found*
Pituitary	All	321,000
	UK	17,800
Cushing's	All	42,700
	UK	2,950
Acromegaly	All	21,300
	UK	1,590
Sandostatin	All	5,980
	UK	275
Prolactinoma	All	4,760
	UK	366
Diabetes Insipidus	All	29,500
	UK	1,400

[a]As of January 2003.

How Caregivers Can Help

Guide your patient to the same sources of information you would like to be given under the same circumstances. Imagine hearing that you have a pituitary tumor. What would you want to know? Remember that although you may have made the diagnosis and given information hundreds of times, it's the first time the patient has heard it.

Some specific actions the doctor and support staff can take:

- Remember that it's really difficult to follow what's being said when your brain is whirling, and you are possibly in a state of shock. Give written information where possible.
- Hand out leaflets along with the diagnosis.
- Point patients in the direction of support organizations, reliable websites, etc.

- Encourage patient questions, and perhaps have a Questions-and-Answers sheet to give.
- Be aware of the possible lay interpretation of the words used:
  - "tumor' is associated with malignancies
  - "base of brain" is anatomically correct but ...

"I still had little idea of the condition and its implications. I'd been told that the pituitary was situated at the base of my brain. I probably thought I had some form of brain tumor. My colleagues and some friends certainly did and were wonderfully supportive. I now know that the terminology is anatomically correct, but it was confusing at this crucial time."

- Explain what you are doing during the diagnosis.

"I went to see the specialist armed with information about my diabetes so I was completely astonished when he started to ask me whether I'd noticed any increase in the size of my hands and feet. What was the size of my hands to do with diabetes? He then waved his hands around asking if I could see his fingers moving. I really wondered whether I was in the right consulting room. Seeing my confusion, he explained that he suspected a condition called acromegaly, associated with an excess of human growth hormone caused by a benign tumor on the pituitary gland, and would arrange some tests to confirm this."

DEALING WITH THE VARIOUS MEDICAL SPECIALISTS

General

Patients meet many different specialists during the course of treatment, some of whom they'll be in contact with for a long time. Some are associated with dramatic events such as surgery and radiotherapy. Patients need to understand why they are seeing different people, and why it is relevant to their treatment! All these relationships are important, especially the long term ones.

Initially, the patient may not know where the pituitary gland is, what it does, how the operation is done, or about the specialist's particular area of involvement. They may not know what questions to ask.

They may come to an endocrinologist after years of nondiagnosis, perhaps even treatment for other things.

"My first diagnosis came after many years of treatment by my GP [general practitioner] for depression, tiredness, loss of libido, and a general loss of interest in everything, resulting in sleeping tablets, antidepressants etc.—all to no avail."

Patient/Doctor Relationships

Most of the following comments are not unique to pituitary disease, but a major difference in this situation is that, initially, most patients and their supporters will have little or no knowledge of the condition and its implications.

The patient's attitude toward the caregiver may reflect their anxiety, how they are feeling, their confusion, distress, even anger, or their reaction to treatment. Help them by establishing and building the relationship. Encourage them to know and understand why they are seeing you and what the treatment is likely to be.

Your attitude to the patient is crucial. We have a right to be respected: this means being told about the condition in understandable terms and to have a second opinion if needed. Many patients are experts in their own nonmedical, fields and will usually respond positively when a physician or other caregiver takes the trouble to treat them as intelligent beings with a vested interest in what is going on.

Sometimes, doctors forget this.

Patient's View of the Different Specialists

Here are some thumbnail sketches.

Endocrinologist/Consultant Physician

- Is a major influence on how well the patient copes with the condition.
- Makes or confirms the initial diagnosis, possibly the first physician from whom the patient first hears about the pituitary gland.
- Arranges initial treatment.
- Provides ongoing treatment; monitors and modifies as appropriate.

Neurosurgeon

- Operates inside the patient's head close to the brain and optic nerves.
- Is a critical factor in subsequent recovery.

Neuroradiologist

- Interprets the MRI scans but probably won't meet the patient.

Radiotherapists

- Meets the patient for consultations and preparation, then again during treatment.
- Should be aware that radiotherapy is another very scary time for the patient.

"The prospect of radiotherapy was daunting and I was especially concerned about my eyesight."

- The technician who makes the mask should be prepared for a patient who may find it an unpleasant and frightening experience.

- A pituitary patient will be a fairly rare visitor to their clinic.

  "Having met the radiographer and learnt more about what was in store, I was quickly in the system. Having the facemask made is a strange experience, but I tried to tell myself to imagine I was having a facemask in an expensive beauty salon and tried to enjoy it."

  "The technician was brilliant, describing what he was doing all the time, constantly telling me what part of the room he was in, which was so reassuring when you can't see anything and are lying flat on a bench with cotton wool in your mouth and nose and pink gunge over your face. He said some people find fitting the mask the worst part of their radiotherapy."

Endocrine Specialist Nurses

- Build relationships with patients by spending time with them for tests and treatment.
- Viewed by patients as an important source of information— and of reassurance.
- May be the recipients of key information from patients about their condition, things that the doctors may not be told.

Other Specialists

- Are met when the patient has treatments such as ultrasound, colonoscopy, bone density scans, gallbladder scans—depending on their condition.
- They need to be able to explain to the patient why they are having the treatment; the patient may not know.

The General Practitioner in the UK or Family Doctor /Primary Care Physician in North America

- May have a poor relationship with the patient as a result of experiences leading up to a diagnosis, often a lengthy process, sometimes traumatic.
- May not have as up-to-date information about treatment as the patient does.
- May not be regularly updated with details of treatment and test results. (This needs to be managed by the hospital.)
- May not see the patient often.
- May have to authorize the use of expensive drugs and meet the cost from his budget for treatment he knows little about.

How Caregivers Can Help

- Put yourself in the patient's shoes. What would you be concerned about and want to know? What would you be feeling? Tell patients the answers to these perhaps unspoken questions.
- Before sending a patient to another specialist, tell them why they are going.

- When seeing new patients, check that they know why you are examining/ treating them. Explain what will happen and when results will be available. They may have been told these things already, but memories are unreliable when anxiety levels are high, and with several different people to see patients can easily become confused.
- By encouraging patients to learn as much as possible about their condition, to ask questions, and to talk about what concerns them.
- By encouraging patients to ask for recommended sources of information. Give it in any case.
- By building a partnership with your patients.

QUESTIONS FOR ENDOCRINOLOGISTS, SURGEONS, AND RADIOTHERAPISTS

"Do you encourage patients to come with a list of questions, or does your heart sink when they produce a list?"

Why Encourage Questions? Why Your Answers Are Important

It is important to the patient to know what is happening to them and to get accurate, considered answers to their questions. They have a right to this and it will facilitate the development of a good patient/doctor relationship.

"At the time it is very difficult to ask questions for a number of reasons, which can include things like shock and denial. However I think that the main problem is that in order to ask informed questions you need to have a certain knowledge of the situation or condition that you are dealing with."

"To a certain extent I also expected all the information that I would need to know to come from the specialist. This was a person with knowledge of the disease and having dealt with the situation time and time again should provide the information a typical patient needed to know. It wasn't until I started finding out things for myself that the specialist hadn't told me about that I started to research things more and ask questions."

"I found that it wasn't until I started learning more about the condition and its consequences that I came across questions that I wanted answers to. For example, until I was aware of the pituitary gland and its influence on the other glands in the body, I didn't think of asking questions about things like fertility."

What Sort of Questions Need Answers?

Here are some examples of questions I asked at the time, some that I wished I'd known to ask earlier, and some that other patients have contributed.

For the Endocrinologist

- Why are you doing these tests? What do the results mean?
- What's likely to happen over the next few months, years, and beyond (follow-ups, medication, endocrine changes as a result of treatment)?
- How will this problem affect my life expectancy? What counts as a cure?

"The trickiest part is understanding why it takes so long for the treatment to become fully effective."

- Why do these tumors grow? What is meant by "benign"? Will my children inherit the condition?
- How soon are post-op patients likely to return to work?
- Why is radiotherapy recommended? What are my options? What benefits will it bring? How experienced are the staff with these procedures?
- About the surgeon: How experienced is he in this procedure?
- What happens to bits they can't remove? Will they regrow?
- What about new drugs and trials?
- How do I know when I need to increase my hydrocortisone dosage? How often can I safely do this? What happens if I take too much? Will it affect my bones?
- How will my treatment be shared between you and my GP?
- How will my GP be informed of what is happening?
- What if my GP or local health authority will not fund the drugs?
- What are some other sources of reliable information?

For the Surgeon

- How is the operation done? How often do you perform this operation?

"I went to see the recommended surgeon who, I was reassured to hear, did lots of these operations. He explained how he would access the pituitary to remove the tumor. I had been wondering and it was the most frequent question asked of me."

- How long will I be in the hospital?
- Show me and explain the MRI scans.
- What should I expect immediately post-op and after a few weeks?
- Does the nursing staff treat pituitary patients very often?

For Radiotherapists

- What happens before, during, and after the treatment?
- What if I move during the treatment (e.g., sneeze because of hay fever)?
- What are the risks? How are treatment and potential side effects monitored?
- What experience does this medical center have in treating pituitary disease?
- What will I feel? Can I wash my hair afterwards? Will my hair fall out? Will I have sore patches?
- Do you have any information I can read?

For Endocrine Specialist Nurses

- About the tests being performed: What will happen? What are they for? When will I know the results?
- What should I do in emergencies? This is especially important when the patient is on steroids (e.g., when and how to use an emergency injection).
- I wasn't able to follow the doctor's explanation completely. Can you explain what the doctor meant by.....? I forgot to ask the doctor about ..... Do you know?
- About anything else that concerns you.

How Caregivers Can Help

- Put the patient's hat on and anticipate what questions you would want answered.
- Remember that it is difficult to ask questions when you do not know what to ask, especially in the early days of diagnosis and treatment. Please give patients the type of information detailed in the previous sections, even if the questions are not voiced.

"I found asking questions very difficult, not knowing what was important and what was irrelevant. Fortunately the staff and consultants at [the hospital] have always been prepared to listen and have never trivialized any of the questions that I have asked."

- Welcome the presence of a relative or friend at the consultation; two brains can remember more of what has been said.
- Ask any companion whether they have any questions or comments.
- Listen to patient's descriptions of how they have been (beyond "I'm fine"!).
- Lots of questions will occur to the patient after they leave the clinic. Make sure they know how to find answers to these questions, too.
- Patients will differ in their needs and desires to know about their condition. Encourage them to ask.
- Don't be surprised if they ask the same question of several people until the answers make sense to them.
- Be sensitive to the patient's response to your answer and actively seek to clarify it, if that seems appropriate.
- Ask open-ended questions to encourage dialogue.

EXPERIENCING VARIOUS TESTS AND TREATMENTS

For the Rest of Their Lives: Adjusting to Long Term Care

"My life seems to be one set of tests after another."

Pituitary disease is a chronic condition, and most patients will be involved with some form of tests and treatment for the remainder of their lives. Each medical treatment can take up a fair amount of time, involve time off from work, and/or require long-distance travel.

"At the time I had no idea that this would affect me for the rest of my life."

It is possible that some patients may reject treatment at some stage (compare with adolescent diabetes mellitus patients), or they may not be aware of its continuing necessity, so it is important that caregivers secure the patient's cooperation with and understanding of the ongoing nature of the tests and treatment as early in the process as possible.

A Patient's View of Some of the Tests and Treatment

Initial Diagnostic Tests

- The patient may have no idea what is being investigated or may think the test is for a different condition. As a consequence, the experience may be rather a puzzle. What's being done and why?
- The tests will depend on the condition being investigated.

"I remember having to drink a pretty disgusting sweet drink; somehow it seemed a desperate act for a diabetic!"

- MRI scans can be a traumatic experience for some.

"Whilst I didn't find the Xray, bone density scan, and blood tests a problem, the MRI scan was altogether something different and left me giddy, head pounding, and totally confused. Being clamped to the unit and given an alarm button to press in case I wanted to get out quick was daunting and claustrophobic enough, but I was not prepared for the noise of the equipment. I have always had very sensitive hearing, but the noise of the MRI scanner in operation nearly blew my mind. A subsequent MRI scan was a vast improvement. No change to equipment, but much more detail supplied by the nurse at every point of the procedure. The offer of ear plugs was much appreciated, cutting down the noise to a far more comfortable level."

Initial Treatment

- With good preparation the surgery is usually OK (even for the person who has had three!), but the thought of someone inside your head is an odd one.

"I was well prepared for the operation, so my apprehension level was nothing above normal. The op went well."

"What they don't tell you about is the removal of the nose plugs. "Painful" seems an inadequate description."

- Radiotherapy can be more traumatic. It is a daunting prospect knowing the beams will be so near your brain, eyes, and ears. As radiotherapy is closely associated with cancer treatment, other people may assume you have cancer, even though you deny it. The extended treatment time becomes very tiring, especially with a long journey, and can cause problems at work.

"Although not painful, only making me feel rather tired, it was the treatment I have found most difficult. I just didn't like the thought of the beams going into my head, but that's just me. Other people I have spoken to have not felt that way."

Ongoing Tests

- Some tests (e.g., growth-hormone [GH] day curves) involve considerable time at the hospital and can be very tiring, especially if a long journey is involved.
- When blood is to be drawn, finding a good vein when it is elusive is a horrible experience, both for the patient and the person trying to get samples. Being cold and tired from early fasting and a long journey does not help matters. Heated sheepskin blankets are wonderful. Needless to say, people who have needle phobias call for special care.
- You need to be feeling well for the concentration required by visual fields tests. I had one when my blood sugar levels were low and the results were appalling.
- Some tests are unpleasant (e.g., water deprivation tests and insulin tolerance tests).

"The worst test is an ITT. I dread it so much that I try very hard to talk myself out of it with the specialist nurses. (To me it feels like how it might be when one is dying.) I wish I could evade the tests and carry on with my life as normal."

"I was initially confused about the purpose of the ITT. The mention of the word insulin immediately made me think of diabetes mellitus and then there was confusion about whether it was being carried out to test for cortisol or GH. The first insulin tolerance test was pretty much harmless. After finishing it I went on to complete half a day plus of work. The second was very different and as a result of the food and several bottles of lucozade not raising my blood sugar levels I needed iv glucose, after which I went into shock. The test started at 9 AM, I left hospital after 12 PM (they had wanted to keep me in longer,) and I was still feeling ill at 5 PM."

Ongoing Treatment

- Injections are employed for many conditions, some self-administered, some needing medical expertise.

"The only problem I've had [with daily injections] was during a period when the injections got so painful that I was unable to continue for several days."

- Several injections are very expensive and require a special technique. If the administrator is not practiced or confident their nervousness may affect the patient.
- Some of the oil-based injections can be very uncomfortable.
- Implants and patches, such as those used for testosterone replacement, involve a medical procedure—more journeys and time off work. The wound can be uncomfortable and the area badly bruised.
- Taking tablet medication seems inevitable, and some foresight and organization are needed to make sure you have enough in stock. Remembering to take them can be a problem, especially when you have a change of routine.
- Changes in routine may upset other things too.

"I commenced treatment (metered nasal spray [Desmopressin]) on leaving hospital after the operation, and it took many months to get used to the treatment. I found that the dose I was initially advised to take was too much so I reduced it down and down again until I was taking none, but this meant a return to waking during the night. I then increased the dose gradually and am now taking the dose that was prescribed at the beginning and this has been stable for a number of years. However, my reaction to this dose can be erratic and some days it appears to wear out by 12 PM but on other days can last until the evening. When I went to Greece during the summer I also found that I required 50–100% extra spray than when I was at home."

- Steroid treatment requires good management by both the patient and clinic. The clinic is responsible for ensuring that the patient understands when to take the medication and by how much and under what circumstances to increase dosages. The patient has to understand how the medication works, when they need to take it, when they will need to take more, and what to do in an emergency.

" I was initially put on too high a dose hydrocortisone and although I had a lot of energy I was also experiencing psychological disturbances. Although I didn't associate them with the hydrocortisone at the time they became less frequent when the dose was reduced and now I am on an appropriate maintenance dose for my body they have gone altogether. Unfortunately due to these experiences I am very reluctant to increase the dosage for any length of time during periods of stress or illness and tend to try and battle on regardless."

How Caregivers Can Help

- Encourage questions.
- Explain what tests and treatment are for, what's involved, how the patient might feel afterward, and when results will be available.
- Ensure that a patient taking steroids has a thorough understanding of the regimen, especially how to handle illness and emergencies. Encourage the

patient to wear a Medic-Alert bracelet (or similar identification). A take-home information sheet would be useful.

- Let patients know the anticipated regimen of tests, so they know and can explain to others (e.g., employers).
- Let patients know the results when available and explain the results during consultations.

SOCIAL PROBLEMS

What Aspects of the Patient's Life May Be Affected by Pituitary Disease?

Driving

- Patients may have experienced frightening changes in their visual fields and even have lost their driving privileges and once recovered will need retesting to regain a license.
- The effects of their drugs may affect their driving, and they should ask the pharmacist for advice.

"My confidence is not as it was and so at times I am reluctant to drive. When the tinnitus and dizziness is particularly bad I do not drive."

Insurance and Mortgages

- Ignorance of the implications of pituitary disease may complicate applications for insurance and mortgages. A specialist broker can help.
- Life insurance rates might be higher. Some insurers confuse diabetes insipidus with diabetes mellitus. "ADH deficiency" may be a better description.
- An annuity might give a better rate!
- Travel insurance is likely to involve an interrogation but shouldn't be a problem. Patients should check the documentation as spelling can be incorrect.

"A lot of the companies had not heard of hypopituitarism which caused a problem. I addressed this by contacting the DVLA [British driving license authority] and getting a letter from them saying that my licence is unaffected by my illness."

Employment

- Effects vary with employer and the individual's response to treatment.
- Prediagnosis behavior (e.g., lack of get up and go) can have, and continue to have, a detrimental effect on relationships at work. In some cases a letter from a specialist for a personnel file may help.

"I had been feeling tired but so did most of my friends. We had demanding jobs involving stress, long hours, and travelling. I'd lost my characteristic

willingness to take on anything thrown at me by my boss—as he had recently pointed out to me."

- Patients will need time off for regular clinic visits, tests, and treatment, depending on their individual condition. They may need help explaining the situation to employers and colleagues.
- The patient may lose a job as a result of continued tiredness or the time required for long treatments like radiotherapy.

Benefits Agency

UK Social Services provide invalidity benefits under certain circumstances.

- The Benefits Agency interview involves convincing a doctor, who may never have come across your condition before, that you are unfit to work.
- In many cases appearances will be deceptive and you will look fine. Pituitary disease is an "invisible illness."
- It is really difficult trying to quantify the impact of chronic fatigue on one's ability to work. (Who is not tired these days?)
- This is a prime example of where knowledgeable patients can really help themselves.

Other

- Travelling with injections can cause problems in some parts of the world.

How Caregivers Can Help

Provide general advice, support, and information as appropriate, such as:

- If the patient's visual fields are inadequate, advise them not to drive.
- Advise the patient about any likely reaction to drugs (such as drowsiness).
- Write to an employer if requested.
- Support an application, or an appeal, to the Benefits Agency (UK).
- Suggest that the patient contact a support organization that may be able to help with insurance or information for employers.

PSYCHOLOGICAL ASPECTS AND PROBLEMS WITHIN THE FAMILY

Having This Condition

Being faced with a condition that has life-long implications is strange. It's not like having your appendix out. Everyone knows what's involved there—after an uncomfortable few weeks you can resume a healthy, medical-free life.

With a pituitary condition however, even if hormone levels are restored to "normal" with adequate suppression or replacement regimens, there may not be a parallel feeling of being fit and well again. Patients may still feel a reduced overall capacity.

"I wish I could carry on with my life as normal."

"I had my tumor removed two years ago, have not had radiotherapy, and am not on drugs. I am "cured" but still get extreme fatigue on any exertion. I have just returned from holiday and am exhausted. I just wonder if it is a thing I will have all my life. I am now 58. Life is an uphill struggle."

Pituitary disease can make you feel under par for a long time.

A special feeling of "flatness" often arises shortly before medication is due. You may feel that key elements of your character (like having boundless energy) have changed. You may not feel like "me" any more.

Fundamental unknowns enter your life. The future becomes uncertain and dreams may evaporate. Why did I get this? Why me? Is it inherited? Will my children get it? Will it regrow? Will I see my children grow up?

In many cases diagnosis may have taken a long time. This may have strained relationships within the family, at work, and with the local family doctor. At home, simple things may have become major irritants, like the snoring that may accompany acromegaly, or depression associated with high levels of cortisol, or tiredness associated with growth hormone deficiency. Sexual relationships may also have deteriorated.

Depression is common, although patients may be reluctant to admit it.

"I have suffered from depression in the past, and I now believe this may have been related to the Cushing's."

"Psychologically, I suffered quite badly before the diagnosis. Although I had always been sure that something was physically wrong with me, I had been treated continually for stress/mental/depression-related disorders. The actual diagnosis of a "microprolactinoma" (whatever that was) was a great relief and confirmed what I had thought for years."

Coping With the Physical Changes

Changes in appearance may cause distress, sometimes depression.

- Changes to the shape of an acromegalic's face are common. The jaw and chin may protrude in a manner like that portrayed in many fairy stories about witches.

  "I go to great lengths to avoid a sideways-on photograph."

- With Cushing's the face shape changes and facial hair often has to be contended with.

"I am left with the problems of being overweight and having facial hair."

- Acromegalics have difficulty finding shoes, gloves, and hats to fit, which can be very frustrating, time consuming, and distressing. You are "abnormal."
- Weight gain is common, even without the impact of steroids.
- Learning to cope with the ups and downs of cortisol replacement is not easy. Handling stressful situations, such as being ill, and needing at times to carry emergency steroids can be frightening.
- Other changes caused by this condition that can add to the distress are urinary urgency and the inconvenience and embarrassment provoked by diabetes insipidus.
- Infertility may be a real distress.
- The occurrence of sexual problems may not be volunteered but it may have a major impact on relationships. Treatment and reassurance can be provided for impotence or loss of libido.
- When you do feel out-of-sorts it is easy to blame your endocrine situation or to start worrying that something might be wrong, when in fact you may be having an "off-day" like everyone else does.

Patient Problems in Response to Particular Treatments

Many aspects of treatment may cause problems for some patients. Here are some examples that others have shared with me.

- The thought of having treatment so close to the brain and optic nerves, both surgery and radiotherapy.

  "It's an invasion inside your head."

  "I have experienced and now suffer with dizziness, tinnitus, and hearing problems since the RT treatment. I feel angry that the RT has done this. I could not cope with treatment and cannot accept what it has done to me."

- When the patient has needle phobia.

  "I have and do suffer from psychological problems, needle phobia being the most inconvenient because of the nature of the tests. Also, I am GH-deficient and inject daily. It took me and the specialist nurse almost a year before I was able to get round to injecting myself."

  "On the plus side, my needle phobia is cured: I used to faint with injections, but I now inject myself daily!"

- When local health authorities will not pay for essential drugs.
- The prospect of becoming hormone deficient after radiotherapy.
- Worrying about taking too much hydrocortisone.
- Worrying about not taking tablets (especially hydrocortisone).

- The claustrophobia experienced with MRI scans and with the radiotherapy mask.

  "Brain scans [MRI] are absolutely frightening. The experience of going through that tunnel leaves me cold."

- During radiotherapy relationships build up with other patients also waiting for treatment. They mainly have cancer; they may think you have a brain tumor.
- Having to have all this treatment at all, even though there are positive aspects of life long-dependency on drugs and having regular checkups.
- When expectations of treatment are not met.

A Sense of Loss

The feeling of loss can arise from many aspects of the condition and may become a very unwelcome burden. Here are some aspects of our lives that may be lost.

- Of feeling fit and well.
- Of hope that you'll ever recover.
- Of joie de vivre, of energy, of confidence.
- Of ability to do things you did before or were planning to do.
- Of dreams.

  "My plans for walking in the Picos de Europa are now on hold. Some days the Thames Path seems like Helvellyn."

- Of employment, contacts, stimulation, and income.
- Of ability to drive and its practical and social implications.
- Of ability to handle stress.
- Of relationships, of fertility.

  "My husband and I were already diagnosed as infertile so we already deal with a sense of loss and now I deal with a sense of loss of my career in childcare (which I studied to replace this sense of loss). I found I could not cope as well as I had done and I miss being part of a team."

Effect on the Patient's World

Any chronic condition will have an impact on the patient's world.

Family relationships may change, because of employment, energy levels, libido, depression, and so forth.

"My fiancé was desperate to have children. We parted as I was infertile."

"I am likely to be infertile, but so far this hasn't been a problem. Of course, you never know how things change. A few years ago I watched a TV programme on premature menopause where other women were effectively in

mourning for the children that they were never going to have and saying that they felt unfeminine because they didn't have periods. After watching this I wondered whether I was "normal" because I have never felt any sense of loss for my fertility or femininity. I've always regarded the lack of periods to be the plus side of hypopituitarism."

The impact may differ during the initial acute period and later chronic-care stage. Patients and supporters may have different needs regarding information; some may try to ignore what has happened. Parents may experience guilt that they may have passed the condition onto children. Several patients report that their relationships with their children suffered as a result of irritability, depression, tiredness, and so forth.

"My children asked if they could live with a friend who had the energy to play with them."

Family and friends may be frightened if the patient overdoes things with insufficient cortisol. This can result in rapidly becoming ill and becoming delirious, even unconscious. Although recovery is quick once an emergency injection is administered it is a very shocking event for others. Family members should know how to give the emergency jab, and where it is kept.

Loss of a job can be devastating. Employment can give you a place in the world and questions such as "What do you do?" or "What are you?" are common when meeting new people. So how should you answer? Are you retired? Do you explain that you're ill (when you look OK)? Work also provides a social community because most people work with others. Being at home all the time can be lonely and boring unless a replacement activity is found.

Reduced income is difficult to deal with.

"I never ask people what they do, as it's a question I find difficult to answer myself."

Coping Strategies

With all these potential problems it's a wonder that any of us are sane! Patients have mentioned the following strategies:

- Trying to keep it in perspective—loss of employment may result in a reduced income but it does give more time for hobbies and other interests.
- Increasing their knowledge of the condition and meeting others (for example at a patient support organization).
- Finding alternative activities that are a better match for reduced capacity.
- Recognizing that they may need help and by seeking it.
- Involving the family in the treatment.

"I believe that having a serious illness, and coping with it, is a bit like climbing Mount Everest. I feel it has made me more confident, and I have noticed this phenomenon in others."

How Caregivers Can Help

- By providing clear and adequate information to let patients and their supporters know what's happening and what may happen.
- By building up a realistic picture of the time needed for a full recovery. It is not *"three weeks"*!
- By acknowledging and understanding the extent to which a patient's life may be impacted.
- By reinforcing the "benign" aspects of the diseases and conditions, their nature as rarely inherited conditions, and the life expectancy that treatment can confer.
- By arranging support and treatment for depression.
- By helping patients deal with specific aspects (such as weight gain).
- By letting the patient know about support organizations.

THE VALUE OF PATIENT ORGANIZATIONS AND SUPPORT GROUPS

What Patient Organizations and Support Groups Provide

- A feeling that you are not alone.
- Contacts and conversations with other patients and supporters that can have a practical impact on day-to-day quality of life.
- The opportunity to exchange experiences, although these may not always be positive ones or reflect current treatment.
- Information via literature, videos, and help lines.
- The reassurance of seeing others who have survived and are coping successfully.
- The opportunity of helping others.

"All the medical staff that I had spoken to about the problem had advised that the diagnosis was rare, which gave a feeling of being alone with the problem. The [support organization's] booklet I picked up at the clinic was very enlightening, so I wrote to them for more detail, registered myself on their files and have not looked back since. Via the local support group and the national help line I found a feeling of support and realisation that I am not alone."

"I have found patient support groups valuable, especially meeting fellow patients. But lately I have not attended because I cannot cope with meeting patients, maybe older than myself, who are struggling. I'm almost in denial. I feel I do not want to be reminded what is happening to my body either now or may in the future because of the nature of the disease."

"Patient support organizations are a useful source of information. It is also good to know that you are not alone and to gain reassurance from other people that others also experience the same symptoms, both physical and mental."

How Caregivers Can Help

- By being aware of the patient support organizations available nationally and locally.
- By making sure that secretarial or administrative staff know, too.
- By giving patients—at time of diagnosis—contact details for these organizations.
- By supporting the local groups, where possible.

FINAL WORDS

All pituitary patients have different experiences of diagnosis, treatment, and how the condition affects their lives. Some are good and some are bad. Common to everyone's account has been the search both to learn about pituitary tumors in general and their own condition specifically. Many patients have said how much this has helped them deal with the illness.

I believe that the more caregivers help with this aspect of treatment, the better will be the overall prognosis for their patients.

Index

MIX
Papier aus verantwortungsvollen Quellen
Paper from responsible sources
FSC® C105338
FSC
www.fsc.org

If you have any concerns about our products,
you can contact us on
ProductSafety@springernature.com

In case Publisher is established outside the EU,
the EU authorized representative is:
Springer Nature Customer Service Center GmbH
Europaplatz 3, 69115 Heidelberg, Germany

Printed by Libri Plureos GmbH
in Hamburg, Germany